THE AMERIC
OF ADDICTI(
HANDBOOK OF
ADDICTION MEDICINE

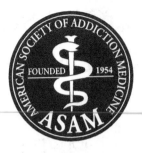

The American Society of Addiction Medicine Handbook of Addiction Medicine

Darius A. Rastegar
Associate Professor of Medicine
Johns Hopkins School of Medicine
Johns Hopkins Bayview Medical Center

Michael I. Fingerhood
Associate Professor of Medicine
Johns Hopkins School of Medicine
Johns Hopkins Bayview Medical Center

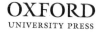

OXFORD
UNIVERSITY PRESS

OXFORD
UNIVERSITY PRESS

Oxford University Press is a department of the University of
Oxford. It furthers the University's objective of excellence in research,
scholarship, and education by publishing worldwide.

Oxford   New York
Auckland   Cape Town   Dar es Salaam   Hong Kong   Karachi
Kuala Lumpur   Madrid   Melbourne   Mexico City   Nairobi
New Delhi   Shanghai   Taipei   Toronto

With offices in
Argentina   Austria   Brazil   Chile   Czech Republic   France   Greece
Guatemala   Hungary   Italy   Japan   Poland   Portugal   Singapore
South Korea   Switzerland   Thailand   Turkey   Ukraine   Vietnam

Oxford is a registered trademark of Oxford University Press
in the UK and certain other countries.

Published in the United States of America by
Oxford University Press
198 Madison Avenue, New York, NY 10016

Library of Congress Cataloging-in-Publication Data
Rastegar, Darius A., 1962– , author.
[Addiction medicine]
The American Society of Addiction Medicine Handbook of Addiction Medicine / Darius Rastegar,
Michael Fingerhood.
p. ; cm.
Preceded by: Addiction medicine / Darius A. Rastegar, Michael I. Fingerhood. Lippincott
Williams & Wilkins, c2005.
At head of title: American Society of Addiction Medicine.
Includes bibliographical references.
ISBN 978–0–19–021464–7 (alk. paper)
I. Fingerhood, Michael I., 1960– , author.   II. American Society of Addiction Medicine.   III. Title.
[DNLM: 1. Substance-Related Disorders.   2. Behavior, Addictive.
3. Evidence-Based Medicine. WM 270]
RC564
616.86—dc23
2015005771

9 8 7 6 5 4 3 2 1
Printed in the United States of America
on acid-free paper

CONTENTS

Preface

Our goal with this handbook is to provide a practical, evidence-based resource for generalists and addiction specialists. Addiction is a common medical problem and one of the leading causes of preventable morbidity and mortality worldwide. We hope that this book will help clinicians feel more comfortable with, and be more competent in, evaluating and treating their patients with substance use disorders.

As primary care physicians, we have incorporated addiction treatment into our own practice, and this has provided us with a unique perspective. We have also been involved in teaching medical students and house staff about substance use disorders for many years and have found that trainees' attitude toward and comfort with treating individuals with these problems can improve with experience and positive role-modeling. We hope this experience has helped us to present this issue in a manner that is useful for other clinicians. While patients with substance use disorders are sometimes thought of as "difficult," we have found that treating these individuals is gratifying and that these patients are appreciative of clinicians who show interest in them, are knowledgeable about the treatment of their problems, and treat them with respect.

This handbook is an update of our 2004 handbook, *Addiction Medicine: An Evidence-Based Handbook*. In writing this handbook, we have had the opportunity to improve upon the previous edition and to update the content. As with the previous edition, we have strived to make it evidence based; by this we mean that the information we present is based on primary data, whenever possible. We have conducted an extensive review of the literature for each of the topic areas covered. Furthermore, we have done our best to explicitly present our sources and to critically evaluate them. For this reason we have provided numerous references and have included additional details in the form of annotations for many of them. We have also used the *ASAM Principles of Addiction Medicine* textbook and the *ASAM Criteria* as resources; we recommend both to our readers for more in-depth information and guidance on the topics covered in this handbook. Another valuable resource, the newsletter *Alcohol, Other Drugs and Health: Current Evidence*, is available free of cost at www.bu.edu/aodhealth and provides summaries of clinically relevant studies in the field. *ASAM Weekly*, a summary of the top research, treatment, and policy news in addiction medicine, is another resource that is available free of cost at www.ASAMweekly.com.

We would like to thank the American Society of Addiction Medicine and, in particular, Lori Karan and the rest of ASAM's Publications Council for providing us with this opportunity to compile and publish this handbook. We would also like to thank Brendan McEntee and Emily McMartin at ASAM, and Christopher Reid at Oxford University Press for their support and assistance. We would also like to thank our colleague, Kenneth Stoller, for providing the perspective of an addiction psychiatrist in Chapter 15. This book would not have been possible without the inspiration of our mentor, Donald R. Jasinski, who introduced us to the field of addiction treatment. Finally, the support of our families was essential, as always.

Darius Rastegar and Michael Fingerhood

Introduction: Addiction from a Clinical Perspective

Overview of Substance Use Disorders

The use of a variety of psychoactive substances is very common. In fact, if one includes caffeine, it is an almost universal experience. Box 1.1 provides an overview of general categories of substances that are taken for psychoactive effects. There are different ways to categorize these substances. Generally, substances are categorized by their effects, but there is some overlap between them and some substances can have multiple effects or different effects at various dosages or levels of use.

BOX 1.1 Categories of Psychoactive Drugs

CNS Depressants

Alcohol, benzodiazepines, barbiturates, meprobamate, carisoprodol, gamma hydroxybutyrate (GHB), volatile organic compounds

Opioids

Morphine, hydromorphone, heroin, oxycodone, hydrocodone, meperidine, codeine, methadone, fentanyl, buprenorphine

Stimulants

Cocaine, amphetamines, cathinones, methylphenidate, caffeine, nicotine

Hallucinogens

Marijuana, synthetic cannabinoids, LSD, mescaline, PCP, MDMA (ecstasy), belladonna alkaloids (atropine, scopolamine)

Dissociatives/Anesthetics

Phencyclidine (PCP), ketamine, dextromethorphan, volatile anesthetics (propofol, nitrous oxide)

According to the U.S. 2013 National Household Survey of Drug Use and Health (NSDUH),[1] 21.6 million Americans are dependent on or abuse an illicit drug or alcohol; this is 8.2% of the population aged 12 or older. Table 1.1 provides data on specific substances. As the name suggests, the NSDUH is a survey of households, so it does not include homeless or institutionalized adults and likely underestimates the true prevalence of these problems. A brief review of the data shows that—by far—tobacco dependence is the most common problem. After tobacco, alcohol is the most common substance of dependence or abuse in the United States. The use of illicit drugs, including

TABLE 1.1 Substance Use and Dependence/Abuse Among Americans Aged 12 and Older: 2013 Estimates*

Substance	Lifetime Use	Recent Use (Past Month)	Dependence or Abuse (Past Year)
Tobacco	175,654 (66.8)	66,879 (25.5)	33,200 (12.7)[†]
Alcohol	213,013 (81.5)	136,868 (52.2)	17,298 (6.6)
Tranquilizers**	23,493 (9.0)	1,705 (0.6)	423 (0.2)
Sedatives[††]	7,480 (2.9)	251 (0.1)	99 (0.0)
Marijuana	114,712 (43.7)	19,810 (7.5)	4,206 (1.6)
Hallucinogens	39,736 (15.1)	1,134 (0.5)	277 (0.1)
Opioids			
Heroin	4,812 (1.8)	289 (0.1)	517 (0.2)
Prescription pain relievers (nonmedical)	35,473 (13.5)	4,862 (1.7)	1,879 (0.7)
Stimulants			
Cocaine	37,634 (14.3)	1,549 (0.6)	855 (0.3)
Methamphetamine and others (nonmedical)	21,656 (8.3)	1,365 (0.5)	469 (0.2)
Inhalants	21,068 (8.0)	496 (0.2)	132 (0.1)

*Numbers are in thousands, percentages in parentheses.
[†]Daily cigarette smokers.
**Includes benzodiazepines, muscle relaxants, prescription antihistamines.
[††]Includes barbiturates, temazepam, chloral hydrate.
Source: 2013 National Survey on Drug Use and Health (NSDUH).

marijuana, opioids, stimulants, and a variety of other agents, is less common, but important nonetheless. The nonmedical use of prescription drugs has overtaken most illicit drugs in the past few decades. Substance use disorders are also responsible for a tremendous amount of preventable morbidity and mortality; smoking alone is believed to cause millions of premature deaths worldwide each year.

Addiction as a Chronic Disease

Historically, addiction has been seen as a sign of moral weakness or failure that was best addressed through punitive actions. Addiction is increasingly understood as a chronic disorder that involves a complex interplay of genetics, physiology, environment, and behavior. The same can be said for many other chronic illnesses. For example, type II diabetes mellitus involves physiological derangements that are largely a consequence of an individual's behavior and choices (diet, exercise, etc.), as well as genetic and environmental factors. Addiction, like type II diabetes, cannot be "cured," but there are effective treatments that can help reduce the complications.

The disease concept dampens negative attitudes toward individuals with addiction and promotes the dedication of resources toward treatment and research in addiction. For healthcare providers, the disease model is useful in taking away blame from patients who commonly experience low self-esteem, shame, and guilt. However, this must be balanced with the need to have patients take control of their lives and accept responsibility for making changes. The message needs to be conveyed that genetics and environment are not destiny and that change can happen, but this requires a carefully agreed upon plan, often using multiple modalities of treatment.

Physiological Factors

The disease model is supported by brain imaging studies that show changes contributing to the abnormal functioning of brain circuits in individuals who have substance use disorders.[2] Evidence suggests that the frontal cortex of the brain, critical in inhibitory control over reward-related behavior, is dysfunctional in individuals with drug addiction.[3,4]

Individuals use drugs for a variety of reasons—for pleasurable effect, to relieve distress, or to improve performance. Rapid onset and high intensity of drug effect increase the abuse potential of drugs. Continued drug use causes changes in the central nervous system that lead to tolerance, dependence, and craving. Use is typically driven by craving for the pleasurable response initially but is often replaced by fear of—or aversion to—the withdrawal symptoms that arise with abstinence.

While addictive drugs act on a variety of neurotransmitters, the reinforcing effects are thought to be primarily due to an increase in dopamine in the nucleus accumbens.[5,6] During drug withdrawal, dopamine levels decrease substantially in the nucleus accumbens.[7] Addictive drugs can cause brain alterations that persist even after long periods of abstinence. These changes contribute to "priming" or "kindling"—the observation that re-exposure to a formerly used substance can precipitate a rapid resumption of drug use at high levels. After only a few days, an individual who relapses to alcohol use can quickly drink large amounts of alcohol and may have severe withdrawal when attempting to stop.

Drugs associated with addiction have acute psychoactive effects that become reinforcing. Eventually, environmental cues, even in the absence of the drug, cause a conditioned response—craving. Craving may overwhelm decision-making and the ability to perceive the negative consequences of continued drug use. Personality traits and mental disorders are also factors in drug addiction. Individuals with addiction tend to be risk takers and less concerned about the potential for negative impact from drug use.[8] Addiction is often seen in individuals with psychiatric disorders (co-occurring disorders); this is probably due mainly to shared risk factors, rather than a simple cause-and-effect relationship (see Chapter 15).

Genetic Factors

The concept of addiction as a disease is further supported by the fact that genetic factors contribute to the development of addiction.

Children of alcoholic parents adopted at birth by nonalcoholic parents have shown an increased likelihood of alcoholism.[9] Specific genes have been associated with alcohol dependence,[10,11,12] as well as with opioid and cocaine addiction.[13,14,15] Additional studies have found that changes in genes contribute to nicotine dependence[16] and drug dependence in general.[17,18] Imaging genetics studies attempt to explain individual differences in vulnerability to addiction.[19] For example, opioids produce predominantly euphoric effects in those who become addicted, whereas they produce mostly sedative effects among those who do not.[20]

Psychosocial Factors

The disease model does not dismiss the role that environment plays in the development and maintenance of addiction. The availability of drugs and use of drugs by peers are significant contributors. Low socioeconomic class and poor parental support also play a role. Environmental factors may even lead to changes in gene expression that can contribute to the development of addiction.[2] Stress may also play a role in the development of substance use disorders through its effect on corticotropin-releasing factor (CRF).[21]

While addiction is characterized by a lack of control over drug use, initiation of drug use is voluntary. Individuals may decide to experiment with drugs because of impulsivity, novelty seeking, stress, socioeconomic deprivation, or peer pressure. Often, individuals see themselves as "different" from those who are addicted and underestimate their own risk. Addiction may begin as the inadvertent effect of repeated self-medication by a vulnerable individual who is trying to relieve physical or psychological distress. Drugs of abuse can be potent and effective short-term alleviators of these symptoms.

Terminology and Definitions

The field of substance use disorders is hampered by confusing and overlapping terminology: *drug abuse, substance abuse/dependence*, and *addiction* are a few examples. This is further complicated by the fact that alcohol use disorders have their own terminology, such as *alcoholism*, *problem drinking*, *hazardous drinking*, *harmful drinking*, *binge drinking*, and *heavy drinking*. Moreover, nicotine dependence (in the form of cigarette use) is generally referred to as *smoking* in the literature.

For the purposes of this book, we will generally use the term *substance use disorder* when referring to the spectrum of problematic use. We may use the term *addiction* when referring to the more severe end of the spectrum. When referring to studies that used DSM-IV definitions, we will use the terms *substance abuse* or *substance dependence* if those were the original terms/definitions used.

DSM-5

The *Diagnostic and Statistical Manual of Mental Disorders* (DSM) has traditionally provided definitions and criteria for these disorders. The fourth edition, DSM-IV, first published in 1994 and updated in 2000, recognized two broad categories: "substance abuse" and "substance dependence."[22] "Substance abuse" referred to a "maladaptive pattern of substance use that leads to clinically significant impairment or distress" or "in situations in which it is physically hazardous," but did not meet the criteria for "substance dependence." "Substance dependence" referred to a more severe and persistent substance problem and was used interchangeably with "addiction."

There were a number of problems with the DSM-IV definitions: the dividing line between abuse and dependence was not clear, substance dependence was often confused with physical dependence, and the term *abuse* has pejorative connotations. The DSM-5, published in May of 2013, no longer uses the terms *abuse* and *dependence* and has replaced these with a single term: "substance use disorder," which encompasses the spectrum of problematic substance use.[23] The diagnosis of a substance use disorder is based on the presence of at least 2 of 11 criteria; these can be divided into four clusters or groups, summarized as follows:

Group I: Impaired Control
1. Substance use in larger amounts or over a longer period of time than was originally intended

2. Persistent desire to cut down on use or multiple unsuccessful attempts at cutting down or stopping use
3. Great deal of time spent using substance or recovering from its effects
4. Intense desire to use or craving for the substance

Group II: Social Impairment
5. Substance use resulting in failure to fulfill obligations at work, school, or home
6. Substance use causing or exacerbating interpersonal problems
7. Important social, occupational, or recreational activities given up or reduced due to substance use

Group III: Risky Use
8. Recurrent use of substance in physically hazardous situations
9. Continued use despite negative physical or psychological consequences

Group IV: Pharmacological Dependence
10. Tolerance to the effects of the substance
11. Withdrawal symptoms with cessation of substance use

One important caveat is that persons who are prescribed certain medications, for example, opioids or benzodiazepines, will develop pharmacological dependence (the last two criteria) but would not be considered to have a substance use disorder based on this alone and would need to meet at least one other criteria.

The severity of the substance use disorder can be estimated from the number of criteria: the presence of two to three would suggest a *mild* substance use disorder; four to five, *moderate*; and six or more, *severe*. "Mild substance use disorder" roughly correlates to "substance abuse" and "moderate-severe substance use disorder" to "substance dependence."

Despite the development of the new DSM-5 terminology and definitions, it is important to be aware of the DSM-IV terminology and definitions because of much of the research conducted in that era used that terminology to select and categorize subjects. Table 1.2 provides a comparison of the DSM-IV criteria for substance abuse and dependence with the DSM-5 criteria for substance use disorders. The DSM-5 uses many of the same criteria that were previously used by DSM-IV, but there were two major changes: (1) recurrent legal problems, which was a criterion for substance abuse, was removed; (2) a new criterion has been added: craving or strong desire/urge to use a substance. There were also some changes made to the wording of specific criteria.

The DSM-5 also includes criteria for a range of substance-induced disorders from substance intoxication to substance withdrawal, substance-induced delirium, dementia, psychosis, mood or anxiety disorders, sexual dysfunction, and sleep disorder. These are discussed further in Chapters 4–12, on specific substances.

ICD-10

Another important source of terminology and diagnostic criteria is the World Health Organization's *International Classification of Diseases* (ICD), the latest version of which is the ICD-10. Diagnostic codes for "mental and behavioural disorders" begin with the letter *F* and those due to "psychoactive substance use" begin with F10–F19, depending on the substance involved.[24] The substances are as follows: F10, alcohol; F11, opioids; F12, cannabinoids; F13, sedative hypnotics; F14, cocaine; F15, other stimulants, including caffeine; F16, hallucinogens; F17, tobacco; F18, volatile solvents; and F19, other psychoactive substances

The codes are then categorized as follows:

F1x.0 *is acute intoxication*, defined as a "transient condition following the administration of alcohol or other psychoactive substance, resulting in disturbances in level of consciousness, cognition, perception, affect or behaviour, or other psychophysiological functions and responses."

F1x.1 is *harmful use*, defined as a "pattern of psychoactive substance use that is causing damage to health. The damage may

TABLE 1.2 Comparison of DSM-IV Criteria for Substance Abuse (SA) and Substance Dependence (SD) with DSM-5 Criteria for Substance Use Disorder (SUD)

Criteria	SA—IV	SD—IV	SUD—5
1. Using more than intended		√	√
2. Not able to cut down/unsuccessful quit attempts		√	√
3. Spending a great deal of time using/recovering		√	√
4. Intense desire to use or craving			√
5. Failure to fulfill major obligations due to substance use	√		√
6. Social or interpersonal problems due to substance use			√
7. Important activities given up due to substance use		√	√
8. Recurrent use in physically hazardous situations	√		√
9. Continued use despite negative health consequences	√	√	√
10. Tolerance to the effects of the substance		√	√
11. Withdrawal when not using the substance		√	√
xx. Continued use despite legal problems	√		

Adapted from American Psychiatric Association: *Diagnostic and Statistical Manual of Mental Disorders,* Fourth Edition, Text Revision. Washington, DC, American Psychiatric Association, 2000, and American Psychiatric Association: *Diagnostic and Statistical Manual of Mental Disorders*, Fifth Edition. Arlington, VA, American Psychiatric Association, 2013.

be physical (as in cases of hepatitis from the self-administration of injected drugs) or mental (e.g., episodes of depressive disorder secondary to heavy consumption of alcohol)." This correlates with "mild substance use disorder" in DSM-5.

F1x.2 is *dependence syndrome*, defined as "a cluster of physiological, behavioural, and cognitive phenomena in which the use of a substance or a class of substances takes on a much higher priority for a given individual than other behaviours that once had greater value." This correlates with "moderate-severe substance use disorder" in DSM-5. The diagnosis of substance dependence syndrome requires the presence of three or more of the six following criteria in the previous year:

1. A strong desire or sense of compulsion to take the substance
2. Difficulties in controlling substance-taking behavior in terms of its onset, termination, or levels of use
3. A physiological withdrawal state when substance use has ceased or been reduced, as evidenced by the characteristic withdrawal syndrome for the substance, or use of the same (or a closely related) substance with the intention of relieving or avoiding withdrawal symptoms
4. Evidence of tolerance, such that increased doses of the psychoactive substances are required in order to achieve effects originally produced by lower doses
5. Progressive neglect of alternative pleasures or interests because of psychoactive substance use or increased amount of time necessary to obtain or take the substance or to recover from its effects
6. Persisting with substance use despite clear evidence of overtly harmful consequences, such as harm to the liver through excessive drinking, depressive mood states consequent to periods of heavy substance use, or drug-related impairment of cognitive functioning. Efforts should be made to determine that the user was actually or could be expected to be aware of the nature and extent of the harm.

The remaining categories are as follows:

F1x.3 Withdrawal state
F1x.4 Withdrawal state with delirium
F1x.5 Psychotic disorder
F1x.6 Amnesic syndrome
F1x.7 Residual and late-onset psychotic disorder
F1x.8 Other mental and behavioural disorders
F1x.9 Unspecified mental and behavioural disorders

These are further divided into subcategories; for example, someone with hallucinogen-associated flashbacks would have an ICD-10 code of F16.70; F16 is the code for hallucinogens and .70 is the code for "flashbacks," under "residual and late onset psychotic disorder" (F1x.7). This is covered further in Chapters 4–12, which discuss specific substances.

Notes

1. Substance Abuse and Mental Health Services Administration. *Results from the 2013 National Survey on Drug Use and Health: National Findings.* NSDUH Series H-48, HHS Publication No. (SMA) 14-4863. Rockville, MD: Substance Abuse and Mental Health Services Administration; 2014.

2. Volkow ND, Warren KR. Drug addiction: the neurobiology of behavior gone awry. In Ries RK, Fiellin DA, Miller SC, Saitz R, eds. *The ASAM Principles of Addiction Medicine,* 5th ed. Philadelphia: Wolters Kluwer; 2014:3–18.

3. Lubman DI, Yucel M, Pantelis C. Addiction, a condition of compulsive behavior? Neuroimaging and neuropsychological evidence of inhibitory dysregulation. Addiction 2004;99:1491–502.

4. Goldstein RZ, Volkow ND. Drug addiction and its underlying neurobiological basis: neuroimaging evidence for the involvement of the frontal cortex. Am J Psychiatry 2002;159:1642–52.

5. Cami J, Farre M. Drug addiction. N Engl J Med 2003;349:975–86.

6. Hyman SE, Malenka RC. Addiction and the brain: the neurobiology of compulsion and its persistence. Nat Rev Neurosci 2001;2:695–703.

7. Nestler EJ. Molecular basis of long-term plasticity underlying addiction. Nat Rev Neurosci 2001;2:119–28.

8. Conway KP, Kane RJ, Ball SA, et al. Personality, substance of choice, and polysubstance involvement among substance dependent patients. Drug Alcohol Depend 2003;71:65–75.

9. Crabbe JC. Genetic contributions to addiction. Annu Rev Psychol 2002;53:435–62.

10. Blum K, Noble EP, Sheridan PJ, et al. Allelic association of human dopamine D2 receptor gene in alcoholism. JAMA 1990:263:2055–60.

11. Palmer RHC, McGeary JE, Francazio S, et al. The genetics of alcohol dependence: advancing towards systems-based approaches. Drug Alcohol Depend 2012;125:179–91.

12. Mulligan MK, Ponomarev I, Hitzemann RJ. Toward understanding the genetics of alcohol drinking through transcriptome meta-analysis. Proc Natl Acad Sci U S A 2006;103:6368–73.

13. Clarke TK, Ambrose-Lanci L, Ferraro TN, et al. Genetic association and analyses of PDYN polymorphisms with heroin and cocaine addiction. Genes Brain Behav 2012;11:415–23.

14. Yuferov V, Levran O, Proudnikov D, et al. Search for genetic markers and functional variants involved in the development of opiate and cocaine addiction and treatment. Ann N Y Acad Sci 2010;1187:184–207.

15. Kreek MJ. Drug addictions: molecular and cellular endpoints. Ann N Y Acad Sci 2001;937:27–49.

16. Rao Y, Hoffmann E, Zia M, et al. Duplications and defects in the CYP2A6 gene: identification, genotyping, and in vivo effects on smoking. Mol Pharmacol 2000;58:747–55.

17. Nestler EJ, Aghajanian GK. Molecular and cellular basis of addiction. Science 1997;278:58–63.

18. Uhl GR, Liu QR, Naiman D. Substance abuse vulnerability loci: converging genome scanning data. Trends Genet 2002;18:420–5.

19. Sweitzer MM, Donny EC, Hariri AR. Imaging genetics and the neurobiological basis of individual differences in vulnerability to addiction. Drug Alcohol Depend 2012;123(Suppl 1):S59-S71.

20. Smith GM, Beecher HK. Subjective effects of heroin and morphine in normal subjects. J Pharmacol Exp Ther 1962;136:47–52.

21. Sarnyai Z, Shaham Y, Heinrichs SC. The role of corticotropin-releasing factor in drug addiction. Pharmacol Rev 2001;53:209–43.

22. American Psychiatric Association: *Diagnostic and Statistical Manual of Mental Disorders*, Fourth Edition, Text Revision. Washington, DC: American Psychiatric Association; 2000.

23. American Psychiatric Association: *Diagnostic and Statistical Manual of Mental Disorders*, Fifth Edition. Arlington, VA: American Psychiatric Association; 2013.

24. World Health Organization. *International Statistical Classification of Diseases and Related Health Problems*, 10th Revision (ICD-10) Version for 2010. http://www.who.int/substance_abuse/terminology/ICD10ClinicalDiagnosis.pdf. Accessed January 20, 2015.

2

Screening and Brief Intervention

Background

Recognition of a substance use disorder begins with screening, followed by consideration of the diagnosis based on history, physical examination, and laboratory testing. While patients are generally open about their use of alcohol or other drugs, in some circumstances, recognition may occur because of a medical complication or a positive drug test obtained through the workplace or a legal setting.

For the patient with a substance use disorder, the role of the primary care practitioner is to (1) recognize the problem, (2) facilitate the patient's acceptance of the problem, (3) motivate the patient to accept treatment, (4) create a treatment plan, (5) provide ongoing care for the patient's medical problems, and (6) motivate the patient to remain in recovery. All these steps depend on skillful medical interviewing that builds rapport and trust between the practitioner and patient.

Screening and brief interventions (SBI) are recommended in the guidelines of a number of professional organizations. The U.S. Preventive Services Task Force recommends SBI to reduce alcohol misuse[1] and tobacco use,[2] but has concluded that the evidence is insufficient to recommend SBI for illicit drug use.[3] SBI are often incorporated into an approach including referral to treatment (SBIRT) for those with a moderate-severe substance use disorder.

Screening for Substance Use Disorders

When taking a substance use history, details related to drug use should be determined within the context of the general medical history, using a nonjudgmental approach. Questions should be direct, and qualified answers and rationalizations should be challenged. The style of questioning should be persistent but empathic and friendly. With the patient's consent, it may be helpful to obtain information from a family member or close friend.

There are a number of instruments that can be used for screening, some designed specifically for alcohol, others for substance use in general or for specific populations. Screening instruments for alcohol are reviewed in Chapter 4, and screening for drug use in adolescents is discussed in Chapter 16. There are a few general instruments that are potentially useful for screening adults for alcohol and other drug misuse in primary care[4]:

1. Alcohol, Smoking and Substance Involvement Screening Test (ASSIST). This is an eight-item screening instrument designed to detect recent or lifetime drug misuse in adults and is completed by the clinician. This instrument and instructions on its use can be found at the World Health Organization (WHO) website.[5]
2. Cut down, Annoyed, Guilty, Eye-opener—Adapted to Include Drugs (CAGE-AID). This is a four-item screening instrument designed to screen for lifetime drug misuse in adults and is completed by the clinician.
3. Drug Abuse Screening Test (DAST). This is a 28-items instrument adapted from the Michigan Alcoholism Screening Test (MAST) and is completed by the patient.

Another approach is to begin with a single question regarding past-year alcohol, tobacco, or illicit drug use and nonmedical use of prescription drugs, and then to follow up with more detailed questions or instruments if the initial response is positive. This approach has been shown to be effective in primary care settings when screening for illicit drug use and nonmedical use of prescription drugs.[6]

Drug Testing

Drug testing is a potentially useful tool for detecting recent drug use but has limited utility as a screening tool. A positive drug test does not necessarily mean that the patient has a substance use disorder, even if he or she has used the substance, and a negative result does not rule out the possibility of a substance use disorder. Moreover, a drug test may be falsely positive—particularly if the pretest probability is low—and may raise unnecessary suspicions. Drug testing should be done in an open manner; although it may seem like an easy and objective way of "catching" someone in denial, this can prove problematic. Obviously, patients already know if they are using drugs, and testing, particularly when not done openly, may undermine a patient's trust in a clinician or the healthcare system. The most important element of the clinician–patient relationship is facilitating the ability of patients to be open about their problem (if there is one).

Drug testing is probably best limited to certain clinical situations: (1) medical scenarios where knowledge of recent alcohol or other drug use would have an impact on patient care (e.g., a comatose or delirious patient); (2) monitoring patients who are actively participating in drug treatment (e.g., someone on methadone maintenance); and (3) monitoring patients who are prescribed controlled substances (e.g., a patient prescribed oxycodone for chronic pain).

Urine drug testing is the most commonly used test method for detecting recent drug use. Saliva, hair, or nail clippings can also be used for drug testing but have limited utility in most clinical settings. Saliva can reveal drug use earlier than urine, while hair and nail analyses provide evidence of drug use over an extended period of time rather than being limited to recent usage. Breath or serum testing can be used to detect volatile substances, such as alcohol, which are not accurately detected in urine; this is discussed further in Chapter 4.

There are two types of urine drug tests: (1) enzyme-linked immunoassay (EIA) and (2) gas chromatography/mass spectrometry (GC/MS). EIA is generally used for initial screening, and GC/MS can be used for confirmation of positive EIA results. EIA testing identifies the presence of a specific substance at levels above a threshold. GC/MS can provide more specific information on the type of substance and its concentration. For example, EIA testing may identify the presence of benzodiazepines in a urine specimen, and GC/MS can be used to identify the specific benzodiazepine. The EIA test is sufficient for most clinical situations. GC/MS is much more expensive and should be reserved for special cases—for example, if there is suspicion of a false-positive result or if the stakes are very high, such as when the test has employment or legal ramifications. The window for detection of a substance varies depending on a number of factors, including the specific substance used, the duration and amount of the substance use, the sensitivity of the test and the cutoff for a positive test result, as well as dilution of the urine and variations in metabolism. Table 2.1 provides approximate maximal ranges for detection of various substances.

TABLE 2.1 Maximal Detection Times for Urine Drug Testing

Drug	Maximal Detection Time (Days)
Amphetamines	3
Benzodiazepines	7 (duration is generally related to half-life of specific benzodiazepine)
Barbiturates	4 (short-acting) 14 or more (long-acting)
Marijuana	7 (light use) 27 (heavy use)
Cocaine	3 (light use) 22 (heavy use)
Heroin	3
LSD	5
PCP	7 (single dose) 21 (chronic use)

Adapted from Warner E, Lorch E. Laboratory diagnosis. In Ries RK, Fiellin DA, Miller SC, Saitz R, eds. *The ASAM Principles of Addiction Medicine*, 5th ed. Philadelphia: Wolters Kluwer; 2014:332–43 (and other sources).

Another factor to consider when using urine drug testing is the possibility of false-positive results. A number of substances may trigger positive EIA results. Table 2.2 provides a list of *some* that have been reported. It should be noted that these substances do not always cause positive results and that false-positive EIA rates often depend on the type of assay used. As with any test, the results should be interpreted in the context of the clinical situation. When an unexpected result occurs (either positive or negative), this should lead to a nonjudgmental discussion with the patient about the results. If there is a suspicion of a false-positive result, GC/MS testing can be performed to confirm the EIA results.

TABLE 2.2 Medications or Substances That May Trigger False-Positive Results on Urine Drug Immunoassays

Drug	Other Drugs and Substances
Opiates	Poppy seeds, quinolones, rifampin
Methadone	Diphenhydramine, verapamil, quetiapine, promethazine, thioridazine
Buprenorphine	Tramadol
Cocaine	Coca leaf tea, topical anesthetics containing cocaine
Amphetamines	Pseudoephedrine, buproprion, ranitidine, phenylpropanolamine, amantadine, desipramine, trazodone, chlorpromazine, selegiline, phentermine, benzphetamine
PCP	Dextramethorphan, tramadol, venlafaxine
Cannabinoids	Dronabinol, efavirenz
Benzodiazepines	Sertraline

Adapted from Moeller KE, et al. Urine drug screening: practical guide for clinicians. Mayo Clin Report 2008;83:66–76 (and other reports).

Brief Intervention

Brief intervention is a motivational process of assessing alcohol or other drug use, giving feedback, setting goals, arriving at a strategy for change, and providing a plan for follow-up. The process was developed and validated among individuals with alcohol use disorders, but it can be applied to all individuals with substance use disorders.[7] In most published clinical trials, someone other than the individual's primary care practitioner performed the brief intervention; the effectiveness may be even greater when motivational interviewing is performed by a primary care practitioner who has a good relationship and rapport with the patient. Furthermore, overall primary care quality may be associated with lower addiction severity among patients with substance use disorders.[8] Thus primary care practitioners need to receive specific training in the use of motivation interviewing when caring for patients with substance use disorders.

Implicit in the motivational process is imparting clear advice to the patient to change, and the patient accepting responsibility for enacting change. Therapeutic empathy describes the recommended counseling style. The goal of brief intervention may not be abstinence but rather reducing use in a nondependent drug user. While brief intervention procedures used in studies vary, most involve one to six counseling sessions. Typical follow-up sessions are usually 15 minutes long. Even a single brief 5-to 10-minute intervention may have an impact on high-risk drinkers,[9] but most patients will require more than this.

Stages of Addiction and Recovery

When considering a brief intervention, it is helpful to first assess the individual's readiness for change. In a model described by Prochaska, DiClemente, and Norcross, individuals with addiction go through stages as they move toward recovery (Figure 2.1).[10]

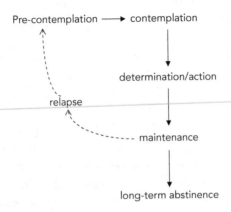

FIGURE 2.1 *Stages of Change in Addiction.*

Adapted from Prochaska JO, DiClemente CC, Norcross JC. In search of how people change. Applications to addictive behaviors. Am Psychol 1992;47:1102–14.

Precontemplation is the stage in which there is no plan for change and individuals lack insight into the problems arising from their substance use. Patients in precontemplation are resistant to consider addressing their problem. As a clinician, it is generally fruitless to try to initiate change in someone who is precontemplative. Instead, the goal should be to facilitate patient movement from precontemplation to contemplation.

An individual enters *contemplation* when family members, friends, coworkers, and health providers have helped convince the individual that a problem exists. It is a stage that people often stay in for long periods of time. During this stage, patients are weighing the pros and cons (benefits and risks) of continued use of drugs.

This is followed by *preparation* or *determination*, in which individuals come to the conclusion that they want to change and are willing to set a plan. Some small behavioral changes may occur during this stage; for example, a smoker may decrease his smoking. However, the full step to attempted abstinence or recovery has not yet occurred.

Action is the stage during which individuals take the formal step to make a change. This may include changing environment, acquaintances, and activities, as well as ceasing use of a drug. This stage may last from 1 day up to several months or more. During this time, patients continue to attempt to strengthen strategies that have been helpful in maintaining abstinence and define and overcome obstacles that make them vulnerable to relapse.

After the action stage, successful individuals enter the *maintenance* stage. During this stage, patients actively pursue continued recovery. Continued efforts to stabilize relationships (family, friends, and acquaintances) and life circumstances (work and free time) are aimed at avoiding relapse. Optimally, the maintenance stage should not be viewed as static but rather as a continued stage of action.

When this model of change was first introduced, it contained only four stages. However, most individuals with substance use disorders do not successfully maintain abstinence/recovery on their initial attempt. For example, most smokers attempt to stop three or four times before they are successful. *Relapse* is therefore an expected stage for most individuals with a substance use disorder, with the hope that, with time, the amount of time spent in relapse gets shorter and periods of recovery grow longer.

Patients appropriate for motivational interviewing are those who are precontemplative or contemplative about making a change. For those who are precontemplative, the goal is to get them to the stage of contemplation; for those who are contemplative, the goal is get them to the stage of preparation or determination to make a change. Despite some understanding of benefit from change, a patient may "enjoy" alcohol or drug effects and be fearful of increased anxiety from stopping use of drugs such as sedatives or alcohol.

The aim of motivational interviewing is to help individuals see the discrepancy between their goals and their current situation and, by doing so, lead them to consider change. One way of conceptualizing the process is to divide it into six steps, as shown in Figure 2.2. The acronym FRAMES (**F**eedback, **R**esponsibility, **A**dvice, **M**enu, **E**mpathy, and **S**elf-efficacy) can help in remembering these steps.

1—Feedback of personal risk (patient-focused review of the specific evidence for problems related to drug use)

2—Emphasis on personal Responsibility for change (empowering the patient to take control of the decision for change—"This is not your fault, but you must take responsibility for making things better.")

3—Clear Advice for change ("Based on all we have discussed, you need to make a change.")

4—Offering a Menu of alternative options ("Here are some ways you can make a change.")

5—Therapeutic Empathy as an innate part of the intervention ("I know this may be difficult.")

6—Enhancement of patient Self-efficacy ("This is not hopeless; with change, things will get better for you.")

FIGURE 2.2 *The Six Components of Motivational Interviewing: FRAME.*

One goal of motivational interviewing is to try to elicit "change talk"; the elements can be remembered by use of the acronym DARN-C:

- Desire: Why would you want to make this change?
- Ability: How would you do it if you decided?
- Reasons: What are the reasons for change?
- Need: How important is it, and why?
- Commitment: What do you plan to do?

Dealing with Denial

Denial, the direct or implied message that there is no problem, is a major obstacle to a patient initiating change or accepting treatment. Denial is complex and may be caused by (1) conscious lying, (2) an attempt to avoid shame, (3) an inability to overcome the problem, (4) euphoric recall of remembering only the good times experienced when drinking or using drugs, (5) the fact that no one else has pointed out problems related to substance use, or (6) toxic effects of drugs on information processing and memory. Denial presents as rationalizations ("I get high because it is the only way I can relax"); glibness ("I drink less than all my friends—are they alcoholics too?"); hostility ("I came to you about my stomach pain and I would appreciate it if you could stay out of my personal life"); comparison of oneself with a "real problem drinker" ("I have a family, a job that I enjoy ... I have nothing in common with those poor guys who have lost everything ... those are your alcoholics"); reticence to discuss drinking or substance use; and assertions that friends and family members do not perceive a problem. These responses are a source of frustration for providers during screening and are a barrier to efforts to get the patient to accept the need for change and agree to treatment.

Three motivational techniques are fundamental for breaking down denial in patients and, if necessary, in their family members: confrontation, showing empathy, and offering hope. These techniques are equally important in the medical interview. Confrontation consists of telling the patient the evidence for a substance use problem. The patient may deny that there is a problem and may even get angry. However, with persistent and nonjudgmental confrontation, most patients will eventually admit that they have a problem. It is important in confrontation to avoid arguing with a patient and to instead simply restate the facts and show care and concern. Specific details of confrontation are outlined in the next section.

Statements that convey empathy and offer hope are important in diminishing a patient's denial. Empathy is conveyed by acknowledging the patient's feelings ("I can see this is upsetting you") and by conveying concern ("I am very concerned about you"). Offering hope is essential; patients must be able to "hear" that there is a way to change and improve their lives. After a diagnosis of a substance use disorder has been made, the objectives of care are to have the patient accept the diagnosis and agree to treatment.

The initial goal of treatment in individuals with dependence is generally abstinence, or engagement in a structured treatment program. Patients must accept help in the difficult process of recovery, even though many will say "I can do it on my own." In addition to regular follow-up by a supportive practitioner who believes the patient can recover, the most important elements are a plan for achieving abstinence (including medically supervised withdrawal, if necessary), participation in self-help groups (Alcoholics/Narcotics Anonymous) or group therapy, and family involvement. Possible treatment options should be explained to the patient and the family. If the patient is in a crisis and not enough time is available during the first visit, a return appointment should be scheduled within a few days, or the patient should be immediately referred to a reliable treatment program.

Confrontation

One must be direct in confronting a patient with a substance use disorder. It is important, however, to include questions or statements that give the patient some sense of control during what can be a one-sided interaction. Because many patients (especially those with alcoholism) have negative emotional responses (e.g., anger and disbelief) to being told they have a problem, they may not internalize what they are being told. Therefore, brevity and directness are essential. Statements of concern, optimism, and support are indicated. Such statements help patients while they are hearing a diagnosis that often brings shame. It is also important to not simply put all the blame on their disease; patients need to be specifically told that they must accept responsibility for making a change and seeking treatment. Figure 2.3 summarizes a recommended approach to confrontation. This approach may be incorporated into the interview at a single visit or over multiple visits.

Despite concerned families and healthcare practitioners, not all patients respond to efforts to motivate them to accept treatment. In this situation, family members and peers can be used to help overcome resistance. There are a number of different approaches,[11] one being a formal *intervention*.[12,13] The aim of the intervention is to present, in a formal meeting, the situation as a crisis that motivates the patient to accept treatment. The intervention team is composed of as many people as possible that are emotionally important to the patient. Before the actual intervention, this team may meet to

1. State the diagnosis (e.g., "I think you have a problem with drinking alcohol and I am very concerned about you.").
2. Acknowledge the patient's reaction (e.g., "I know this is making you uncomfortable.").
3. Ask the patient about his or her view of the situation.
4. Explain the evidence for the problem—avoid blame and offer hope.
5. Ask the patient what he or she knows about treatment.
6. Tell the patient about treatment options, including the likely need for abstinence.
7. Assign responsibility to the patient to make a change and accept treatment.
8. Get the patient to select a treatment plan.
9. Take action to initiate treatment plan.
10. Establish your role as an ally with the patient and schedule follow-up in a short time interval.

FIGURE 2.3 *Recommended Approach for Confrontation of a Patient with a Substance Use Disorder.*

discuss how best to convince the patient that there is a problem and that he or she needs treatment. The team may rehearse their confrontation, even scripting the order of speaking.

The process is initiated by having each participant describe specific details of how the patient's addiction has led to anger, fear, disappointment, sadness, or embarrassment for the participant or to some other negative impact. Each person begins their confrontation with an expression of concern for the patient, followed by statements related to the impact the patient's drug use has had on him or her. Each participant ends their confrontation with specific measures they will take if the patient does not agree to treatment (e.g., loss of job, no further visits, being forced out of their home). As part of a formal intervention, arrangements may be made in advance to have the person admitted for drug treatment. Financing of treatment, arranging for absence from work, and other details are best worked out by the team before the intervention.

For many patients, employment or legal problems are an important trigger to seeking addiction treatment. Sometimes such treatment is coercive, with treatment required for the person to maintain employment or avoid imprisonment. Many employers have recognized the economic and human costs of substance use disorders and have developed employee assistance programs to motivate and help employees get into treatment. Courts have increasingly recognized that incarcerating drug users is not a solution for their problems. Physicians can work with employee assistance programs, as well as courts and parole officers, to help patients get appropriate treatment. This approach uses the motivation to keep a job or avoid incarceration as leverage for getting treatment and following through with recovery.

Dealing with Relapse

The relapse process generally begins long before the person actually uses the drug again.[14] An analysis of 48 episodes of relapse revealed that most relapses were associated with three high-risk situations: (1) frustration and anger, (2) social pressure, and (3) interpersonal temptation.[15] The relapse process often progresses in the following sequence: reactivation of denial, progressive isolation and defensiveness, building a crisis to justify symptom progression, immobilization, confusion and overreaction, depression, loss of control over behavior, recognition of loss of control, and finally relapse to drug use.

Although it should not be telegraphed to the patient, relapse is part of the natural history of successful recovery for most individuals with addiction. For example, in one cohort study, 90% of alcoholics had at least one relapse during a 4-year follow-up period.[16] One should not become discouraged when relapse happens; instead, the patient should be immediately recruited back into treatment using the same motivational techniques employed initially. Relapse is a time for both patient and practitioner to learn from mistakes and to correct them by strengthening treatment.

Research on Screening, Brief Intervention, and Referral to Treatment (SBIRT)

Studies of brief interventions as part of screening, brief intervention, and referral to treatment (SBIRT) for reducing substance use have yielded mixed results. A comprehensive review of the extensive literature on this subject is beyond the scope of this handbook; we refer readers to *The ASAM Principles of Addiction Medicine* for more details on this topic.[17]

Earlier studies showed brief interventions to be effective in reducing alcohol consumption in problem drinkers.[18,19,20,21] Clinical trials also showed benefit of brief intervention for alcohol use among pregnant women,[22] for alcohol-misusing patients in an emergency department,[23] for alcohol use in participants in a needle exchange program,[24] and for alcohol and drug use among adolescents.[25,26] One study showed that a single brief intervention in the primary care setting can help motivated patients achieve abstinence from heroin and cocaine.[27] Randomized clinical trials of the cost-benefit of brief provider intervention for problem drinking have shown benefit at 12 months[28] and 48 months.[29] Follow-up of brief intervention for at-risk alcohol drinkers has shown the impact to be long-lasting, with continued impact on alcohol intake at 9 years.[30]

More recent studies, however, have failed to show effectiveness among non-treatment-seeking, screen-detected populations in general[31] and in the primary care setting,[32,33,34] as well as among medical inpatients.[35] Limitations of SBIRT appear to be due to poor success with patients following through with referral to treatment, and limited effectiveness of SBIRT for those with more severe substance use disorders. These interventions are probably more effective among those seeking help from their primary care clinician; most trials excluded these individuals. It is hoped that ongoing and future research will help us better understand how to engage those who are not seeking help.

Notes

1. Jonas DE, Garbutt JC, Amick HR, et al. Behavioral counseling after screening for alcohol misuse in primary care: a systematic review and meta-analysis for the U.S. Preventive Services Task Force. Ann Intern Med 2012;157:645–54.

2. U.S. Preventive Services Task Force. Counseling and interventions to prevent tobacco use and tobacco-caused disease in adults and pregnant women: U.S. Preventive Services Task Force Reaffirmation Recommendation Statement. Ann Intern Med 2009;150:551–5.

3. U.S. Preventive Services Task Force. Drug use, illicit: screening. January 2008. www.uspreventiveservicestaskforce.org. Accessed December 28, 2014.

4. Lanier D, Ko S. *Screening in Primary Care Settings for Illicit Drug Use: Assessment of Screening Instruments—A Supplemental Evidence Update for the U.S. Preventive Services Task Force.* Evidence Synthesis No. 58, Part 2. AHRQ Publication No. 08-05108-EF-2. Rockville, MD: Agency for Healthcare Research and Quality; January 2008.

5. Humeniuk RE, Henry-Edwards S, Ali RL, Poznyak V, Monteiro M (2010). *The Alcohol, Smoking and Substance Involvement Screening Test (ASSIST): Manual for Use in Primary Care.* Geneva: World Health Organization. http://www.who.int/substance_abuse/activities/assist/en/. Accessed December 28, 2014.

6. Smith PC, Schmidt SM, Allensworth-Davies D, Saitz R. A single-question screening test for drug use in primary care. Arch Intern Med 2010;170:1155–60.

7. Miller WR. Motivational interviewing: research, practice and puzzles. Addict Behav 1996;21:835–42.

8. Kim TW, Samet JH, Cheng DM, et al. Primary care quality and addiction severity: a prospective cohort study. Health Serv Res 2007;42:755–72.

9. **Reiff-Hekking S, Ockene JK, Hurley TG, Reed GW. Brief physician and nurse practitioner-delivered counseling for high risk drinking. Results of a 12-month follow-up. J Gen Intern Med 2005;20:7–13.** *In a randomized trial of 530 high-risk drinkers, a single 5- to 10-minute special intervention (SI) was compared with usual care (UC) in four academic primary care practices. At 12-month follow-up, after controlling for baseline differences in alcohol consumption, SI participants had significantly larger changes in weekly alcohol intake (SI = –5.7 drinks per week; UC = –3.1 drinks per week), and of those who changed to safe drinking at 6 months, more SI than UC participants maintained that change at 12 months.*

10. Prochaska JO, DiClemente CC, Norcross JC. In search of how people change. Applications to addictive behaviors. Am Psychol 1992;47:1102–14.

11. Fernandez AC, Begley EA, Marlatt GA. Family and peer interventions for adults: past approaches and future directions. Psychol Addict Behav 2006;20:207–13.

12. Landau J, Garrett J, Shea RR, et al. Strength in numbers: the ARISE method for mobilizing family and network to engage substance abusers in treatment. A relational intervention sequence for engagement. Am J Drug Alcohol Abuse 2000;26:379–98.

13. Landau J, Stanton MD, Brinkman-Sull D, et al. Outcomes with the ARISE approach to engaging reluctant drug- and alcohol-dependent individuals in treatment. Am J Drug Alcohol Abuse 2004;30:711–48.

14. Bradley BP, Phillips G, Green L, Gossop M. Circumstances surrounding the initial lapse to opiate use following detoxification. Br J Psychiatry 1989;154:354–9.

15. Marlatt GA. Craving for alcohol, loss of control, and relapse: a cognitive-behavioral analysis. In Nathan PE, Marlatt GA, Loberg T, eds. *Alcoholism: New Directions in Behavioral Research and Treatment*. New York: Plenum Press; 1978:271–314.

16. Polich JM, Armor DJ, Braiker HB. Stability and change in drinking patterns. In *The Course of Alcoholism: Four Years After Treatment*. New York: John Wiley & Sons; 1981:159–200.

17. Zgierska A, Fleming MF. Screening and brief intervention. In Ries RK, Fiellin DA, Miller SC, Saitz R, eds. *The ASAM Principles of Addiction Medicine*, 5th ed. Philadelphia: Wolters Kluwer; 2014:297–331.

18. **Fleming MF, Barry KL, Manwell LB, et al. Brief physician advice for problem alcohol drinkers: a randomized controlled trial in community-based primary care practices. JAMA 1997;277:1039–45.** *In this trial, 482 men and 292 women were randomized to a control or an experimental group who had two 10- to 15-minute counseling visits delivered by physicians. At 12-month follow-up, there were significant reductions in 7-day alcohol use (mean number of drinks in previous 7 days decreased from 19 to 12 for the experimental group vs. 19 to 16 for controls, p < 0.001), episodes of binge drinking (mean number of binge drinking episodes during previous 30 days decreased from 5.7 to 3.1 for the experimental group vs. 5.3 to 4.2 for controls, p < 0.001), and frequency of excessive drinking (percentage drinking excessively in previous 7 days decreased from 48% to 18% for the experimental group vs. 48% to 33% for control, p < 0.001).*

19. Wilk AI, Jensen NM, Havighurst TC. Meta-analysis of randomized control trials addressing brief interventions in heavy alcohol drinkers. J Gen Intern Med 1997;12:274–83.

20. Grossberg PM, Brown DD, Fleming MF. Brief physician advice for high-risk drinking among young adults. Ann Fam Med 2004;2:474–80. *In this randomized trial, 226 young adults (aged 18–30) were assigned to either usual care or brief intervention. Over the 4-year follow-up, there were significant reductions in number of persons drinking >3 drinks/day, average 7-day alcohol use, number of persons drinking ≥6 drinks/occasion, and number of binge drinking episodes in the previous 30 days. There were also significant differences in emergency department visits (103 vs. 177), motor vehicle crashes (9 vs. 20), total motor vehicle events (114 vs. 149), and arrests for controlled substance or liquor violation (0 vs. 8).*

21. Manwell LB, Fleming MF, Mundt MP, et al. Treatment of problem alcohol use in women of childbearing age: results of a brief intervention trial. Alcohol Clin Exp Res. 2000;10:1517–24. *In this randomized trial, 205 females (ages 18–40) with problem drinking were assigned to a brief intervention or a control group; 85% completed the 48-month follow-up. There was a significant treatment effect in reducing both 7-day alcohol use (p = 0.004) and binge drinking episodes (p = 0.002). Women in the intervention group who became pregnant during the follow-up had the most dramatic decreases in alcohol use. A logistic regression model based on a ≥20% reduction in drinking found an odds ratio (OR) of 1.9 (95% CI, 1.1–3.5) among those who received the brief intervention.*

22. Chang G, Wilkins-Haug L, Berman S, Goetz MA. Brief intervention for alcohol use in pregnancy: a randomized trial. Addiction 1999;94:1499–508. *This randomized controlled trial assessed alcohol use in 258 women initiating prenatal care, comparing assessment only (AO) versus brief intervention (BI). Among women with prenatal alcohol consumption before assessment, there was no difference between groups, but for women who were abstinent preassessment, those who received BI maintained higher rates of abstinence (86% vs. 72%).*

23. Crawford MJ, Patton R, Touquet R, et al. Screening and referral for brief intervention of alcohol-misusing patients in an emergency department: a pragmatic randomized controlled trial. Lancet 2004;364:1334–9.

24. Stein MD, Charuvastra A, Maksad J, Anderson BJ. A randomized trial of a brief alcohol intervention for needle exchangers (BRAINE). Addiction 2002;97:691–700. *In this randomized controlled trial of 187 needle exchange program clients, motivational intervention (MI) for alcohol use (two 1-hour sessions 1 month apart) was compared with no intervention. The MI group was more likely to have ≥7 consecutive days abstinent, with an OR of 2.6 (95% CI, 2.0–2.9).*

25. **Spirito A, Monti PM, Barnett NP, et al. A randomized clinical trial of a brief motivational intervention for alcohol-positive adolescents treated in an emergency department.** J Pediatr 2004;145:396–402. *This randomized controlled trial studied 152 alcohol-using adolescents in an emergency department, comparing a motivational intervention (MI) with standard intervention. MI produced significant improvement in average number of drinking days/month and frequency of high-volume drinking.*

26. **McCambridge J, Strang.** The efficacy of single session motivational interviewing in reducing drug consumption and perceptions of drug-related risk and harm among young people: results from a multi-site cluster randomized trial. Addiction 2004;99:39–52.

27. **Bernstein J, Bernstein E, Tassiopoulos K, et al. Brief motivational intervention at a clinic visit reduces cocaine and heroin use.** Drug Alcohol Depend 2005;77:49–59. *This randomized trial of 1,175 patients in urban teaching hospital outpatient clinics compared a single-session motivational intervention (MI) for heroin and cocaine use with standard intervention. At 6 months, the MI group was more likely to be abstinent for cocaine alone (22% vs. 17%, OR 1.51, CI 1.01–2.24), heroin alone (40% vs. 31%, OR 1.57, CI 1.00–2.47), and both drugs (17% vs. 13%, OR 1.51, CI 0.98–2.26).*

28. **Fleming MF, Mundt MP, French MT, et al. Benefit-cost analysis of brief physician advice with problem drinkers in primary care settings.** Med Care 2000;38:7–18. *In this trial, 482 men and 292 women who reported drinking above a threshold limit were randomized into control or intervention groups. At 6- and 12-month follow-up, outcomes examined included alcohol use, emergency department visits, and number of hospital days, legal events, and motor vehicle accidents. The total economic benefit of the brief intervention was $423,519 (95% CI: $35,947, $884,848), composed of $195,448 (95% CI: $36,734, $389,160) in savings in emergency department and hospital use, and $228,071 (95% CI: –$191,419, $757,303) in avoided costs of crime and motor vehicle accidents. The average (per subject) benefit was $1,151 (95% CI: $92, $2,257). The estimated total economic cost of the intervention was $80,210, or $205 per subject. The benefit-cost ratio was 5.6:1 (95% CI: 0.4–11.0), or $56,263 in total benefit for every $10,000 invested.*

29. **Fleming MF, Mundt MP, French MT, et al. Brief physician advice for problem drinkers: long-term efficacy and benefit-cost analysis.** Alcohol Clin Exp Res 2002;26:36–43. *This randomized controlled trial consisted of 482 men and 292 women who reported drinking above a threshold limit. At 48-month follow-up, subjects who received the intervention*

exhibited significant reductions in 7-day alcohol use, number of binge drinking episodes, and frequency of excessive drinking, all with p < 0.01. The treatment sample also had fewer days of hospitalization (p = 0.05) and fewer emergency department visits (p = 0.08). Seven deaths occurred in the control group and three in the treatment group. Benefit-cost analysis showed a $43,000 reduction in future health care costs for every $10,000 invested in brief intervention for problem drinking.

30. Nilssen O. Long-term effect of brief intervention in at-risk alcohol drinkers: a 9-year follow-up study. Alcohol Alcoholism 2004;39:548–51.

31. Young MM, Stevens A, Galipeau J, et al. Effectiveness of brief interventions as part of screening, brief intervention and referral to treatment (SBIRT) for reducing the nonmedical use of psychoactive substances: a systematic review. Syst Rev 2014;3:50.

32. **Saitz R, Palfai TPA, Cheng DM, et al. Screening and brief intervention for drug use in primary care–The ASPIRE randomized clinical trial. JAMA 2014;312:502–13.** *This randomized trial compared a brief 10- to 15-minute interview by a health educator (BNI), and a 30- to 45-minute intervention with a 20- to 30-minute booster conducted by a counselor (MOTIV), with no brief intervention. At 6 months, mean adjusted number of days using the main drug at 6 months was 12 for no brief intervention versus 11 for the BNI group (incidence rate ratio [IRR], 0.97; 95% CI, 0.77–1.22) and 12 for the MOTIV group (IRR, 1.05; 95% CI, 0.84–1.32; p = 0.81 for both comparisons vs. no brief intervention). There were no significant effects of BNI or MOTIV on any other outcome stratified by main drug or drug use severity.*

33. Roy-Byrne P, Bumgardner K, Krupski A, et al. Brief interventions for problem drug in safety-net primary care settings—a randomized clinical trial. JAMA 2014;312:492–501.

34. Kaner E, Bland M, Cassidy P. Effectiveness of screening and brief alcohol intervention in primary care (SIPS trial): pragmatic randomized controlled trial. BMJ 2013;346:e8501.

35. **Saitz R, Palfai TP, Cheng DM. Brief intervention for medical inpatients with unhealthy alcohol use—a randomized controlled trial. Ann Intern Med 2007;146:167–76.** *This randomized controlled trial involved 12-month follow-up of 341 medical inpatients drinking risky amounts of alcohol who received a 30-minute session of motivational counseling by a trained counselor or usual care. The intervention was not associated with receipt of alcohol assistance by 3 months, or drinks/day at 12 months.*

3

General Treatment Principles

Background

A wide variety of treatment modalities exist for treatment of substance use disorders (SUDs). Despite the tremendous variation in substances, there are common themes in treatment and many similarities in the therapeutic approaches. In this chapter, we will address the treatment setting and then briefly review types of treatment and their applications. Further details and references can be found in the corresponding chapters on specific substances.

Most SUD treatments can be roughly divided into two types of modalities: (1) *psychosocial treatment,* which includes brief intervention, self-help groups, counseling, cognitive-behavioral therapy, and analytic psychotherapy, and (2) *pharmacotherapy,* which includes drug antagonists or agonists and other agents. Of course, these treatments are not mutually exclusive, and the best approach in many cases is a combination of therapeutic modalities.

At the end of this chapter, we will briefly discuss how to evaluate treatment studies and outline some of the common problems and why they are of concern.

Treatment Setting

When treating an individual with an SUD, one of the first decisions that needs to be made is the optimal treatment setting. This decision is often limited by availability, insurance limitations, and patient preference. The American Society of Addiction Medicine (ASAM) has developed patient placement criteria to help guide this decision.[1] These are available in textbook format and through online software (www.asamsoftware.com). The criteria have been shown to have high interrater reliability[2] and study data support their utility. One observational study of alcohol-dependent individuals admitted to different levels of care reported that those who were *undertreated* (i.e., were placed at a lower level of care than would be recommended by placement criteria) did worse than those who were appropriately matched; moreover, *overtreatment* was not associated with better outcomes.[3] However, another observational study reported that outcomes between "matched" and "mismatched" patients were not significantly different.[4] Moreover, there are often barriers to matching patients to the recommended level of care.[5] Nevertheless, these criteria are widely used, and many insurance companies use them to determine medical necessity.

A detailed description of the ASAM criteria is beyond the scope of this handbook; we encourage readers to refer to the original text. What follows is a very brief outline.

The ASAM criteria involve six dimensions to assess patients:

1. Acute intoxication and/or withdrawal potential
2. Biomedical conditions and complications
3. Emotional, behavioral, or cognitive conditions and complications
4. Readiness to change
5. Relapse, continued use, or continued problem potential
6. Recovery/living environment

The ASAM placement criteria for adults divide patients into four general treatment levels: (1) outpatient treatment, (2) intensive outpatient treatment or partial hospitalization, (3) residential treatment, and (4) medically managed intensive inpatient treatment; levels 2 and 3 are, respectively, subdivided into two and four further levels. The appropriate level is determined by the patient's status in the six dimensions just listed. The criteria can be summarized thus:

Level 1 (outpatient) is appropriate for patients who (1) have minimal risk of severe withdrawal, (2/3) have no unstable biomedical or emotional conditions, (4) are cooperative, (5) have adequate coping skills, and (6) are in a supportive environment.

Level 2 (intensive outpatient or partial hospitalization) is appropriate for patients who (1) have minimal to moderate risk of severe withdrawal, (2/3) mild or manageable biomedical or emotional conditions, (4) are somewhat resistant to change, (5) have a high risk of relapse, and (6) are in an unsupportive environment. Level 2 is further subdivided into Level 2.1 (intensive outpatient) and 2.5 (partial hospitalization).

Level 3 (residential services) is appropriate for patients who (1) have minimal to moderate risk of withdrawal that can be managed at this level, (2/3) have medical or emotional conditions that require monitoring and structure (but not intensive treatment), (4) are resistant to treatment, (5) are unable to control their use, and (6) are in an environment that is dangerous for recovery. Level 3 is further subdivided into Level 3.1 (clinically managed low-intensity residential), 3.3 (clinically managed population-specific high-intensity residential), 3.5 (clinically managed high-intensity residential), and 3.7 (medically monitored intensive inpatient).

Level 4 (medically managed intensive inpatient services) is appropriate for patients who (1) have a severe withdrawal risk or (2/3) require 24-hour medical or psychiatric and nursing care for medical or emotional conditions (dimensions 4 through 6 have no impact on determining this level).

The ASAM placement criteria also include a separate category of opioid treatment program (OTP).

Psychosocial Treatment

A variety of psychosocial modalities have been used in treatment of substance use disorders. Providing brief advice or counseling in primary care settings appears to be effective for some individuals. Participation in self-help groups is associated with improved outcomes and drug counseling (group or individual) may also be helpful. A number of behavioral approaches also appear to be modestly effective.

Brief Interventions

The simplest and most straightforward form of treatment is to screen patients for tobacco, alcohol, and other drug use and to counsel those for whom this likely is a problem. Brief interventions or advice generally take the form of giving advice on the health effects of the drug, assessing the patient's readiness for change, and providing information and assistance on treatment options. These interventions can be performed in primary care settings, emergency departments, and inpatient units by physicians, nurse practitioners, nurses, or trained counselors. Although the evidence is not consistent,[6] brief interventions have been reported to be modestly effective for smokers, problem drinkers, as well as heroin and cocaine users, but there may be factors that influence outcomes, including the type of intervention, the motivation of the individual, and the severity of the problem.

Motivational Enhancement

For many individuals, lack of motivation to change appears to be an important barrier; for this reason, *motivational interviewing* and *motivational enhancement therapy* have been developed as treatment options. These treatments typically involve one to four patient-centered sessions in which the patient's goals and the role that their substance use plays in their life are explored and the negative consequences of this problem are discussed. This is followed by help and encouragement for further treatment. Strategies employed include expressing empathy for the patient and acceptance of their ambivalence for change, pointing out discrepancies between the patient's goals and their current situation, providing new perspectives when resistance is encountered, and expressing confidence in the patient's ability to change. A number of studies suggest that this approach is effective for some, though the evidence to support this approach is not strong.[7] This topic is covered in more detail in Chapter 2.

Self-Help Groups

Self-help groups (also known as "mutual help groups" or "mutual self-help groups") are one of the oldest and most commonly used forms of SUD treatment. Alcoholics Anonymous (AA) is perhaps the best-known example of this approach; Narcotics Anonymous (NA) and Cocaine Anonymous (CA) are analogous groups for those addicted to opioids or stimulants. These groups are organized and led by individuals in recovery, not by treatment professionals, and many use a 12-step approach (these are outlined in Chapter 4, on alcohol). The data on the effectiveness of these groups (primarily from observational studies) are limited, but suggest that participation is associated with better outcomes.[8] However, it is difficult to gauge the impact of this type of treatment from observational data, and experimental evidence is sparse.[9]

Drug Counseling

After self-help groups, drug counseling is probably the most commonly used treatment modality; this can be done in a group or individual setting. In contrast to self-help groups, group drug counseling sessions are typically led by trained drug counselors. However, the philosophy and approach of these groups is often quite similar, with a focus on the stages of recovery and providing a supportive atmosphere for maintaining abstinence and making lifestyle changes.

Individual drug counseling is a more intensive one-on-one treatment led by a trained counselor; like group counseling, it often focuses on stages of recovery and the development of tasks and goals based on the 12-step philosophy. Therapists often assist individuals with social, family, and legal problems. A number of studies suggest that both of these modalities are modestly effective in the short term (i.e., while individuals participate), but there are limited data on longer-term effectiveness.

Behavioral Therapy

There are a wide variety of behavioral approaches available that appear to be effective for treating SUDs. In general, behavioral therapy focuses on particular behaviors that affect an individual's functioning (e.g., drug use); the therapist works with the patient to find effective strategies to reduce these "target behaviors." A distorted perception of self and the surrounding environment is thought to lead to negative thoughts and hopelessness that contribute to drug use. One strategy is to examine the thought processes that underlie specific behaviors in order to help the individual recognize these "dysfunctional" patterns of thinking and develop strategies to counter them; this approach is referred to as *cognitive-behavioral therapy*. A variant is referred to as *coping skills therapy*, the aim of which is to foster coping skills to reduce the risk of use. Such skills include assertiveness training, focusing on the consequences of use, finding alternative behaviors, and learning ways to avoid or escape situations that lead to use. Another, similar approach is sometimes referred to as *relapse prevention therapy*; this uses a variety of cognitive and coping strategies to deal with high-risk situations and early signs of impending relapse. Individuals are encouraged to find healthy activities that decrease their need for substances and to prepare for possible lapses in abstinence in order to prevent them from developing into a full-blown relapse. In *network therapy* behavioral techniques are used and family members and friends enlisted to reinforce compliance and undermine denial.

Recently, there has been increasing interest in *mindfulness-based treatment* for substance use disorders. Although there are varying definitions, mindfulness generally involves attention to the present moment experience and cultivating a nonjudgmental, nonreactive state of awareness. It has been reported to be effective in a 2014 review[10] and in a 2014 clinical trial published after the review.[11]

Yet another behavioral strategy is to provide rewards for desirable behaviors or punishment for undesirable ones; this practice is often referred to as *contingency management*. Most studies of contingency management use vouchers as a reward for drug-free urine drug tests, often in the setting of methadone maintenance programs. In another treatment modality, "alternate reinforcers" and a healthier lifestyle are promoted, by combining cognitive-behavioral therapy with vocational rehabilitation, as well as with contingency management and other behavioral modalities; this is sometimes referred to as *community reinforcement*. These approaches appear to be modestly effective while in place, but the effect seems to dissipate once the rewards and other external factors are removed.

Drug Courts

Persons with SUD often become involved with the criminal justice system. Drug courts are, in the United States at least, a common way of dealing with illicit-drug users who break the law. This approach is quite similar to contingency management, with an emphasis on sanctions rather than on rewards. Typically, offenders in these programs are required to enter an addiction treatment program, undergo frequent testing (generally urine drug testing) to verify abstinence, and appear frequently in court to be monitored by judges; those who do not comply with the program requirements face the threat of sanctions, including imprisonment. Studies suggest that these programs can reduce drug use and recidivism, at least while participants are under court supervision.[12] However, evidence of long-term effectiveness is lacking.[13]

Analytic Psychotherapy

Analytic psychotherapy uses a variety of strategies to help individuals deal with their problems (including addiction). While behavioral therapy focuses on problem behaviors, analytic psychotherapy focuses on understanding the thoughts and feelings that lead to these behaviors. *Expressive-supportive therapy* is one such analytically based treatment modality. In the expressive mode, the patient focuses on interpersonal relationships and transference to others; in the supportive mode, the patient forms a therapeutic alliance and tries to strengthen coping skills and defenses to reestablish equilibrium. Techniques used include confrontation, clarification, partial interpretation, and suggestion (advice); in contrast to traditional psychoanalysis, there is limited free association and less focus on interpretation and developing insight into the origins of a problem. *Interpersonal psychotherapy* is a time-limited treatment that focuses on current events and problems and tries to alleviate symptoms and social dysfunction. In general, this type of approach seems to have limited effectiveness for addiction treatment but may offer some benefits, especially for those with a co-occurring psychiatric disorder.

Residential Treatment

Residential programs are another heterogeneous treatment modality that can range from halfway houses that are little more than a place to stay, to more intensive treatment facilities. In general, observational data suggest that most who enter this type of treatment do not complete it, but those who stay tend to have better outcomes.

Therapeutic communities are a variant of residential treatment, which are typically organized and led by individuals who are in recovery, though many such communities employ professional staff, who are often in recovery themselves. In these communities, the focus is on members' behaviors; their lives are often tightly controlled and monitored by the group, and, in general, contact outside of the community is limited. Older members serve as role models, and undesirable behaviors are sanctioned, often through peer confrontation. These types of programs are probably more effective than their less structured counterparts, but they typically have high attrition rates.

Modified therapeutic communities are a more recently developed model of care that are less intense and more flexible and focus more on individualized treatment. These programs emphasize positive reinforcement and conflict resolution instead of confrontation and sanctions. There is some research that supports their effectiveness, particularly for individuals with concurrent psychiatric illness and SUD.

Pharmacotherapy

There are a number of medications that can help individuals with substance use disorders. Pharmacotherapy can be provided in a variety of settings, including office-based practice. In this setting, it is typically accompanied by *medical management*, which focuses on adherence, side effects, and progress toward goals in an empathic, supportive, and nonjudgmental manner.

Drug Antagonists

The use of specific agents to block the effect of an abused substance is an attractive option that has been long pursued in search of an effective treatment for SUD. So far, this approach has largely failed. The best-studied example is the use of opioid antagonists, such as naltrexone, to block the effect of opioids. While opioid antagonists are very effective for treatment of acute overdose, these agents have not been found to be very effective for SUD treatment in general—except perhaps in a subset of highly motivated individuals or in settings where drug agonist treatment is not available.

An analogous approach is to use a drug that antagonizes some of the central nervous system (CNS) effects of a substance, such as using dopamine antagonists (e.g., olanzapine) for treatment of stimulant (specifically cocaine) use disorders; this has not been found to be effective. However, the search for effective drug antagonists has not been abandoned. Injectable or implantable long-acting formulations of opioid antagonists may prove to be effective, and there is active research into the development of vaccines to specific drugs.

Drug Agonists

In contrast to drug antagonists, drug agonists have been shown to be effective in SUD treatment. These agents have been used for treatment of SUDs in two ways: (1) for withdrawal management (detoxification) and (2) for maintenance therapy. The benzodiazepine sedative-hypnotics are effective treatment for alcohol withdrawal. Likewise, methadone, an opioid agonist and buprenorphine, a partial agonist, are effective for treating the symptoms of opioid withdrawal. Nicotine replacement and nicotine receptor agonists have been shown to help smokers quit.

Maintenance therapy has become an important treatment modality for opioid dependence. Methadone and buprenorphine maintenance treatment are both effective at reducing illicit opioid use and the risk of complications (especially overdose). Long-acting stimulants may likewise help reduce illicit cocaine (and methamphetamine) use, but there is much less experience with this approach. Using alternative nicotine-delivery systems, such as use of electronic cigarettes, has been proposed as a way to reduce the morbidity and mortality associated with smoking.

Other Agents

A wide variety of other agents have been studied for SUD treatment, and a few have been modestly effective or show promise. While these agents do not directly mimic or block the effect of the target drug, they generally have effects on other neurotransmitters that may affect craving or reward. The antidepressants bupropion and nortriptyline have been found to help smokers quit (but other antidepressants do not). Naltrexone and accamprosate appear to be modestly effective for alcoholism. Studies suggest that the antiepileptic agents topiramate and gabapentin may also be effective treating for alcoholism.

Aversion Therapy

Another treatment strategy is to pair an unpleasant stimulus with the use of a particular substance; this is referred to as "aversion therapy," or "aversive conditioning." The best-studied example of this is the use of disulfiram (antabuse), which causes an unpleasant reaction when combined with alcohol use. A variety of aversive treatments have been tried to help smokers quit, including rapid puffing, smoke-holding, excessive smoking, and silver acetate. Disulfiram may help selected individuals, but, in general, this therapeutic approach has not been shown to be very effective.

Alternative Therapies

A number of so-called alternative therapies are used for SUD treatment. The one that has been studied best is acupuncture (specifically for smoking and cocaine dependence), but it has not been shown to be effective. Hypnotherapy has been used for smoking cessation and for other SUDs; like acupuncture, there is limited evidence to support its effectiveness. Other proposed treatment modalities include meditation, biofeedback, and relaxation therapy. The research in this area of therapy is still in its infancy. There may yet prove to be a role for them in the treatment of SUDs.

Evaluating Addiction Treatment Research

Performing high-quality research on SUDs is a difficult task. This problem is compounded by the relatively low priority given to research in this area, despite its importance. A number of issues limit the strength of many of the available research studies.[14] While these are not unique to addiction research, they must nonetheless be taken into account. Box 3.1 offers some general guidelines for evaluating therapeutic studies. We will offer a brief overview of some of these issues and why they are important. Many readers will already be familiar with these general principles from evidence-based medicine, but it may be helpful to review them in the context of addiction treatment research.

Observational Studies and Lack of Control Group

Many research studies on addiction treatment are observational studies and lack a control group for comparison. These often take the form of a "before and after" analysis in which the subjects' drug use (or other measures) after a specific treatment are compared with their "baseline" status before treatment to establish the effectiveness of an intervention. While finding an improvement in a particular outcome measure (such as drug use) during or after a certain

---

BOX 3.1 Suggested Guidelines for Assessing
Treatment Studies

Was the assignment of patients to treatments randomized?
Were all patients who entered the study accounted for at its
conclusion?
Was the analysis performed on an intention-to-treat basis?
Were the study patients recognizably similar to my own?
Were all clinically relevant outcomes reported?
Were both statistical and clinical significance considered?
Is the treatment feasible in my practice setting?

Adapted from Sackett DL, Haynes RB, Guyatt GH, et al. *Clinical
Epidemiology: A Basic Science for Clinical Medicine*, 2nd ed. Boston: Little,
Brown; 1991.

---

treatment is certainly evidence in support of that intervention, it is
limited at best. Given the cyclical nature of addiction, if one were to
take a group of individuals who wished to stop or cut down on their
substance use and followed them over time (without any intervention), it is likely that one would observe a relative improvement. This
is further reinforced by the observation that when studies do have a
control group, they often have a significant improvement from baseline.[15] Without a comparable control group (preferably selected by
randomization), it is impossible to know whether the treatment was
really effective and if it was effective, to what extent. On the other
hand, simply screening for an alcohol use disorder seems to have an
effect on subsequent outcomes and will attenuate the relative impact
of brief interventions when the control group was screened.[16]

Exclusion of Dropouts

Even when a clinical trial uses a randomly assigned control group for
comparison, the study is often limited by dropouts; this weakens the
ability of a trial to detect a significant difference and tends to dilute

the measured effect of a treatment (if there is one). This is a particular problem in SUD research, since these studies typically have high dropout rates. There are two general ways of dealing with this problem.[17] One is to include everyone enrolled in the study—even those who did not remain in treatment—in the analysis of the outcomes and to count all of those for whom there is no outcomes data as treatment failures; this is called "intention-to-treat analysis" and is the most rigorous way of analyzing the data. If a study can demonstrate a benefit even when using intention-to-treat analysis, this is strong evidence in support of that treatment. Unfortunately, this is hard to do, and many studies of SUD treatment exclude those who drop out and rely instead on an "as-treated analysis." This approach may introduce a bias because those who drop out are typically different in many ways from those who stay in treatment. Furthermore, even if the treatment is truly effective (for those who remain), this type of analysis tends to make the treatment appear to be more effective than it really is (for all those who enter treatment).

Limited Generalizability

When evaluating the relevance of a clinical trial to one's own practice, it is important to carefully look at who the subjects were and whether they are comparable to the individuals you are caring for. Many SUD research studies are conducted on relatively healthy and motivated volunteers. Individuals with polysubstance dependence or serious medical or psychiatric comorbidities are often excluded.[18] This makes it difficult to generalize the results and apply them to the many individuals who do not fit this profile. One way to gauge this is to look at the number of subjects who were screened, to find those who were included in the trial; unfortunately, some reports do not give this information.

Varied Outcome Measures

What is the goal of SUD treatment? Long-term abstinence is the simplest and most obvious answer to this question, but "cure" is rarely achieved in practice, and there are many other benefits of addiction treatment. These potential benefits include reducing substance use, preventing medical complications, and ameliorating the societal impact (e.g., crime, homelessness, unemployment). The individual's own satisfaction and sense of well-being are also important outcomes. Moreover, there are numerous ways to measure each of these outcomes, and it is not unusual for a study to use multiple measures for each.[19] The wide variety of possible outcome measures speaks to the importance of SUDs, but it also creates problems for researchers and those evaluating their research. It is only natural that researchers will tend to emphasize those measures for which positive outcomes were found—especially in the abstracts of their articles—but this obviously is fertile ground for the introduction of bias.[20] The wide variety of outcome measures also makes it difficult to compare one study with another. Some have developed composite measures of addiction; a commonly used example is the Addiction Severity Index (ASI), which includes questions on medical and psychiatric status, employment status, drug/alcohol use, legal status, and family/social relationships, but these measures are not consistently used.

Clinical Significance

Even when a well-designed study shows a *statistically* significant improvement in an outcome measure, the clinician must always ask whether this difference is *clinically* significant. Studies on SUDs generally focus on measures of substance use as their primary outcome and less commonly report on clinical outcomes such as morbidity or mortality. It is difficult to gauge the clinical impact of statistically significant but relatively modest changes in substance use associated with a specific treatment. Furthermore, many trials look at treatment outcomes over a relatively short period of time (typically 12 to 24 weeks), and it is impossible to determine the long-term significance of their findings. Clinicians need to keep this in mind when deciding whether to use a treatment for a specific patient. On the other hand, there is always a range of responses, so even when the average response is not impressive, there will be some individuals who may have a clinically significant response to a specific treatment (as well as those who do not respond at all).

Limited Applicability

Last (but not least) the practitioner must ask whether the treatment can be applied where they practice. Most addiction treatment studies are not conducted in office-based practices and may not be feasible in that setting. For example, there are many studies of different treatment strategies in the setting of methadone maintenance programs, which take advantage of having a "captive audience," and probably could not be employed in the typical primary care office.

Notes

1. Mee-Lee D, Shulman GD, Fishman MJ, Gastfriend DR, Miller MM, eds. The *ASAM Criteria: Treatment Criteria for Addictive, Substance-Related, and Co-Occurring Conditions*, 3rd ed. Carson City, NV: Change Companies; 2013.

2. Baker SL, Gastfriend DR. Reliability of multidimensional substance abuse treatment matching: implementing the ASAM Patient Placement Criteria. J Addict Dis 2003;22(Suppl 1):45–60.

3. Magura S, Staines G, Kosanke N, et al. Predictive validity of the ASAM patient placement criteria for naturalistically matched vs. mismatched alcoholism patients. Am J Addict 2003;12:386–97.

4. McKay JR, Cacciola JS, McLellan AT, et al. An initial evaluation of the psychosocial dimensions of the American Society for Addiction Medicine criteria for inpatient versus intensive outpatient substance abuse rehabilitation. J Stud Alcohol 1997;58:239–52.

5. Kosanke N, Magura S, Staines G, et al. Feasibility of matching alcohol patients to ASAM levels of care. Am J Addict 2002;11:124–34.

6. Field CA, Baird J, Saitz R, Caetano R, Mont PM. The mixed evidence for brief intervention in emergency departments, trauma care centers, and inpatient hospital settings: what should we do? Alcohol Clin Exp Res 2010;34:2004–10.

7. Smedslund G, Berg RC, Hammerstrom KT, et al. Motivational interviewing for substance abuse. Cochrane Database Syst Rev 2011;5:CD008063.

8. Gossop M, Stewart D, Mardsen J. Attendance at Narcotics Anonymous and Alcoholics Anonymous meetings, frequency of attendance and substance use outcomes after residential treatment for drug dependence: a 5-year follow-up study. Addiction 2008;103:119–25.

9. Ferri M, Amato L, Davoli M. Alcoholics Anonymous and other 12-step programs for alcohol dependence. Cochrane Database Syst Rev 2006;3:CD005032.

10. Chiesa A, Serretti A. Are mindfulness-based interventions effective for substance use disorders? A systematic review of the evidence. Subst Use Misuse 2014;49:492–512.

11. Bowen S, Witkiewitz K, Clifasefi SL, et al. Relative efficacy of mindfulness-based relapse prevention, standard relapse prevention, and treatment as usual for substance use disorders: a randomized clinical trial. JAMA Psychiatry 2014;71:547–56.

12. Brown RT. Systematic review of the impact of adult drug-treatment courts. Transl Res 2010;155:263–74.

13. Perry A, Coulton S, Glanville J, et al. Interventions for drug-using offenders in the courts, secure establishments and the community. Cochrane Database Syst Rev 2006;(3):CD005193.

14. Moyer A, Finney JW, Swearingen CE. Methodological characteristics and quality of alcohol treatment outcome studies, 1970-98: an expanded evaluation. Addiction 2002;97:253–63.

15. Moyer A, Finney JW. Outcomes for untreated individuals involved in randomized trials of alcohol treatment. J Subst Abuse Treat 2002;23:247–52.

16. McCambridge J, Kypri K. Can simply answering research questions change behaviour? A systematic review and meta analyses of brief alcohol intervention trials. PLoS One 2011;6:e23748.

17. Nich C, Carroll KM. Intention-to-treat meets missing data: implications of alternate strategies for analyzing clinical trials data. Drug Alcohol Depend 2002;68:121–30.

18. Humphreys K, Weisner C. Use of exclusion criteria in selecting research subjects and its effect on the generalizability of alcohol treatment outcome studies. Am J Psychiatry 2000;157:588–94.

19. Finney JW, Moyer A, Swearingen CE. Outcome variables and their assessment in alcohol treatment studies: 1968-1998. Alcohol Clin Exp Res 2003;27:1671–9.

20. Chan AW, Altman DG. Identifying outcome reporting bias in randomised trials in PubMed: review of publications and survey of authors. BMJ 2005;330:753–6.

4

Alcohol

Background

The use of alcoholic beverages dates back thousands of years to a biblical reference to Noah drinking wine and getting drunk. Distillation of alcohol into whiskey started during the Middle Ages when alcohol was first used for medicinal purposes and as an anxiolytic. Not long after that, the detrimental effects of alcohol were first recognized.

Alcoholic beverages are fermented (wine and beer) or distilled. The concentration of alcohol (ethanol) in wine ranges from 10% to 22% by volume, while most beer contains 4–6% alcohol by volume. Distilled alcoholic beverages (e.g., whiskey, brandy, rum, gin, and vodka) contain a higher percentage of alcohol. "Proof" (in the United States) is double the percentage of alcohol by volume—for example, 90 proof is equivalent to 45% alcohol by volume. The generally used unit of consumption for alcohol is a "drink," which is equivalent to a shot glass of distilled alcohol (1 fluid oz.), one glass of wine (4 oz.), or one bottle/can of beer (12 oz.); each contains approximately 12 grams of alcohol. Patients may report their consumption in terms of number of containers. Table 4.1 lists common alcohol containers and approximate equivalence in drinks.

Epidemiology

According to the 2013 U.S. National Survey of Drug Use and Health (NSDUH),[1] an estimated 137 million of Americans are current drinkers of alcohol (52% of those aged 12 or older); 60 million (23%) are binge drinkers (five or more drinks on at least 1 day in the past 30 days). Heavy drinking (five or more drinks on the same occasion 5 or more days in the past 30 days) was reported by 17 million people (6.3%). Rates of binge drinking are greatest for those aged 18–25, with resultant higher rates of motor vehicle accidents in this population.

The estimated cost of excessive alcohol consumption in the United States in 2006 was $224 billion, or about $1.90 per drink.[2]

TABLE 4.1 Common Alcohol Containers: Volume and Number of Drinks*

Type of Alcohol	Container	Volume (Metric)	Approximate Drinks†
Beer (3–5% alcohol)	12 oz bottle/can	340 mL	1
	22 oz	620 mL	2
	40 oz	1133 mL	3–4
Wine (10–15% alcohol)	Glass	140 mL	1
	Standard bottle	750 mL	5–6
Distilled alcohol (40–50% alcohol)	Shot	30 mL	1
	Miniature	50 mL	2
	Half-pint	237 mL	8–9
	Pint	473 mL	16–18
	Fifth	757 mL	25–30
	Quart	946 mL	31–37
	Half-gallon	1892 mL	63–73

*One drink contains approximately 12 grams of alcohol.
†Actual conversion will depend on alcohol content.

From 2006 to 2010 an annual average of 88,000 alcohol-attributable deaths occurred in the United States and excessive drinking accounted for 1 in 10 deaths among working-age adults in the United States.[3]

The causes of alcoholism are multifactorial. Genetic predisposition to alcoholism appears to be present in at least half of all alcoholics.[4] Social conditioning, enabling behavior by others close to the individual, and being a child in a dysfunctional family are important nongenetic factors. Other psychiatric disorders (antisocial personality disorder, other substance use disorders, or an affective disorder) may also play a role. For elderly alcoholics, isolation is often associated with the onset of problem drinking. Individuals who have had bariatric surgery, especially Roux-en-y gastric bypass, may be at increased risk of developing an alcohol use disorder as well.[5]

Drug Effects

Alcohol is generally classified as central nervous system (CNS) depressant but has complex effects on a variety of neurotransmitters, the most important of which appear to be stimulation of gamma-aminobutyric acid (GABA) and inhibition of glutamate. A comprehensive review of the effects is beyond the scope of this handbook; we refer readers to ASAM *Principles of Addiction Medicine* for more details.[6]

Acute Effects

The acute effects of a given amount of alcohol on an individual will vary depending on a number of factors:

1. Weight (higher weight, less impact)
2. Gender (women tend to be affected more)
3. Genetics (variations in absorption and metabolism)
4. Rapidity of consumption (faster consumption leads to higher levels)
5. Presence of food in the stomach (slows absorption)
6. Tolerance (those who consume alcohol regularly develop a tolerance to the effects and metabolize alcohol more rapidly)

As a result, it is difficult to predict the effect of the consumption of a given amount of alcohol on a particular individual. Blood alcohol levels are reported in a number of different ways. The most common method in the media is the blood alcohol content (BAC), which is expressed as a percentage of grams of alcohol per grams of blood;

alcohol level can also be expressed as mg/dL, which is equivalent to the BAC × 1000. The concentration of alcohol in the breath correlates with blood alcohol levels but is lower by a factor of approximately 2100; "breathalyzer" readings are an estimate of the blood alcohol level using this factor.

In the United States (and Canada), a person with a BAC of 0.08% (80 mg/dL) or higher is considered intoxicated. A very general rule of thumb is that a standard drink will increase the average person's blood alcohol concentration by roughly 25 mg/dL (0.025%); therefore, legal intoxication generally requires the consumption of at least four drinks. The rate of metabolism of alcohol varies but is approximately 10–15 mg/dL per hour. Those who drink large quantities of alcohol chronically may metabolize it at a higher rate, about 20–30 mg/dL per hour.

The distribution of alcohol throughout the body is uniform, with equivalent plasma and CNS concentrations. At the cellular level, ethanol is a depressant, similar to anesthetics. At low levels, alcohol preferentially depresses neurons that are inhibitory, resulting in a stimulatory effect on behavior. However, this same inhibition accounts for the decline in coordination and reaction time that occurs with even small doses of alcohol. At higher doses of ethanol, impaired memory and changes in mood occur. There is individual variance in regard to the euphoria-producing and hallucinogenic effects of alcohol. Some individuals become dysphoric with even low doses of alcohol. For all individuals, the depressant/sedative effects of alcohol predominate at higher doses. Table 4.2 lists some of the expected signs and symptoms associated with different blood alcohol concentrations; the behavioral changes vary widely and are dependent on personality and circumstances. It should also be noted that these apply to nondependent individuals as well.

Acute Toxicity and Overdose

Alcohol overdose or intoxication is characterized by an initial period of excitement and euphoria followed by depression and sleep, and may progress to coma and death. The American Psychiatric

TABLE 4.2 Effects of Alcohol by Blood Concentration

Blood Alcohol Concentration (mg/dL)	Signs and Symptoms*
<25	Sense of warmth and well-being; talkativeness
25–50	Euphoria, clumsiness. Minor impairment of judgment and control
50–100	Impaired sensorium, slowed reaction time, decreased reflexes. Ataxia, worsening coordination
100–250	Cerebellar and vestibular dysfunction (ataxia, diplopia, nystagmus, visual impairment, slurred speech). Emotional lability, confusion, stupor. Nausea and vomiting. Legally intoxicated in all states
250–400	Stupor or coma. Little response to stimuli. Incontinence. Respiratory depression
>400	Respiratory paralysis. Loss of protective reflexes. Hypothermia. Death

*For nondependent individuals; there is a wide variation in the association between levels and signs/symptoms.
Adapted from Kleinschmidt KC. Ethanol. In Shannon M, Barrow SW, Burns M, eds. *Clinical Management of Poisoning and Drug Overdose*, 4th ed. Philadelphia: Saunders; 2007:5.

Association (APA), in its *Diagnostic and Statistical Manual of Mental Disorders*, Fifth Edition (DSM-5), provides criteria for alcohol intoxication: the presence of "clinically significant problematic behavior or psychological changes" plus of one (or more) of the following signs or symptoms after alcohol use: (1) slurred speech, (2) incoordination, (3) unsteady gait, (4) nystagmus, (5) impairment in attention or memory, and (6) stupor or coma.[7] In the ICD-10, the code depends on whether there is a perceptual disturbance or a comorbid use disorder, as well as the severity of the disorder. Other symptoms may include lowered inhibitions, poor judgment, labile mood, nausea, and vomiting. Blackouts and amnesia for events that occurred during intoxication are common. Alcohol idiosyncratic intoxication (pathological intoxication) is an uncommon syndrome characterized by an aggressive or violent reaction to drinking alcohol, followed by amnesia for the episode.

The duration and magnitude of intoxication depend on the amount and the rapidity with which the alcohol was consumed and other factors noted earlier. Individuals may develop substantial tolerance, appearing sober at blood alcohol levels of 150 mg/dL or more, whereas most people without tolerance become intoxicated at levels between 100 and 200 mg/dL. While there is a risk of death with blood alcohol concentrations over 300 mg/dL, the median lethal concentration (LC50) for the nondependent population is 450 mg/dL. There have been reports of alcoholics surviving with concentrations as high as 1500 mg/dL.

Withdrawal

Alcohol withdrawal is generally divided into three clusters of symptoms:[8]

1. Autonomic hyperactivity—tremulousness, sweating, tachycardia, nausea, vomiting, anxiety and agitation. These symptoms typically appear within a few hours of the last drink and peak within 24–48 hours.
2. Neuronal excitation—this includes seizures, which typically appear within 12–48 hours of abstinence.
3. Delirium tremens (or alcohol withdrawal delirium)—this includes confusion, impaired consciousness, and hallucinations (visual, tactile, and occasionally auditory), along with severe autonomic hyperactivity. This typically occurs 48–72 hours after the last consumed drink.

The DSM-5 criteria for alcohol withdrawal include the presence of at least two of the following eight symptoms, in a setting of cessation or reduction of alcohol consumption: (1) autonomic hyperactivity (sweating or tachycardia), (2) tremor, (3) insomnia, (4) nausea or vomiting, (5) transient visual, tactile, or auditory hallucinations or illusions, (6) psychomotor agitation, (7) anxiety, and (8) generalized tonic-clonic seizures.[7] The ICD-10 code for alcohol withdrawal depends on whether there is a perceptual disturbance (F10.232) or none (F10.239).

The assessment of the severity of alcohol withdrawal, as well as the treatment of alcohol withdrawal, is covered further in the section "Medically Supervised Withdrawal," later in this chapter

Alcohol Hangover

Although not technically a withdrawal syndrome, some individuals experience unpleasant symptoms as the effects of heavy drinking wear off; this is generally referred to as an "alcohol hangover." Typical symptoms include headache, fatigue, concentration problems, thirst, dizziness, nausea, cognitive impairment, and mood changes.[9] The etiology of this syndrome is not well understood, but there appears to be a genetic predisposition.[10] While there are many apocryphal cures for hangover, there is insufficient evidence to recommend anything other than simple analgesics.[11]

Assessment

Diagnosis of an alcohol use disorder requires skillful interviewing and careful evaluation. A useful, broad definition of *alcoholism* is a condition in which drinking alcohol leads to recurring trouble in one or more of several domains—interpersonal (family and friends), educational, legal, financial, medical, or occupational. Physiological manifestations—tolerance (the need for increased amounts of a substance to achieve intoxication or desired effect) and withdrawal—might not occur until later.

The National Council on Alcoholism and Drug Dependence, the American Medical Association, and the American Society of Addiction Medicine jointly define alcoholism as "a primary, chronic disease with genetic, psychosocial, and environmental factors influencing its development and manifestations. The disease is often progressive and fatal. It is characterized by impaired control over drinking, preoccupation with the drug alcohol despite adverse consequences, and distortions in thinking, most notably denial. Each of these symptoms may be continuous or periodic."[12]

The DSM-5 considers alcoholism under the category "Substance Use Disorders" and the diagnostic criteria for an alcohol use disorder are the same as for other substances—see Chapter 1 for more details.[7] The ICD-10 code for a mild alcohol use disorder is F10.10 and F10.20 for moderate-severe.

The National Institute on Alcohol Abuse and Alcoholism (NIAAA) defines *at-risk drinking* as more than 14 drinks/week or more than 4 drinks/occasion for men and more than 7 drinks/week or more than 3 drinks/occasion for women.[13] The terms *problem drinking, hazardous drinking, at-risk drinking*, and *unhealthy alcohol use* have also been used in the literature.[14] The goal is to identify individuals who may not meet DSM-5 criteria for alcohol use disorder but are at increased risk for alcohol-related problems or have had isolated problems related to drinking alcohol, such as a driving under the influence (DUI). These individuals do not necessarily need structured treatment, but may benefit from primary care intervention to prevent negative consequences from drinking,[15] such as behavioral counseling interventions, which have been shown to improve outcomes for adults with risky drinking.[16]

Screening and Diagnostic Tools

Alcohol use disorders are common and often not volunteered; therefore all patients should be screened as recommended by the U.S. Preventive Services Task Force.[17] There are a number of alcohol screening tools. The four-question CAGE is one of the simplest and most studied tools; an approach outlined in Box 4.1 incorporates the four CAGE questions into screening for alcoholism.[18,19] Inquiry begins with an open-ended question that prompts patients to respond with more than a simple yes or no or with a quantitative

BOX 4.1 Using the CAGE Questionnaire

1. Integrate alcohol use inquiry into the interview so that it follows inquiry about less sensitive habits:

   "We have talked about your usual diet and your smoking. Can you tell me how you use alcoholic beverages?"

2. For patients who report present or past use of alcohol, screen for evidence of alcoholism:

   "Has your use of alcohol caused any kinds of problems for you?" or "Have you ever been concerned about your drinking?"

3. CAGE Questions: If the patient has not disclosed a problem with drinking, use these four focused questions and probe for clarification of positive or ambivalent responses.

   "I would like to ask you a few more questions about alcohol that I ask all of my patients":

   C Have you ever felt you ought to CUT DOWN on your drinking?

   A Have people ANNOYED you by criticizing your drinking?

   G Have you ever felt bad or GUILTY about your drinking?

   E Have you ever had a drink first thing in the morning (EYE OPENER) to steady your nerves or get rid of a hangover?

reply. Among patients who report current use of alcohol, discomfort or glibness may suggest that a problem exists.[20] CAGE questions must be interpreted within a recent time frame; for example, someone now in his fifties may have had problems with alcohol while in college and not had a problem since. In a study of adult outpatients in an urban clinic, a CAGE score of 2 or more was associated with a sensitivity and specificity of 74% and 91%, respectively.[21] Probabilities of an alcohol problem were 7%, 46%, 72%, 88%, and 99% for CAGE scores 0 through 4, respectively. A positive

"C" answer is the most sensitive one (i.e., lowest false-negative rate), while a positive "E" answer is the most specific (i.e., lowest false-positive rate). In clinical practice, one positive answer should always lead to further probing.

Another screening tool, the 10-item AUDIT, developed by the World Health Organization, focuses on alcohol consumption and, as such, can be regarded as a screening tool for problem drinking (Box 4.2).[22] It is important to note that in many studies evaluating the lengthier screening tools, such as the AUDIT, the questions were asked by research assistants, not by clinicians as part of routine

---

BOX 4.2 The AUDIT Questionnaire

1. How often do you have a drink containing alcohol?

   (0) Never   (1) Monthly or less   (2) Two to four times a month   (3) Two to three times a week   (4) Four or more times a week

2. How many drinks containing alcohol do you have on a typical day when you are drinking?
   [Code number of standard drinks.]

   (0) 1 or 2   (1) 3 or 4   (2) 5 or 6   (3) 7 to 9   (4) 10 or more

3. How often do you have six or more drinks on one occasion?

   (0) Never   (1) Less than monthly   (2) Monthly (3) Weekly   (4) Daily or almost daily

4. How often during the last year have you found that you were not able to stop drinking once you had started?

   (0) Never   (1) Less than monthly   (2) Monthly (3) Weekly   (4) Daily or almost daily

5. How often during the last year have you failed to do what was normally expected from you because of drinking?

   (0) Never   (1) Less than daily   (2) Monthly   (3) Weekly (4) Daily or almost daily

6. How often during the last year have you needed a first drink in the morning to get yourself going after a heaving drinking session?

   (0) Never   (1) Less than monthly   (2) Monthly
   (3) Weekly   (4) Daily or almost daily

7. How often during the last year have you had a feeling of guilt or remorse after drinking?

   (0) Never   (1) Less than monthly   (2) Monthly   (3) Weekly   (4) Daily or almost daily

8. How often during the last year have you been unable to remember what happened the night before because you had been drinking?

   (0) Never   (1) Less than monthly   (2) Monthly
   (3) Weekly   (4) Daily or almost daily

9. Have you or someone else been injured as a result of your drinking?

   (0) No   (2) Yes, but not in the last year   (4) Yes, during the last year

10. Has a relative or friend or a doctor or other health worker been concerned about your drinking or suggested you cut down?

    (0) No   (2) Yes, but not in the last year   (4) Yes, during the last year

---

A score of 8 or more indicates a strong likelihood of harmful alcohol consumption.

From Saunders JB. Development of the Alcohol Use Disorders Identification Test (AUDIT). Addiction 1993;88:791–804.

practice. A shorter variant of the AUDIT, incorporating only its first three questions (AUDIT-C), appears to perform well as a screening tool.[23] A single question, a variant on the third question on the AUDIT, can also be used to screen for an alcohol use disorder: "How many times in the past year have you had X or more drinks in a day?" (where X is 5 for men and 4 for women, and a response of 1 or more is considered positive). The use of this tool in primary care settings has been validated[24] and is recommended by the NIAAA.[25] A positive screen on this single question should lead to further delving into alcohol use pattern and specific inquiry related to drinking and driving.

Some studies have suggested that the AUDIT is a better tool than the CAGE in specific populations, such as women[26,27] and minorities.[28] Two other screening tests, the TWEAK (to screen for alcohol use in pregnant women) and the CRAFFT (to screen for alcohol and drug use in adolescents) are discussed in Chapter 16. Another screening tool, the Michigan Alcoholism Screening Test (MAST), is a 24-question standardized instrument that has been used extensively, generally in the setting of research studies.[29]

Findings on history, physical exam, and laboratory testing that may aid in the diagnosis of alcohol use disorder are found in Table 4.3. While laboratory tests such as gamma-glutamyl transpeptidase (GGT), other liver enzymes, and red blood cell mean corpuscular volume may suggest an alcohol use disorder, none perform as well as the CAGE.[30] Nevertheless, abnormalities in these tests may be helpful in supporting persistent inquiry and discussion. Carbohydrate-deficient transferrin (CDT) testing can be used to identify heavy alcohol intake and may help in monitoring an individual's abstinence.[31] It is not as useful for women, or for individuals with significant liver disease or obesity,[32] and it has not yet been shown to be useful in screening general medical patients for alcoholism. Blood phosphatidylethanol (PEth) level may be useful in detecting alcohol use in patients with liver disease but has limited utility in quantifying use.[33]

Medical Complications

The association between alcohol and mortality follows a J-shaped curve, with moderate alcohol consumption (1–2 drinks/day for

TABLE 4.3 Findings on History, Physical Examination, and Laboratory Testing Suggestive (unmarked to*) to Highly Suggestive (** to***) or Diagnostic (****) of Alcoholism

Presenting History

****	Drinking problem, recurring	*	Legal problem
***	Blackouts with drinking	*	Noncompliance in treatment
***	Spouse/other complains of patient's drinking	*	School learning problem
***	Driving while intoxicated (DWI) record	*	Hypertension
**	Gastrointestinal bleeding, especially upper		Headache
**	Traumatic injuries		Palpitations
**	Parent, grandparent, or relative is alcoholic		Abdominal pain
**	Friends are alcoholic or have other chemical dependence		Amenorrhea
**	Family or other violence		Weight loss
**	First seizure in an adult		Vague complaints
**	Job performance problem		Insomnia
*	Unexplained syncope		Anxiety
*	Depression		Marital discord
*	Suicide attempt		Financial problem
*	Sexual dysfunction		

Past Medical History

****	Hepatitis, alcoholic
***	Pancreatitis, acute or chronic
***	Cirrhosis
***	Portal hypertension
***	Wernicke-Korsakoff syndrome
***	Frequent trauma
***	Cold injury
***	Nose and throat cancer
**	Other chemical dependence
**	Near-drownings
**	Burns, especially third degree
**	Leaves hospital against medical advice
**	Attempted suicide
**	Gastritis
**	Refractory hypertension
**	Cerebellar degeneration
**	Peripheral neuropathy
**	Aspiration pneumonia
*	Gout
*	Cardiomyopathy
*	Tuberculosis
*	Anxiety
*	Depression
*	Marital discord or family problem

Physical Examination

***	Odor of beverage alcohol on breath
***	Parotid gland enlargement, bilateral
***	Spider nevi or angioma
*	Borderline tachycardia
*	Splenomegaly
*	Hypertension

(continued)

TABLE 4.3 (Continued)

Physical Examination

*** Tremulousness, hallucinosis	Diaphoresis
** Breath mints odor	Alopecia
** Hepatomegaly	Abdominal tenderness
** Gynecomastia	Cerebellar signs (e.g., nystagmus)
** Small testicles	
** Unexplained bruises, abrasions, or cuts	

Laboratory Abnormalities

**** Blood alcohol level >300 mg/100 mL	** Hyperuricemia
*** Blood alcohol level >100 mg/100 mL without impairment	* Creatine kinase elevation
	* Hypophosphatemia or
*** High serum ammonia	Hypomagnesemia
*** Gamma-glutamyl transpeptidase elevation	Hyponatremia
** Blood alcohol level positive, any amount	Hypokalemia
** High amylase (nonspecific for pancreas)	Thrombocytopenia
** Abnormal liver function tests (especially AST > ALT)	Hyperlipoproteinemia, type 4 or 5
** Anemia, macrocytic or megaloblastic, microcytic, or mixed	

women and 2–4 drinks/day for men) associated with lower mortality than abstinence or higher levels of consumption.[34] There are a number of potential health benefits of moderate alcohol consumption, including reducing the risks of heart disease,[35,36] cerebrovascular disease,[37,38] kidney disease,[39] and diabetes mellitus.[40]

Despite the possible health benefits of moderate alcohol consumption, there are significant health hazards; prospective studies show that alcoholics have higher rates of mortality and medical morbidity than others.[41,42] The most common causes of early death in alcoholics are cirrhosis of the liver, cancers of the respiratory and gastrointestinal tracts, accidents, suicide, and ischemic heart disease. Importantly, alcoholic men who achieve long-term abstinence have a comparable mortality rate to that of their nonalcoholic peers.[43]

Pulmonary Complications

Most of the pulmonary complications seen in individuals with an alcohol use disorder are related to the fact that virtually all such patients also smoke. Lung cancer is the most common cancer diagnosed in alcoholics,[44] though alcohol consumption does not appear to increase the risk of lung cancer in never-smokers.[45] Patients who drink and smoke also have high rates of chronic obstructive lung disease. Individuals who drink to intoxication are at risk for aspiration pneumonia. Finally, alcoholism and homelessness and incarceration increase the risk for tuberculosis, particularly drug-resistant tuberculosis.[46]

Cardiovascular Complications

An association between hypertension and heavy alcohol consumption has been has been found in many clinical studies.[47,48,49] Drinking may also make hypertension more difficult to treat, as medication noncompliance is common. Clinical guidelines for treatment of hypertension recommend consideration of alcohol intake as a contributing factor.[50]

Alcohol increases the risk of stroke, partly due to its effects on blood pressure, although there may be an increased risk of stroke in heavy drinkers independent of blood pressure.[51] Even "moderate" alcohol consumption may increase the risk of stroke; in one study, men who drank more than two drinks/day were at higher risk for ischemic stroke.[52] In contrast, among men with hypertension, moderate alcohol consumption has been shown to be associated with a decreased risk for myocardial infarction, but not with decreased overall risk for death or death due to cardiovascular disease.[53]

Cases of dilated cardiomyopathy among alcoholics have been observed, with reports of the reversal of cardiomyopathy with abstinence.[54] Most reported cases of alcoholic cardiomyopathy occur in individuals who have been drinking for decades.[55] However, an analysis of data from the Framingham cohort found no association between heart failure and alcohol intake.[56] Moreover, other studies suggest that moderate alcohol intake is associated with a reduced risk of heart failure.[57]

Alcohol consumption is associated with an increased risk of developing atrial fibrillation,[58] particularly in men,[59] even with moderate intake.[60] Among those with atrial fibrillation, heavy alcohol use is associated with an increased risk of thromboembolism and death.[61] Arrhythmias (most commonly atrial fibrillation) have been observed to occur transiently after an alcohol binge among individuals without other risk factors and have been referred to as "holiday heart"; however, it is not clear if there is a true association.[62]

Gastrointestinal Complications

Alcohol affects the digestive system from the oropharynx to the rectum. Poor oral hygiene is common in alcoholics, resulting in both dental and gum disease, with potential risk of consequent bacteremia. Glossitis, cheilitis, and parotid gland enlargement are generally associated with malnutrition and/or liver disease. In the small intestine, absorption is affected, contributing to malabsorption of vitamins and diarrhea.

Alcohol lowers esophageal sphincter pressure and increases the risk of reflux esophagitis, but not Barrett's esophagus.[63] Heavy alcohol consumption is associated with an increased risk of esophageal squamous cell carcinoma, but not adenocarcinoma.[64] Vomiting from alcohol intoxication puts patients at risk for Mallory-Weiss tears. Alcohol leads to mucosal changes in the stomach causing gastritis and increases the risk for peptic ulcer disease, though this may be limited to those with *H. pylori* infection.[65] Alcohol consumption of more than two drinks/day has been also been associated with an increased risk of colon cancer.[66]

Pancreatitis

Pancreatitis from alcohol occurs with varying incidences in different populations, with genetics contributing to risk.[67] Abdominal pain from pancreatitis typically is mid-epigastric and radiates to the back. Laboratory testing reveals elevation in amylase and lipase, and imaging shows evidence of pancreatic inflammation. Management traditionally has consisted of treatment of the pain with opioids and withholding of oral feeding until signs and symptoms improve. However, there is a lack of good evidence to support "bowel rest," and a low-fat oral diet or enteral feeding may be considered.[68] Continued drinking may result in chronic pancreatitis, with endocrine (hyperglycemia) and exocrine complications (steatorrhea and malabsorption).

Liver Disease

Liver disease from alcohol use is largely related to the amount and duration of use. The risk of cirrhosis is greater for women,[69] with cirrhosis occurring at lower amounts of alcohol intake and at an earlier age.[70] Hepatic steatosis (fatty liver) is the earliest effect of alcohol on the liver and it can occur even with moderate drinking. Patients are most often asymptomatic, but they may have enlarged livers and elevated transaminases (AST and ALT). With continued drinking, hepatic steatosis may progress to hepatitis.

Alcoholic hepatitis is a histological diagnosis with hepatocellular necrosis, inflammatory exudates, fibrosis, and Mallory bodies present on biopsy.[71] Patients may be asymptomatic or present acutely with jaundice and ascites. Hepatomegaly is present in most individuals. Laboratory testing reveals elevation in bilirubin, transaminases, and alkaline phosphatase, suggesting cholestasis. Anemia, thrombocytopenia, and coagulopathy are markers of more severe disease. Patients with alcoholic hepatitis should also be assessed for presence of hepatitis C virus; in cohort studies up to 25% of alcoholics tested positive for hepatitis C infection.[72]

Therapy for alcoholic hepatitis is generally supportive, with abstinence from alcohol imperative. Therapies investigated without evidence of clear benefit include propylthiouracil,[73] pentoxifylline,[74] androgens,[75,76] and anti-TNF agents.[77,78] The data from studies of corticosteroids are mixed, with some clinical trials showing benefit[79,80,81] and others showing no benefit.[82,83,84] One study of the combination of corticosteroids and N-acetylcysteine showed increased 1-month survival, but no impact on 6-month survival.[85] Even meta-analyses of these studies provide conflicting results, mostly related to the difference in patient populations in the studies.[86,87,88] The American College of Gastroenterology guideline for the treatment of alcoholic hepatitis recommends the use of corticosteroids (prednisolone 40 mg/day for 4 weeks, followed by a taper over 2–4 weeks) in patients with encephalopathy or "discriminant function" over 32.[89] The discriminant function is calculated by multiplying the number of seconds the prothrombin time is above control times 4.6 and then adding the total bilirubin (mg/dL). Therapy is not recommended for individuals with active infection, renal failure, pancreatitis, or gastrointestinal bleeding. Transplantation for severe acute alcoholic hepatitis is controversial, as most centers require 6 months of sobriety. But one French study showed survival benefit for early liver transplantation in patients with a first episode of severe alcoholic hepatitis not responding to medical therapy.[90]

Cirrhosis occurs in up to one third of chronic alcoholics. Liver biopsy shows fibrosis, scarring with regenerating nodules, and necrosis. Radiographic imaging shows a small, shrunken liver. These pathological changes lead to portal hypertension and hepatocellular dysfunction. Nonspecific symptoms include weakness, anorexia, and fatigue, while specific symptoms and signs related to hepatic dysfunction include jaundice, ascites, confusion (hepatic encephalopathy), spider angiomata, hemorrhoids, palmar erythema, gynecomastia, and testicular atrophy. Laboratory studies show impairment in hepatic synthetic function with elevation in prothrombin time and decreased albumin. Cirrhosis also puts individuals at risk for hepatocellular carcinoma. Most progress to liver failure, and the only effective treatment is liver transplantation. Post-transplant outcomes in patients who undergo transplantation for alcoholic liver disease are comparable to those who undergo transplantation for other causes of end-stage liver disease.[91]

Renal and Electrolyte Complications

Electrolyte abnormalities (hypokalemia, hypomagnesemia, and hypophosphatemia) are common in patients with alcoholism. Most abnormalities are related to poor nutrition, but renal tubular disorders may contribute. Hypophosphatemia may not become apparent until after normal oral intake has resumed.[92] Treatment is electrolyte repletion, either orally or intravenously. Hyponatremia may occur in beer drinkers who have large volume intake of high-calorie, low-sodium beer, accompanied by little other oral intake; the term *beer potomania* is often used to describe this syndrome.[93]

Alcoholic ketoacidosis is an uncommon complication of alcoholism and typically occurs when susceptible individuals have prolonged vomiting and anorexia after drinking heavily.[94] In these individuals, liver metabolites acetaldehyde and acetate trigger liver production of beta-hydroxybutyrate and acetoacetate, resulting in acidosis. Treatment is intravenous saline and glucose.

Acute renal failure may occur in the setting of rhabdomyolysis, discussed later in the chapter. In the setting of cirrhosis with liver failure, the hepatorenal syndrome may occur. Histologically, the kidneys appear normal. Renal insufficiency in this disorder is likely related to splanchnic vasodilatation and renal vasoconstriction.[95] There is no clear treatment, except liver transplantation.

Neurological Complications

Wernicke's encephalopathy, a syndrome of global confusion, ataxia, and impaired eye movement (most commonly, lateral gaze nystagmus and lateral rectus muscle paralysis), is caused by thiamine (vitamin B1) deficiency. The condition does not occur if dietary thiamine intake is adequate. *Korsakoff's psychosis* is the term associated with the confabulatory and amnesia components of the encephalopathy. Acute Wernicke's encephalopathy is a medical emergency. Treatment with parenteral thiamine (100 mg) may improve ocular symptoms within a few hours. Magnesium should also be repleted as it is a cofactor for thiamine transketolase, an enzyme necessary for glucose metabolism. With abstinence from alcohol and good nutrition for several months, some patients recover entirely.[96] However, many individuals remain impaired.

Confusion may also be caused by hepatic encephalopathy occurring in the setting of liver failure. Ammonia and GABA are generated by the action of bacteria in the gut and are normally metabolized by the liver. In the setting of cirrhosis, these two compounds enter the systemic circulation in high amounts, causing confusion, disorientation, and coma. Treatment includes lactulose, which acidifies stool, preventing back diffusion of ammonia, or antibiotics such as neomycin and rifaxamin, which reduce colonic bacteria levels.

Cerebellar degeneration, independent from Wernicke's encephalopathy, may result in ataxia with a wide-based gait. Nutritional factors and direct toxic effects of alcohol have been implicated as causes. With abstinence and nutritional support, patients may improve.

Peripheral neuropathy can be the result of trauma or B vitamin (cyanocobalamin, thiamine, pyridoxine and pantothenic acid) deficiency. When due to nutritional deficiency, lower extremity involvement is more common. Symptoms, which usually include pain, paresthesias, and weakness, are distal and symmetric. Treatment consists of abstinence and B-complex vitamin replacement.

Alcohol withdrawal seizures are typically grand mal, but status epilepticus is rare. Patients with new seizures should be evaluated with computerized tomography (CT) and electroencephalography (EEG), as the etiology could be related to trauma, causing an intracranial bleed. Management of seizures is discussed later in this chapter, under treatment of withdrawal.

Musculoskeletal Complications

Alcohol use disorders are associated with an increased risk of traumatic injuries.[97] Osteonecrosis of the femoral head is associated with alcohol intake, for unclear reasons.[98] Alcohol also has impacts on bone metabolism, with an increased risk of osteoporosis in alcoholic men,[99] whereas moderate amounts of alcohol intake in women appear to actually improve bone density.[100,101]

Acute alcohol myopathy or rhabdomyolysis occurs most commonly in the setting of binge drinking, without history of trauma. Multiple muscle groups are tender and painful. The etiology is unknown, but hypophosphatemia is present in many cases. Rhabdomyolysis may also occur in the setting of intoxication as a result of focal muscle trauma. Treatment in both instances is hydration, correction of metabolic abnormalities, and monitoring for renal damage. A chronic form of alcoholic myopathy may also occur with or without polyneuropathy.[102] This myopathy is painless and progresses with significant muscle atrophy.

Gout has long been associated with alcohol intake.[103] A cohort study of men found that those who drank beer, but not wine, were at increased risk for having an episode of gout.[104]

Psychiatric Complications

Among patients with chronic mental illness, especially depression and anxiety, alcohol use disorder is common. In many patients, alcohol use disorder is the primary problem and treatment of depressive symptoms is not successful unless alcohol treatment is initiated.[105] Co-occurring disorders are covered further in Chapter 15.

Alcoholics may experience hallucinations during withdrawal, but also while drinking—this has sometimes been referred to as "alcoholic hallucinosis." There is some controversy about whether this is a distinct syndrome or symptoms occurring in a mix of individuals with either withdrawal symptoms or an independent psychiatric disorder.[106] Nonetheless, in a study of alcoholic men receiving treatment, 7.5% reported having prior hallucinations (in settings other than withdrawal); those who reported hallucinations had a younger onset of drinking, drank more, and were more likely to use other substances than those who did not.[107]

Other Medical Complications

Alcohol consumption, even at moderate levels, has been associated with an increased risk of breast cancer.[108,109,110] Even light drinking has been attributed to excess deaths from cancers of the orpopharynx, esophagus, and breast.[111]

Hematological abnormalities (elevated mean corpuscular volume of red blood cells, anemia, thrombocytopenia) are related to nutritional deficiencies (B vitamins) as well as to direct toxic effects of alcohol on the gut (malabsorption and/or mucosal injury) and bone marrow. Alcohol-induced hypogonadism results in decreased libido and impotence. Dermatological disorders common in alcoholics include sunburn (with increased risk for skin cancer), rosacea (classically, the large red nose), and porphyria cutanea tarda.

Pregnancy

Alcohol ingestion during pregnancy may lead to morphological abnormalities (especially of the face) and low birth weight of the infant, and developmental and cognitive impairment manifest the fetal alcohol spectrum disorder.[112] The risk of minor abnormalities (e.g., low birth weight) begins with the consumption of one drink per day; this risk increases with increasingly larger amounts of alcohol consumption. Further discussion of alcohol and pregnancy can be found in Chapter 16.

Treatment

Most individuals with an alcohol use disorder never receive treatment.[113] Clinicians play an important role in identifying those with an alcohol use disorder, motivating them toward change, helping them get treatment, and monitoring their progress and adherence with a treatment plan. The goals of treatment in patients will vary depending on the severity of the problem. For those who have a moderate to severe alcohol use disorder, the goal is generally the achievement of abstinence (or progressively longer periods of abstinence) from alcohol with improved health and life functioning. For individuals with less severe alcohol use disorder or problem drinking, decreasing consumption to healthy limits may be a reasonable goal.

There are three general types of treatment for alcohol use disorders: (1) medically supervised withdrawal, or detoxification, which is generally followed by another form of treatment, or aftercare; (2) brief advice and other psychosocial treatments; and (3) pharmacotherapy.

Medically Supervised Withdrawal (Detoxification)

Alcohol withdrawal is a barrier to recovery and can be dangerous; medically supervised withdrawal, or *detoxification*, is a process to help individuals achieve abstinence. The treatment of alcohol withdrawal is also an issue when individuals with alcohol use disorders are hospitalized and may not necessarily be seeking treatment for their alcohol problems.

Assessment of Risk of Withdrawal/Treatment Setting

Individuals with alcohol use disorders may experience withdrawal symptoms that range from mild to life-threatening. Therefore, it is important to identify those at risk for withdrawal, particularly those at risk for severe withdrawal. There are a number of risk factors for severe alcohol withdrawal. A prior history of severe withdrawal appears to be the most significant one; elevated systolic blood pressure on presentation and comorbid medical conditions are also risk factors.[114] In one study of hospitalized patients, an AUDIT-PC (questions 1, 2, 4, 5, 10 of the AUDIT) score of ≥4 had a sensitivity of 91% and specificity of 90% for identifying patients at risk for alcohol withdrawal.[115] In another small pilot study of hospitalized patients, a novel 10-item scale was reported to be highly sensitive and specific for moderate-severe withdrawal.[116]

For individuals who are not already hospitalized and want to stop drinking, a decision needs to be regarding the treatment setting. The ASAM has developed patient placement criteria to help guide this decision;[117] an overview of placement criteria is provided in Chapter 3. Many alcoholics can undergo withdrawal as outpatients.[118] The decision between inpatient and outpatient treatment should be based on comorbid medical or psychiatric conditions and severity of alcohol withdrawal symptoms. Suggested indications for inpatient treatment are listed in Box 4.3. Use of a structured algorithm for determining the need for inpatient treatment of withdrawal may help decrease unnecessary admissions.[119]

For mildly symptomatic patients with a stable home environment and supportive family or friends, outpatient treatment with supervised daily visits to a treatment program or physician's office is as effective as inpatient treatment. Visits can be supplemented with attendance at an AA meeting daily. For moderately symptomatic patients, the choice of outpatient versus inpatient detoxification should be based on what programs are available. Some outpatient programs are intensive, requiring patients to spend entire days being monitored, with patients receiving medication as needed and participating in group counseling, but going home to sleep. Other outpatient programs may consist of brief daily visits with assessment of withdrawal, administration of medication for withdrawal, and supplies of take-home medications for use later in the day.

BOX 4.3 Indications for Inpatient Detoxification

- Evidence of hallucinations, severe tachycardia, severe tremor, fever, extreme agitation (CIWA score >15)
- History of severe withdrawal symptoms
- History of seizure disorder
- Presence of ataxia, nystagmus, confusion, or ophthalmoplegia, which may be indicative of Wernicke's encephalopathy
- Severe nausea and vomiting that would prevent the ingestion of medication
- Evidence of acute or chronic liver disease that may alter the metabolism of drugs used in the treatment of withdrawal
- Presence of cardiovascular disease such as severe hypertension, ischemic heart disease, or arrhythmia, for which increased sympathetic output during withdrawal poses particular risk
- Pregnancy
- Presence of associated medical or surgical condition requiring treatment
- Lack of medical or social support system to allow outpatient detoxification

---

Medications for Withdrawal

Benzodiazepines

Essential to management is early recognition of withdrawal, early treatment, frequent monitoring, and continual treatment. The standard of care for treatment of alcohol withdrawal is benzodiazepines, titrated on the basis of symptoms.[120] All of the benzodiazepines are effective, and there is no evidence of superiority for any individual agent.[121] Diazepam (Valium) has an advantage of having a rapid onset of action and long half-life. Its long half-life permits loading on the first day—we use 10 mg every 1–4 hours until severe symptoms dissipate; some patients may require 20 mg doses if

TABLE 4.4 Benzodiazepines Used for the Treatment of Alcohol Withdrawal

	Onset of Action	Rate of Metabolism	Liver Metabolized	Usual Starting Dose (mg)
Chlordiazepoxide	Intermediate	Long	Yes	50–100
Diazepam	Fast	Long	Yes	10–20
Lorazepam	Intermediate	Intermediate	No	2–4
Oxazepam	Slow	Short	No	30–60

they do not respond adequately to 10 mg doses. This approach will reduce the need for further dosing on subsequent days. Lorazepam (Ativan) does not require hepatic metabolism and is safer in patients with severe liver disease (i.e., prolonged prothrombin time); we generally start with 1 mg doses every 1–4 hours. Shorter-acting agents like lorazepam may also be better for older adults (i.e., age >70).[122] Table 4.4 provides a list of benzodiazepines that can be used and usual starting doses for treatment of withdrawal.

Patients should be monitored for response after initial dosing to make an assessment of indicated dosage and dosing interval. Dosing should be titrated to effect. The aim of drug treatment is to alleviate the most severe symptoms and signs of withdrawal and to prevent seizures. Symptom-driven therapy, compared to fixed schedule therapy, has been shown to decrease treatment duration and the amount of benzodiazepine used.[123] Moreover, providing a fixed dose taper does not eliminate or reduce the need for monitoring and symptom-triggered treatment. Benzodiazepines should be given such that withdrawal symptoms are improved without oversedating the patient. If the patient is being treated as an outpatient, each day's medication should be entrusted to a family member or friend who will be staying with the patient. Most patients need to be medicated for 24 to 72 hours, though some may have prolonged withdrawal (up to a week). Figure 4.1 shows a sample symptom-triggered protocol based on the approach used at our

1. Complete Clinical Institute Withdrawal Assessment for Alcohol (CIWA) and follow instructions below based on the CIWA score.
2. Notify physician if heart rate is >120, systolic blood pressure >180, or diastolic blood pressure >120.
3. Notify physician if patient is unable to take oral medications.
4. Give thiamine 100 mg orally daily.
5. Give folic acid 1 mg orally daily.

For CIWA score <8:
—Give diazepam 5 mg orally as needed for anxiety or mild withdrawal:
  —every 4 hours for up to 6 doses (day 1), then
  —every 6 hours for up to 4 doses (day 2), then
  —every 8 hours for up to 3 doses (day 3).
—Reassess CIWA every 4 hours—every 6 hours if CIWA is <8 for >24 hours.

For CIWA score 8–16:
—Give diazepam 10 mg orally every 4 hours until CIWA is <8 (up to 10 doses).
—Reassess CIWA every 4 hours.

For CIWA score 17–24:
—Give diazepam 20 mg orally every 2 hours until CIWA is <17 (up to 4 doses).
—Reassess CIWA every 2 hours.
—Notify physician if CIWA is still >16 after 4 hours.

For CIWA score >24:
—Give diazepam 20 mg orally and notify physician.

FIGURE 4.1 *Sample Alcohol Withdrawal Protocol with Diazepam.**

*For patients with cirrhosis or age >70, replace diazepam with oral lorazepam at a ratio of 1 mg of lorazepam/10 mg of diazepam.

institution. In this protocol the Clinical Institute Withdrawal Assessment for Alcohol (CIWA-Ar) score is used to monitor symptoms; this is discussed later in the chapter.

Other Drugs for Withdrawal
PHENOBARBITAL

Phenobarbital appears to be an effective treatment for alcohol withdrawal and has the advantage of being long-acting. There are reports of effective treatment protocols using phenobarbital alone[124] or in combination with benzodiazepines,[125] but there is no evidence that they are superior to benzodiazepines alone.

ANTICONVULSANTS

A number of anticonvulsants have been studied for the treatment of alcohol withdrawal, including gabapentin, valproate, and carbamazepine. A 2010 Cochrane review found insufficient evidence in favor of anticonvulsants for treating alcohol withdrawal, but acknowledged that carbamazepine may be effective.[126] Carbamazepine was effective in treating patients with mild alcohol withdrawal in two studies.[127,128] Valproate reduced the severity of alcohol withdrawal in one study, but patients still required treatment with a benzodiazepine.[129] Gabapentin seems to reduce alcohol consumption and craving[130] and may be effective for treatment of mild-moderate withdrawal.[131,132] Pregabalin was ineffective in one trial.[133]

ANTIHYPERTENSIVES

Two classes of antihypertensive have been studied for use in the management of alcohol withdrawal—centrally acting alpha agonists (i.e., clonidine)[134] and beta-blockers.[135,136,137] These drugs alleviate sympathetic markers of withdrawal (hypertension and tachycardia) but do not prevent the more severe aspects of withdrawal (seizures and delirium tremens).

NEUROLEPTICS

Neuroleptics, such as haloperidol, can be used to treat delirium or agitation in patients with alcohol withdrawal, but they do not prevent other complications such as seizures. These drugs should not be used alone to treat withdrawal. There are reports of protocols using neuroleptics along with benzodiazepines;[138] however, this approach has not been shown to be superior to adequately dosed benzodiazepines alone. In our experience, it is generally best to titrate benzodiazepines until the patient is calm, rather than complicating treatment with the addition of another sedative.

ALCOHOL

Alcohol, in either oral or intravenous form, has been used to prevent alcohol withdrawal, particularly when abstinence is not necessarily a goal—for example, in an alcohol-dependent patient with a traumatic injury. There is limited research on this topic in the literature, but there are no protocols that have been shown to be as safe and effective as benzodiazepines.[139]

Measuring Withdrawal Severity

Symptom-triggered treatment requires a tool to measure the severity of alcohol withdrawal; the Clinical Institute Withdrawal Assessment for Alcohol, revised (CIWA-Ar) is the most commonly used scale and is shown in Box 4.4.[140] The maximum score

---

BOX 4.4 Addiction Research Foundation Clinical Institute Withdrawal Assessment for Alcohol (CIWA-Ar)

NAUSEA AND VOMITING—Ask: "Do you feel sick to your stomach? Have you vomited?" Observation.

  0 no nausea and no vomiting
  1 mild nausea with no vomiting
  2
  3
  4 intermittent nausea with dry heaves
  5
  6
  7 constant nausea, frequent dry heaves and vomiting

TREMOR—Arms extended and fingers spread apart. Observation.

  0 no tremor
  1 not visible, but can be felt fingertip to fingertip
  2
  3
  4 moderate, with patient's arms extended

5

6

7   severe, even with arms not extended

PAROXYSMAL SWEATS—Observation.

0   no sweat visible

1   barely perceptible sweating, palms moist

2

3

4   beads of sweat obvious on forehead

5

6

7   drenching sweats

ANXIETY—Ask: "Do you feel nervous?" Observation.

0   no anxiety, at ease

1   mildly anxious

2

3

4   moderately anxious, or guarded, so anxiety is inferred

5

6

7   equivalent to acute panic states, as seen in severe delirium or acute schizophrenic reactions

AGITATION—Observation.

0   normal activity

1   somewhat more than normal activity

2

3

4   moderately fidgety and restless

5

6

7   paces back and forth during most of the interview, or constantly thrashes about

TACTILE DISTURBANCES—Ask: "Have you any itching, pins and needles sensations, any burning, any numbness, or do you feel bugs crawling on or under your skin?" Observation.

0 none
1 very mild itching, pins and needles, burning or numbness
2 mild itching, pins and needles, burning or numbness
3 moderate itching, pins and needles, burning or numbness
4 moderately severe hallucinations
5 severe hallucinations
6 extremely severe hallucinations
7 continuous hallucinations

AUDITORY DISTURBANCES—Ask: "Are you more aware of sounds around you? Are they harsh? Do they frighten you? Are you hearing anything that is disturbing you? Are you hearing things you know are not there?" Observation.

0 not present
1 very mild harshness or ability to frighten
2 mild harshness or ability to frighten
3 moderate harshness or ability to frighten
4 moderately severe hallucinations
5 severe hallucinations
6 extremely severe hallucinations
7 continuous hallucinations

VISUAL DISTURBANCES—Ask: "Does the light appear to be too bright? Is its color different? Does it hurt your eyes? Are you seeing anything that is disturbing to you? Are you seeing things you know are not there?" Observation.

0 not present
1 very mild sensitivity
2 mild sensitivity
3 moderate sensitivity
4 moderately severe hallucinations

5 severe hallucinations
6 extremely severe hallucinations
7 continuous hallucinations

HEADACHE, FULLNESS IN HEAD—Ask: "Does your head feel different? Does it feel like there is a band around your head?" Do not rate for dizziness or lightheadedness. Otherwise, rate severity.

0 not present
1 very mild
2 mild
3 moderate
4 moderately severe
5 severe
6 very severe
7 extremely severe

ORIENTATION AND CLOUDING OF SENSORIUM—Ask: "What day is this? Where are you? Who am I?"

0 oriented and can do serial additions
1 cannot do serial additions or is uncertain about date
2 disoriented for date by no more than 2 calendar days
3 disoriented for date by more than 2 calendar days
4 disoriented for place and/or person

Total CIWA-Ar Score _____ (Maximum Possible Score 67)

From Sullivan JT, Sykora K, Schneiderman J, et al. Assessment of alcohol withdrawal: the revised Clinical Institute Withdrawal Assessment for Alcohol scale (CIWA-Ar). Br J Addict 1989;84:1353–7.

is 67 and pharmacological therapy is generally initiated at scores of 8–10; a score of 16–20 or greater is generally considered to be severe withdrawal. The frequency of assessment depends on the score and response to treatment. Those with scores over 16 should be assessed every 1–2 hours, and those with scores 8–16, every 2–4 hours; a sample protocol using the CIWA is shown in Figure 4.1. It is important that staff be trained in its use. If patients are not directly asked each individual item and are only scored on the basis of what they volunteer, the CIWA-Ar will be consistently underscored. The CIWA-Ar should not be used on intoxicated individuals because they may report nonspecific symptoms such as headache, nausea, and anxiety that may lead to inappropriate administration of sedatives. Finally, the CIWA-Ar is not useful for patients who are experiencing delirium tremens, and it is better to use a sedation-agitation scale to titrate medications.

The CIWA-Ar is somewhat long and may take up to 5 minutes to complete. There is ongoing interest in developing shorter scales,[141] though none have been sufficiently validated to endorse their use at this time.

Prevention of Seizures

Seizures may occur without the presence of any other manifestations of alcohol withdrawal.[142] There is no consensus about the use of antiepileptics to prevent seizures for alcoholics who have seizures in the past, and it is sometime difficult to determine if prior seizures were due to alcohol or an independent disorder. In one study of alcoholics with prior seizures receiving treatment for withdrawal, phenytoin (diphenylhydantoin), at a dosage of 300 mg/day for 5 days, appeared to prevent most withdrawal seizures.[143] However, in subsequent studies of alcoholics who had a seizure, phenytoin did not prevent a recurrent seizure.[144,145]

There is strong evidence that benzodiazepines can prevent seizures.[146] Lorazepam has been shown to prevent recurrent seizures in someone who has had a seizure related to alcohol withdrawal.[147] Therefore, patients who are significantly symptomatic and receiving sufficient pharmacological therapy with a benzodiazepine do not require other antiepileptics. However, mildly symptomatic patients with a history of seizures may benefit from prophylactic phenytoin (or another antiepileptic) if they are not going to be treated with a benzodiazepine.

Treatment of Delirium Tremens

Delirium tremens (DTs) is not commonly seen during withdrawal, especially if individuals have been adequately treated earlier in the course of withdrawal. Patients with DTs are very ill and are best treated in an intensive care setting. As with less severe withdrawal, the treatment of choice is benzodiazepines,[148] but these patients generally require very high doses to achieve sedation and often these need to be administered intravenously. Diazepam can be given in intravenous boluses. Lorazepam can also be given in intravenous boluses or as a continuous infusion.[149] As noted earlier, the CIWA-Ar is not useful in delirious patients; a sedation-agitation scale[150] can be used instead.

Psychosocial Treatments

Psychosocial treatment options range from brief advice to self-help groups, outpatient counseling (individual or group), and residential treatment. These treatments are often employed after patients have undergone medically supervised withdrawal or detoxification as outlined in the previous section. Effective treatment programs are abstinence-oriented; it is often best to use AA or group therapy as a mainstay of treatment, avoid the use of psychoactive drugs in long-term treatment, involve the family, and provide close follow-up. Primary care clinicians can play an important role at follow-up visits in monitoring and reinforcing patient participation in the treatment plan.

Brief Interventions

Primary care clinicians can help patients with risky drinking reduce their alcohol consumption through a brief intervention.[151] However, these interventions seem to be of limited utility in individuals with more severe alcohol use disorder, as they require more extensive treatment.[152,153] Brief interventions are further discussed in Chapter 2.

Self-Help Groups

Peer-led self-help groups or 12-step groups, such as Alcoholics Anonymous (AA), and other programs have traditionally been the mainstay of maintenance of sobriety. These groups can help break down the denial process and effectively deal with the associated guilt and shame through a combination of nonjudgmental acceptance and support. Individuals with a moderate to severe alcohol use disorder should be strongly encouraged to attend self-help groups regularly. Directing patients to attend a specific group may facilitate involvement and improve outcomes.[154] Regular attendance is correlated with long-term recovery and improved functioning.[155,156] Patients who continue to attend self-help groups after inpatient treatment also have improved outcomes.[157]

Many patients are reluctant to attend AA or other self-help groups. When referring a patient, it is important to convey familiarity with how these groups work and to express confidence in the program. Immediate action, taken while the patient is in the office, may consist of having the patient contact a family member or friend who is active in a self-help group, or telephoning the local AA office and having the patient request a contact to take him or her to a convenient meeting. Establishing a direct connection with another person who attends the group has been shown to improve attendance and outcomes.[158] The best way for clinicians to learn about these programs is to attend several different meetings in their community. To locate such meetings, one can call the local AA office or look on the Internet, at www.aa.org. For individuals who are uncomfortable with some of the religious and spiritual connotations of AA, there are "secular" alternatives available, including SMART recovery (smartrecovery.org), Secular Organizations for Sobriety (sossobriety.org), and AA Agnostica (aaagnostica.org).

Counseling

Counseling can be provided in an individual or group setting and generally focuses on facilitating continued motivation toward abstinence. In contrast to self-help groups, these groups are led by trained counselors, rather than peers. Cognitive-behavioral approaches include examination of cognitive processes and emotions as factors that may have an impact on continued drinking (and attempts at abstinence) and use of behavioral methods for promoting change or maintenance of sobriety. Further discussion of cognitive-behavioral therapy can be found in Chapter 3.

Residential Treatment

Residential (or inpatient) treatment for 2 to 6 weeks (or more) may be helpful for some patients.[159] Indications for residential treatment include unsuccessful or too slow recovery despite adequate outpatient treatment; weak support systems; danger to self or others; severe medical, psychiatric, or other problems related to alcoholism; and, possibly, a patient's desire for residential treatment.

Residential programs range from highly structured treatment programs to informal recovery houses. Although treatment goals among residential treatment programs vary, major goals include breaking down denial; educating about alcoholism; providing an introduction to group treatment (self-help groups and group therapy); learning how to ask for help; learning how to communicate directly and honestly; learning how to enjoy life while abstinent; beginning the restoration of relationships; and developing a specific, structured long-term recovery program.

Emerging Technology

There are a number of novel treatments that take advantage of new technologies. Internet-based interventions have been developed and primarily target younger at-risk drinkers.[160] Smartphone applications to support recovery have also been developed and have shown impact in limiting the number of drinking days among patients leaving residential treatment[161] and in reducing problematic alcohol intake among college students.[162]

Pharmacological Treatment

Pharmacological treatment for alcohol dependence should be considered for individuals who relapse despite being able to achieve sobriety for periods of time. Pharmacotherapy should be considered as an adjunct to treatment, rather than the focus of treatment. In the United States, three drugs are approved for use in the treatment of alcohol use disorder—disulfiram, naltrexone, and acamprosate. A 2014 systematic review concluded that both naltrexone and acamprosate are effective.[163] Some drugs can only be prescribed after abstinence has been achieved (e.g., disulfiram), while others can be started while a patient is still actively drinking.

Disulfiram

Disulfiram inhibits acetaldehyde oxidation by interfering with aldehyde dehydrogenase. The symptoms of the alcohol–disulfiram reaction are the result of elevated acetaldehyde levels, and this effect may persist for up to 2 weeks after cessation of disulfiram. Some individuals have typical symptoms after drinking only small amounts of alcohol. A small percentage of patients are able to drink despite taking disulfiram without significant symptoms. An alcohol–disulfiram reaction usually begins within 10 minutes of drinking and may last for up to several hours. Symptoms include flushing, headaches, anxiety, sweating, nausea, vomiting, dizziness, palpitations, hyperventilation, and confusion.

Although controlled studies have failed to show that it increases duration of sobriety,[164,165,166] the use of disulfiram may be considered for some patients. Patients who are motivated to succeed in recovery and who have experienced relapse or dread the likelihood of relapse are candidates for disulfiram. It may also be effective those who have their medications monitored or directly administered. Because disulfiram is taken once daily, it can serve as a reminder that one cannot drink, and the decision not to drink need only be made once a day.

Disulfiram at recommended dosages of 250–500 mg/day is well tolerated by most patients. Contraindications for the use of disulfiram include diabetes, emphysema, seizures, significant liver or renal disease, coronary artery disease, pregnancy, or a history of drinking while taking disulfiram. If alcohol-related liver disease is present, prescribing of disulfiram should be delayed until the liver enzyme levels (AST and ALT) are less than three times the upper range of normal. Disulfiram may impair the metabolism and potentiate the effects of caffeine, warfarin, ritonavir, and phenytoin; it can cause neuropathy and may exacerbate the neurological side effects of isoniazid. It should be used with caution in conjunction with alpha- or beta-adrenergic antagonists, vasodilators, sympathomimetic amines, monoamine oxidase inhibitors, tricyclic antidepressants, and neuroleptics. Patients on disulfiram should avoid medications (cough syrups) and foods (e.g., salad dressings) that contain alcohol.

Naltrexone

Naltrexone is an opioid antagonist, which appears to work by reducing alcohol craving, and may be useful in preventing relapse or reducing drinking in motivated patients. A number of studies suggest that it is effective at reducing alcohol use in the short term. In the COMBINE study, patients receiving naltrexone and support from their primary care practitioner had the best outcomes, even superior to those receiving naltrexone and behavioral intervention from an addiction counselor.[167] There are limited data supporting naltrexone assisting in long-term abstinence; most studies were limited to endpoints of 3–6 months. A large multicenter study of alcoholic veterans did not find a benefit from using naltrexone over 1 year.[168] Nevertheless, a 2010 Cochrane review of the use of opioid antagonists for alcoholism concluded that the evidence supports the use of naltrexone for alcoholism treatment.[169] Long-acting injectable naltrexone may be more effective.[170] There is some evidence that a genetic polymorphism of the μ-opioid receptor gene (OPRM1) is associated with a better response to naltrexone.[171]

Naltrexone is an opiate antagonist and thus cannot be prescribed to patients on opioid analgesics; patients maintained on naltrexone will not obtain pain relief if prescribed an opioid. Naltrexone is well tolerated, with nausea as its main side effect. Patients should be prescribed 25 mg (half tablet) a day for 2 days and 50 mg/day thereafter. Naltrexone can be used in combination with disulfiram. Although there is no clear evidence of hepatotoxicity, the manufacturers of naltrexone advise monitoring of liver function tests (initially at monthly intervals and then less frequently). Naltrexone does not cause physical dependence and can be stopped at any time without withdrawal symptoms. If a patient is going to have elective surgery, oral naltrexone should be stopped at least 72 hours beforehand to allow the use of opioid analgesia. The use of injectable naltrexone in a patient having urgent surgery can make achievement of adequate analgesia with opioids challenging; high doses may be needed, and close monitoring and anesthesia input are warranted.

Acamprosate

Acamprosate has complex effects, but it appears to increase GABA transmission and decrease glutamate.[172] Compliance is often a challenge, as acamprosate must be taken as 666 mg (two pills) three times a day. Most studies of acamprosate examine its utility in patients who have completed detoxification. Results of studies are mixed, with at best modest benefit.[173,174,175] The COMBINE study showed no utility of acamprosate with or without a behavioral intervention.[169] Nevertheless, two systematic reviews of acamprosate concluded that it is an effective adjuvant therapy for alcoholism and has been shown to significantly improve abstinence rate.[176,177]

Anticonvulsants

A number of anticonvulsant agents, most recently topiramate and gabapentin, have been studied for treatment of alcohol dependence. In a 12-week study of alcoholics, topiramate use improved abstinence rates and reduced the amount of alcohol consumed among those who drank.[178] A subsequent larger multicenter study by the same group also showed impact on reducing heavy drinking.[179] In another trial, a lower dose (75 mg/day) of topiramate after inpatient detoxification was associated with a reduction in relapse rate over 16 weeks.[180] The efficacy of topiramate may be genetically affected.[181] Side effects, including parasthesias, psychomotor slowing, and weight loss, are a barrier to its use. In a 2014 trial, gabapentin at a dose of 1800 mg/day was associated with significantly reduced heavy drinking and increased abstinence compared to placebo.[182] However, a 2014 Cochrane review of anticonvulsants for alcohol dependence concluded that "evidence supporting the clinical use of anticonvulsants to treat alcohol dependence is insufficient."[183]

Other Drugs

Ondansetron, a selective 5-HT3 serotonin receptor antagonist, has been reported to be effective (in one study) in a subgroup of subjects with early-onset alcoholism, by increasing days of abstinence. This finding has not been confirmed in other randomized controlled trials. Finally, one 13-week clinical trial found that varenicline was associated with a reduction in alcohol consumption and craving.[184]

Although many alcoholics have symptoms such as anxiety, insomnia, and tremors, the use of benzodiazepines and other sedatives should be avoided, as they interfere with successful recovery. All sedatives are cross-tolerant with alcohol and may trigger relapse. Additionally, combining sedatives with alcohol increases risk of respiratory depression and may impair judgment and the ability to control consumption.

Prevention and Management of Relapse

After overcoming of denial and motivating the patient to change, follow-up is the most difficult part of treatment. Patients often have

TABLE 4.5 Summary of Alcohol Use Disorder Treatment Studies

Intervention	Studies	Outcomes
Medically Supervised Withdrawal (Detoxification)		
Benzodiazepines	RCTs Meta-analysis	Effective; as-needed treatment more effective than fixed dose
Carbamazepine	RCTs	Effective for mild-moderate withdrawal
Gabapentin	RCT	Effective in one RCT
Psychosocial		
Brief advice	RCTs Meta-analysis	Effective for reducing alcohol use among problem drinkers
Self-help groups	Observational	Participation is associated with better outcomes
Counseling	RCTS	Effective (in some studies)
Cognitive-behavioral therapy (CBT)	RCTs	Effective (in some studies)
Residential Treatment	Observational	Participation is associated with better outcomes (in some studies)
Pharmacotherapy		
Disulfiram	RCTs Meta-analysis	Not shown to be effective overall, but may be beneficial in selected individuals
Naltrexone	RCTs Meta-analysis	Effective in short term (3–6 months)

(continued)

TABLE 4.5 (Continued)

Intervention	Studies	Outcomes
Pharmacotherapy		
Acamprosate	RCTs Meta-analysis	Modestly effective in short term (3–6 months)
Topiramate	RCT	Effective in three RCTs (12–13 weeks)
Ondansetron	RCT	Effective in a subgroup of early-onset alcoholics in one RCT
Gabapentin	RCT	Effective in one 12-week RCT

See text for references and more details.
RCT: randomized controlled trial.

a honeymoon period during which they may be lulled into believing that the problem is behind them and regular follow-up is no longer necessary. During the first few weeks after stopping drinking, patients need a great deal of support, as this is the time when they are at highest risk of relapsing. Weekly phone contact may be helpful, with a gradually decreasing frequency of calls thereafter. High-risk times for relapse include special days and occasions, such as vacations, holidays, business trips, birthdays, and anniversaries, or crises such as separation, divorce, death of a close person, or illness in the family.

The relapse process begins before the person drinks. This process often progresses in a predictable manner: reactivation of denial, progressive isolation and defensiveness, building a crisis to justify symptom progression, depressed mood, loss of control over behavior, and, finally, relapse to drinking. Relapse is part of the natural history of recovery for most alcoholics and should not cause one to become discouraged. Instead, the provider should help the patient overcome the shame and frustration, facilitating the patient toward getting back into treatment using the same motivational techniques practiced initially. Relapse is a time for the patient to learn about his or her mistakes and to correct them by strengthening treatment (Table 4.5).

Notes

1. Substance Abuse and Mental Health Services Administration. *Results from the 2013 National Survey on Drug Use and Health: Summary of National Findings*. NSDUH Series H-48, HHS Publication No. (SMA) 14-4863. Rockville, MD: Substance Abuse and Mental Health Services Administration; 2014.

2. Bouchery E, Harwood H, Sacks J, et al. Economic costs of excessive alcohol consumption in the U.S., 2006. Am J Prev Med 2011;41:516–24.

3. Stahre M, Roeber J, Kanny D, et al. Contribution of excessive alcohol consumption to deaths and years of potential life lost in the United States. Prev Chronic Dis 2014;11:e109.

4. Levey DF, Le-Niculescu H, Frank J, et al. Genetic risk prediction and neurobiological understanding of alcoholism. Transl Psychiatry 2014;4:e456.

5. King WC, Chen JY, Mitchell JE. Prevalence of alcohol use disorders before and after bariatric surgery. JAMA 2012;307:2516–25.

6. Woodward JJ. The pharmacology of alcohol. In *The ASAM Principles of Addiction Medicine*, 5th ed. Ries RK, Fiellin DA, Miller SC, Saitz R, eds. Philadelphia: Wolters Kluwer; 2014:100–16.

7. American Psychiatric Association. *Diagnostic and Statistical Manual of Mental Disorders*, Fifth Edition (DSM-5). Washington, DC: American Psychiatric Association; 2013.

8. Hall W, Zador D. The alcohol withdrawal syndrome. Lancet 1997;349:1897–900.

9. Verster JC, Stephens R, Penning R, et al. The alcohol hangover research group consensus statement on best practice in alcohol hangover research. Curr Drug Abuse Rev 2010;3:116–26.

10. Slutske WS, Piasecki TM, Nathanson L, et al. Genetic influences on alcohol-related hangover. Addiction 2014;109:2027–34.

11. Verster JC, Penning R. Treatment and prevention of alcohol hangover. Curr Drug Abuse Rev 2010;3:103–9.

12. Morse RM, Flavin DK. The definition of alcoholism. JAMA 1992;268:1012–4.

13. National Institute on Alcohol Abuse and Alcoholism. *The Physician's Guide to Helping Patients with Alcohol Problems.* NIH publication no. 07-3769. Washington, DC: Government Printing Office; 2007.

14. Merrick E, Horgan CM, Hodgkin D, et al. Unhealthy drinking patterns in older adults: prevalence and associated characteristics. J Am Geriatr Soc 2008;56:214–23.

15. Van Amsterdam J, Van den Brink W. Reduced-risk drinking as a viable treatment goal in problematic alcohol use and alcohol dependence. J Psychopharm 2013;27:987–97.

16. Jonas DE, Garbutt JC, Amick HR, et al. Behavioral counseling after screening for alcohol misuse in primary care: a systematic review and meta-analysis for the U.S. Preventive Services Task Force. Ann Intern Med 2012;157:645–54.

17. U.S. Preventive Services Task Force. Screening and behavioral counseling interventions in primary care to reduce alcohol misuse: U.S. Preventive Services Task Force recommendation statement. Ann Intern Med 2013;159:210–8.

18. Mayfield DG, McLeod G, Hall P. The CAGE questionnaire: validation of a new alcoholism screening instrument. Am J Psychiatry 1974;131:1121–3.

19. Ewing JA. Detecting alcoholism: the CAGE questionnaire. JAMA 1984;252:1905–7.

20. Cyr MG, Wartman SA. The effectiveness of routine screening questions in the detection of alcoholism. JAMA 1988;259:51–4.

21. Buchsbaum DG, Buchanan RG, Centor RM, et al. Screening for alcohol abuse using CAGE scores and likelihood ratios. Ann Intern Med 1991;115:774–7.

22. Saunders JB, Aasland OG, Babor TF, et al. Development of the Alcohol Use Disorders Identification Test (AUDIT). Addiction 1993;88:791–804.

23. Bradley K, DeBenedetti AF, Volk RJ, et al. AUDIT-C as a brief screen for alcohol misuse in primary care. Alcohol Clin Exp Res 2007;31:1208–17.

24. Smith P, Schmidt S, Allensworth-Davies D, Saitz R. Primary care validation of a single-question alcohol screening test. J Gen Intern Med 2009;24:783–800.

25. National Institute on Alcohol Abuse and Alcoholism. (2005) *Helping Patients Who Drink Too Much: A Clinician's Guide.* NIAAA Publication No. 07-3769. Rockville, MD.

26. Bradley KA, Bush KR, Epler AJ, et al. Two brief screening tests from the Alcohol Use Disorders Identification Test (AUDIT). Arch Intern Med 2003;163:821–9.

27. Bradley KA, Boyd-Wickizer J, Powell SH, Burman ML. Alcohol screening questionnaires in women: a critical review. JAMA 1998;280:166–71.

28. Steinbauer JR, Cantor SB, Holzer CE, Volk RJ. Ethnic and sex bias in primary care screening tests for alcohol use disorders. Ann Intern Med 1998;128:353–62.

29. Storgaard H, Nielsen SD, Gluud C. The validity of the Michigan Alcoholism Screening Test (MAST). Alcohol Alcohol 1994;29:493–502.

30. **Beresford TP, Blow FC, Hill E, et al. Comparison of CAGE questionnaire and computer-assisted laboratory profiles in screening for covert alcoholism. Lancet 1990;336:482–5.** *Of 915 adults studied, 244 were alcohol dependent. The CAGE (≥2 positive answers) was 76% sensitive and 94% specific with a positive predictive value of 87%. No laboratory value had a significant predictive value.*

31. **Huseby NE, Nilssen O, Erfurth A, et al. Carbohydrate-deficient transferrin and alcohol dependency: variation in response to alcohol intake among different groups of patients. Alcoholism: Clin Exp Res 1997;21:201–5.** *Sensitivity of carbohydrate-deficient transferrin (CDT) was 75% for patients admitted for alcohol detoxification, but <50% for alcoholics admitted for surgery. In both groups, sensitivity was worse for women and those age <35.*

32. Fagan KJ, Irvine KM, McWhinney BC, et al. Diagnostic sensitivity of carbohydrate deficient transferrin in heavy drinkers. BMC Gastroenterol 2014;14:97.

33. Stewart SH, Koch DG, Willner IR, et al. Validation of blood phosphatidylethanol as an alcohol consumption biomarker in patients with chronic liver disease. Alcohol Clin Exp Res 2014;38:1706–11.

34. DiCastelnouvo A, Costanzo S, Bagnardi V, et al. Alcohol dosing and total mortality in men and women: an updated meta-analysis of 34 prospective studies. Arch Intern Med 2006;166:2437–45.

35. Murkamal KJ, Conigrave KM, Mittleman MA, et al. Role of drinking pattern and type of alcohol consumed in coronary heart disease in men. N Engl J Med 2003;348:109–18.

36. Hvidtfeldt UA, Tolstrup JS, Jakobsen MU. Alcohol intake and risk of coronary heart disease in younger, middle-aged, and older adults. Circulation 2010;121:1589–97.

37. Hart RG, Pearce LA, McBride R, et al. Factors associated with ischemic stroke during aspirin therapy in atrial fibrillation: analysis of 2012 participants in the SPAF I-III clinical trials. Stroke 1999;30:1223–9.

38. Jiminez M, Chiuve SE, Glynn RJ. Alcohol consumption and risk of stroke in women. Stroke 2012;43:939–45.

39. Schaeffner ES, Kurth T, de Jong PE, et al. Alcohol consumption and the risk of renal dysfunction in apparently healthy men. Arch Intern Med 2005;165:1048–53.

40. Howard AA, Arnsten JH, Gourevitch MN. Effect of alcohol consumption on diabetes mellitus: a systematic review. Ann Intern Med 2004;140:211–9.

41. **Klatsky AL, Armstrong MA, Friedman GD. Alcohol and mortality. Ann Intern Med 1992;117:646–54.** *In this cohort of 128,934, comparing those who drank ≥6 drinks/day with non-drinkers, the relative risk of death from noncardiovascular causes was 1.6; for women, it was 2.2 and for those aged <50, 1.9.*

42. Roerecke M, Rehm J. Alcohol use disorders and mortality: a systematic review and meta-analysis. Addiction 2013;108:1562–78.

43. **Bullock KD, Reed RJ, Grant I. Reduced mortality risk in alcoholics who achieve long-term abstinence. JAMA 1992;267:668–72.** *In this 11-year follow-up of cohort of 199 alcoholic veterans, standardized mortality ratios were 5.0 for the relapsed group and 1.3 for the abstinent group.*

44. Hurt RD, Offord KP, Croghan IT, et al. Mortality following inpatient addictions treatment. Role of tobacco use in a community-based cohort. JAMA 1996;275:1097–103.

45. Bagnardi V, Rota M, Botteri E, et al. Alcohol consumption and lung cancer risk in never smokers: a meta-analysis. Ann Oncol 2011;22:2631–9.

46. Kliman K, Altraja A. Predictors of extensively drug-resistant pulmonary tuberculosis. Ann Intern Med 2009;150:766–75.

47. Potter JF, Beevers DG. Pressor effect of alcohol in hypertension. Lancet 1984;1:119–22.

48. Puddey IB, Beilin LJ, Vandongen R. Regular alcohol use raises blood pressure in treated hypertensive subjects: a randomized controlled trial. Lancet 1987;1:647–51.

49. Minami J, Yoshii M, Todooki M, et al. Effects of alcohol restriction on ambulatory blood pressure, heart rate and heart rate variability in Japanese men. Am J Hypertens 2002;15:125–9.

50. James PA, Oparil S, Carter BL, et al. 2014 Evidence-based guideline for the management of high blood pressure in adults: Report from the panel members appointed to the eighth Joint National Committee (JNC 8). JAMA 2014;311:507–20.

51. **Reynolds K, Lewis LB, Nolen JDL, et al. Alcohol consumption and risk of stroke-a meta-analysis. JAMA 2003;289:579–88.** *Based on 35 cohort or case-control studies, consumption of >4–5 drinks/day was associated with a relative risk of 1.6 for all strokes, 1.7 for ischemic stroke, and 2.2 for hemorrhagic stroke.*

52. Mukamal KJ, Ascherio A, Mitleman MA, et al. Alcohol and risk for ischemic stroke in men: the role of drinking patterns and usual beverage. Ann Intern Med 2005;142:11–19.

53. Beulens J, Rimm EB, Ascherio A, et al. Alcohol consumption and risk for coronary heart disease among men with hypertension. Ann Intern Med 2007;146:10–20.

54. Stolberger C, Finsterer J. Reversal of dilated to hypertrophic cardiomyopathy after alcohol abstinence. Clin Cardiol 1998;21:365–7.

55. McKenna CJ, Codd MB, McCann HA, Sugrue DD. Alcohol consumption and idiopathic dilated cardiomyopathy: a case-control study. Am Heart J 1998;135:833–7.

56. Walsh CR, Larson MG, Evans JC. Alcohol consumption and risk for congestive heart failure in the Framingham Study. Ann Intern Med 2002;136:181–91.

57. Larsson SC, Orsini N, Wolk A. Alcohol consumption and risk of heart failure: a dose-response meta-analysis of prospective studies. Eur J Heart Fail 2015;17:367–73.

58. Djousse L, Levy D, Benjamin EJ, et al. Long-term alcohol consumption and the risk of atrial fibrillation in the Framingham Study. Am J Cardiol 2004;93:710–3.

59. Frost L, Vestergaard P. Alcohol and risk of atrial fibrillation or flutter. Arch Intern Med 2004;164:1993–8.

60. Larsson SC, Drca N, Wolk A. Alcohol consumption and risk of atrial fibrillation: a prospective study and dose-response meta-analysis. J Am Coll Cardiol 2014;64:281–9.

61. Overvad TF, Rasmussen LH, Skjoth F, et al. Alcohol intake and prognosis of atrial fibrillation. Heart 2013;99:1093–9.

62. Kupari M, Koskinen P. Time of onset of supraventricular tachyarrhythmia in relation to alcohol consumption. Am J Cardiol 1991;67:718–22.

63. Anderson LA, Cantwell MM, Watson RG, et al. The association between alcohol and reflux esophagitis, Barrett's esophagus and esophageal adenocarcinoma. Gastroenterology 2009;136:799–805.

64. Pandeya N, Williams G, Green AC, et al. Alcohol consumption and the risks of adenocarcinoma and squamous cell carcinoma of the esophagus. Gastroenterology 2009;136:1215–24.

65. Risk factors for peptic ulcer disease: a population based prospective cohort study comprising 2416 Danish adults. Gut 2003;52:186–93.

66. Cho E, Smith-Warner SA, Ritz J, et al. Alcohol intake and colorectal cancer: a pooled analysis of 8 cohort studies. Ann Intern Med 2004;140:603–13.

67. Whitcomb DC, LaRusch J, Krasinskas AM, et al. Common genetic variants in the CLDN2 and PRSS1-PRSS2 loci alter risk for alcohol-related and sporadic pancreatitis. Nat Genet 2012;44:1349–54.

68. Marick PE. What is the best way to feed patients with pancreatitis? Curr Opin Crit Care 2009;15:131–8.

69. Becker U, Deis A, Sørensen TI, et al. Prediction of risk of liver disease by alcohol intake, sex and age: a prospective population study. Hepatology 1996;23:1025–9.

70. Norton R, Batey R, Dwyer T, MacMahon S. Alcohol consumption and the risk of alcohol-related cirrhosis in women. BMJ 1987;295:80–2.

71. Lucey M, Mathurin P, Morgan T. Alcoholic hepatitis. N Engl J Med 2009; 360:2758–69.

72. Fingerhood MI, Sullivan JT, Jasinski DR. Prevalence of hepatitis C in a chemical dependence population. Arch Intern Med 1993;153:2025–30.

73. Orrego H, Blake JE, Blendis LM, et al. Long-term treatment of alcoholic liver disease with propylthiouracil. N Engl J Med 1987;317:1421–7.

74. Akriviadis E, Botla R, Briggs W, et al. Pentoxifylline improves short-term survival in severe acute alcoholic hepatitis: a double-blind, placebo-controlled trial. Gastroenterology 2000;119:1637-48.

75. Mendenhall, CL, Anderson, S, Garcia-Pont, P, et al. Short-term and long-term survival in patients with alcoholic hepatitis treated with oxandrolone and prednisolone. N Engl J Med 1984;311:1464-70.

76. Rambaldi A, Iaquinto G, Gluud C. Anabolic-androgenic steroids for alcoholic liver disease: a Cochrane review. Am J Gastroenterol 2002;97:1674-81.

77. Menon KV, Stadheim L, Kamath PS, et al. A pilot study of the safety and tolerability of etanercept in patients with alcoholic hepatitis. Am J Gastroenterol 2004;99:255-60.

78. Naveau S, Chollet-Martin S, Dharancy S, et al. A double-blind randomized controlled trial of infliximab associated with prednisolone in acute hepatitis. Hepatology 2004;39:1390-7.

79. Maddrey WC, Boitnott JK, Bedine MS, et al. Corticosteroid therapy of alcoholic hepatitis. Gastroenterology 1978;75:193-9.

80. Carithers RL Jr, Herlong HF, Diehl AM, et al. Methylprednisolone therapy in patients with severe alcoholic hepatitis: a randomized multi-center trial. Ann Intern Med 1989;110:685-90.

81. Ramond MJ, Poynard T, Rueff B, et al. A randomized trial of prednisolone in patients with severe alcoholic hepatitis. N Engl J Med 1992;326:507-12.

82. Theodossi A, Eddleston AL, Williams R. Controlled trial of methylprednisolone therapy in severe acute alcoholic hepatitis. Gut 1982;23:75-9.

83. **Mendenhall CL, Anderson, S Garcia-Pont P, et al. Short-term and long-term survival in patients with alcoholic hepatitis treated with oxandrolone and prednisolone. N Engl J Med 1984;311:1464-70.** *In this study, 263 patients with alcoholic hepatitis were randomized to 30 days of treatment with oxandrolone, prednisolone or placebo; there was no difference in 30-day mortality for either treatment group when compared to placebo.*

84. Cabre E, Rodriguez-Iglesias P, Caballeria J. Short- and long-term outcome of severe alcohol-induced hepatitis treated with steroids or enteral nutrition: a multicenter randomized trial. Hepatology 2000;32:36-42.

85. Nguyen-Khac E, Thevenot T, Piquet MA et al. Glucocorticoids plus N-acetylcysteine in severe alcoholic hepatitis. N Engl J Med 2011;365:1781–89.

86. **Imperiale TF, McCullough AJ. Do corticosteroids reduce mortality from alcoholic hepatitis? A meta-analysis of the randomized trials. Ann Intern Med 1990;113:299–307.** *Analysis of 11 studies showed a 37% reduction in mortality with corticosteroids. However, among those with hepatic encephalopathy, no study showed benefit, and patients with gastrointestinal bleeding were almost uniformly excluded.*

87. Christensen E, Gluud C. Glucocorticoids are ineffective in alcoholic hepatitis. A meta-analysis adjusting for confounding variables. Gut 1995; 37:113–8.

88. **Mathurin P, Mendenall CL, Carithers RL, et al. Corticosteroids improve short-term survival in patients with severe alcoholic hepatitis (AH): individual data analysis of the last three randomized placebo controlled trials of corticosteroids in severe AH. J Hepatology 2002;36:480–7.** *In this meta-analysis of three studies of 215 patients with severe alcoholic hepatitis treated with corticosteroids or placebo, 28-day survival was higher in the treated group (85% vs. 65%; p = 0.001).*

89. O'Shea RS, Dasarathy S, McCullough AJ. Practice Guideline Committee of the American Association for the Study of Liver Diseases; Practice Parameters Committee of the American College of Gastroenterology. Alcoholic liver disease. Hepatology 2010;51:307–28.

90. Mathurin P, Moreno C, Samuel D, et al. Early liver transplantation for severe alcoholic hepatitis. N Engl J Med 2011;365:1790–800.

91. Anonymous. Annual Data Report of the US Organ Procurement and Transplantation Network (OPTN) and the Scientific Registry of Transplant Recipients (SRTR). Am J Transplant 2013;13 Suppl 1:8–10.

92. Fung AT, Rimmer J. Hypophosphatemia secondary to oral refeeding syndrome in a patient with long-term alcohol misuse. Med J Aust 2005;183:324–6.

93. Fenves AZ, Thomas S, Knochel JP. Beer potomania: two cases and review of the literature. Clin Nephrol 1996;45:61–4.

94. Levy LJ, Duga J, Girgis. Ketoacidosis associated with alcoholism in non-diabetic subjects. Ann Intern Med 1973;78:213–9.

95. Arroyo V, Guevara M, Gines P. Hepatorenal syndrome in cirrhosis: pathogenesis and treatment. Gastroenterology 2002;122:1658–76.

96. Meyer JS, Tanahashi N, Ishikawa Y, et al. Cerebral atrophy and hypoperfusion improve during treatment of Wernicke-Korsakoff syndrome. J Cereb Blood Flow Metab 1985;5:376–85.

97. Borges G, Mondragón L, Medina-Mora ME, et al. A case-control study of alcohol and substance use disorders as risk factors for non-fatal injury. Alcohol Alcohol 2005;40:257–62.

98. Matsuo K, Hirohata T, Sugioka Y, et al. Influence of alcohol intake, cigarette smoking, and occupational status on idiopathic osteonecrosis of the femoral head. Clin Orthoped 1988;234:115–23.

99. Kelepouris N, Harper KD, Gannon F, et al. Severe osteoporosis in men. Ann Intern Med 1995;123:452–60.

100. Felson DT, Zhanh Y, Hannan MT, et al. Alcohol intake and bone mineral density in elderly men and women. The Framingham study. Am J Epidemiol 1995;142:485–92.

101. Holbrook TL, Barrett O, Connor E. A prospective study of alcohol consumption and bone mineral density. BMJ 1993;306:1506–9.

102. Preedy VR, Adachi J, Ueno Y, et al. Alcoholic skeletal myopathy: definitions, features, contributions of neuropathy, impact and diagnosis. Eur J Neurol 2001;8:677–87.

103. Wang M, Jiang X, Wu W, Zhang D. A meta-analysis of alcohol consumption and the risk of gout. Clin Rheumatol 2013;32:1631–8.

104. **Choi HK, Atkinson K, Karlson EW, et al. Alcohol intake and risk of incident gout in men: a prospective study. Lancet 2004;363:1277–81.** *Relative risk of gout in drinkers compared to non-drinkers was 2.0 for 1–2 drinks/day and 2.5 for ≥2 drinks/day. Beer consumption had the highest risk and wine the least, with no increased risk in those who drank one glass of wine/day.*

105. Nunes EV, Levin FR. Treatment of depression in patients with alcohol or other drug dependence. A meta-analysis. JAMA 2004;291:1887–96.

106. Glass IB. Alcoholic hallucinosis: a psychiatric enigma—1. The development of an idea. Br J Addiction 1989:84:29–41.

107. Tsuang JW, Irwin MR, Smith TL, Schuckit MA. Characteristics of men with alcoholic hallucinosis. Addiction 1994;89:73–8.

108. Smith-Warner SA, Spiegelman D, Yaun S, et al. Alcohol and breast cancer in women: a pooled analysis of cohort studies. JAMA 1998; 279:535–40.

109. Singletary KW, Gapstur SM. Alcohol and breast cancer: review of epidemiologic and experimental evidence and potential mechanisms. JAMA 2001:286:2143–51.

110. Chen WY, Rosner B, Hankinson SE, et al. Moderate alcohol consumption during adult life, drinking patterns, and breast cancer risk. JAMA 2011;306:1884–90.

111. Bagnardi V, Rota M, Botteri E, et al. Light alcohol drinking and cancer: a meta-analysis. Ann Oncol 2012;24:301–8.

112. Sokol RJ, Delaney-Black V, Nordstrom B. Fetal alcohol spectrum disorder. JAMA 2003;290:2996–9.

113. Cohen E, Feinn R, Arias A, Kranzler HR. Alcohol treatment utilization: findings from the National Epidemiologic Survey on Alcohol and Related Conditions. Drug Alcohol Depend 2007;86:214–21.

114. **Fiellin DA, O'Connor PG, Holboe ES, Horwitz RI. Risk for delirium tremens in patients with alcohol withdrawal syndrome. Subst Abuse 2002;23:83–94.** *In this study, 15 patients with delirium tremens (DT) were compared with 45 uncomplicated alcohol withdrawal controls. Cases were more likely to report prior complicated withdrawal (DT or alcohol withdrawal seizure) (53 vs. 27%; OR 3.1), have a systolic blood pressure >145 mmHg on admission (60 vs. 27%; OR 4.1), and have comorbidity scores of at least 1 (60% vs. 18%; OR 6.9).*

115. Pecoraro A, Ewen E, Horton T, et al. Using the AUDIT-PC to predict alcohol withdrawal in hospitalized patients. J Gen Intern Med 2013;29:34–40.

116. Maldonado JR, Sher Y, Ashouri JF, et al. The Prediction of Alcohol Withdrawal Severity Scale (PAWSS): systematic literature review and pilot study of a new scale for the prediction of complicated alcohol withdrawal syndrome. Alcohol 2014;48:375–90.

117. Mee-Lee D, Shulman GD, Fishman MJ, Gastfriend DR, Miller MM, eds. The *ASAM Criteria: Treatment Criteria for Addictive, Substance-Related, and Co-Occurring Conditions*, 3rd ed. Carson City, NV: Change Companies; 2013.

118. Hayashida M, Alterman AI, McLellan T, et al. Comparative effectiveness and costs of inpatient and outpatient detoxification of patients with mild-to-moderate alcohol withdrawal syndrome. N Engl J Med 1989;320:358–65.

119. Stephens JR, Liles EA, Dancel R, et al. Who needs inpatient detox? Development and implementation of a hospitalist protocol for

the evaluation of patients for alcohol detoxification. J Gen Intern Med 2014;29:587–93.

120. Mayo-Smith MF, for the American Society of Addiction Medicine Workshop Group on Pharmacologic Management of Alcohol Withdrawal. Pharmacologic management of alcohol withdrawal. A meta-analysis and evidence-based medicine practice guideline. JAMA 1997; 278:144–51.

121. Minozzi S, Amato L, Vecchi S, Davoli M. Benzodiazepines for alcohol withdrawal. Cochrane Database Syst Rev 2010;17:CD005063.

122. Taheri A, Dahri K, Chan P, et al. Evaluation of a symptom-triggered protocol approach to the management of alcohol withdrawal syndrome in older adults. J Am Geriatr Soc 2014;62:1551–5.

123. **Saitz R, Mayo-Smith MF, Roberts MS, et al. Individualized treatment for alcohol withdrawal. A randomized double-blind controlled trial. JAMA 1994;272:519–23.** *In this trial, 101 consecutive admissions for alcohol withdrawal were randomized to placebo or fixed-dose chlordiazepoxide every 6 hours (50 mg doses × 4, then 25 mg doses × 8). All received symptom-triggered chlordiazepoxide. The fixed-dose group received more medication (mean of 425 mg vs.100 mg; p < 0.001).*

124. Hendley GW, Dery RA, Barnes RL, et al. A prospective, randomized, trial of phenobarbital versus benzodiazepines for acute alcohol withdrawal. Am J Emerg Med 2011:29:382–85.

125. Rosenson J, Clements C, Simon B, et al. Phenobarbital for acute alcohol withdrawal: a prospective randomized double-blind placebo-controlled study. J Emerg Med 2013;44:592–98.

126. Minozzi S, Amato L, Vecchi S, Davoli M. Anticonvulsants for alcohol withdrawal. Cochrane Database Syst Rev 2010;17:CD005064.

127. Malcolm R, Ballenger JC, Sturgis ET, Anton R. Double-blind controlled trial comparing carbamazepine to oxazepam treatment of alcohol withdrawal. Am J Psychiatry 1989;146:617–21.

128. Stuppaeck CH, Pycha R, Miller C, et al. Carbamazepine versus oxazepam in the treatment of alcohol withdrawal: a double-blind study. Alcohol Alcohol 1992;27:153–8.

129. Reoux JP, Saxon AJ, Malte CA, et al. Divalproex sodium in alcohol withdrawal: a randomized double-blind placebo controlled clinical trial. Alcohol Clin Exp Res 2001;23:1324–9.

130. Furieri FA, Nakamura-Palacios EM. Gabapentin reduces alcohol consumption and craving: a randomized placebo-controlled trial. J Clin Psychiatry 2007;68:1691–700.

131. Bonnet U, Banger M, Lewek M, et al. Treatment of acute alcohol withdrawal with gabapentin: results from a controlled two-center trial. J Clin Psychopharmacol 2003;23:514–9. *In this trial, 61 patients were randomized to gabapentin 400 mg four times/day or placebo, in addition to symptom-driven clomethiazole. There was no difference between groups in consumption of clomethiazole, nor in alleviating withdrawal symptoms.*

132. Myrick H, Malcom R, Randall PK, et al. A double-blind trial of gabapentin versus lorazepam in the treatment of alcohol withdrawal. Alcohol Clin Exp Res 2009;33:1582–88. *One hundred individuals seeking treatment for alcohol withdrawal with a CIWA ≥10 were randomized to 4-day treatment with (1) gabapentin 900 mg/day tapering to 600 mg, (2) gabapentin 1200 mg/day tapering to 800 mg, or (3) lorazepam 6 mg/day tapering to 4 mg. The lower-dose gabapentin arm was discontinued after two reported "seizure-like episodes." Withdrawal symptoms and likelihood of drinking were roughly comparable between the high-dose gabapentin and lorazepam.*

133. Forq A, Hein J, Volkmar K, et al. Efficacy and safety of pregabalin in the treatment of alcohol withdrawal syndrome: a randomized placebo-controlled trial. Alcohol Alcohol 2012:47:149–55.

134. Robinson BJ, Robinson GM, Maling TJ, Johnson RH. Is clonidine useful in the treatment of alcohol withdrawal? Alcohol Clin Exp Res 1989;13:95–8.

135. Horwitz RJ, Gottlieb LD, Kraus ML. The efficacy of atenolol in the outpatient management of the alcohol withdrawal syndrome: results of a randomized clinical trial. Arch Intern Med 1989;149:1089–93.

136. Worner TM. Propranolol versus diazepam in the management of the alcohol withdrawal syndrome: double-blind controlled trial. Am J Drug Alcohol Abuse 1994;20:114–24.

137. Kraus ML, Gottlieb LD, Horwitz RI, Anscher M. Randomized clinical trial of atenolol in patients with alcohol withdrawal. N Engl J Med 1985;313:905–9.

138. Stanley KM, Worrall CL, Lunsford SL, et al. Experience with an adult alcohol withdrawal syndrome practice guideline in internal medicine patients. Pharmacotherapy 2005;25:1073–83.

139. Weinberg JA, Magnotti LJ, Fischer PE, et al. Comparison of intravenous ethanol versus diazepam for alcohol withdrawal prophylaxis in the trauma ICU: results of a randomized trial. J Trauma 2008;64:99–104.

140. Sullivan JT, Sykora K, Schneiderman J, et al. Assessment of alcohol withdrawal: the revised Clinical Institute Withdrawal Assessment for Alcohol scale (CIWA-Ar). Br J Addict 1989;84:1353–7.

141. McPherson A, Benson G, Forrest EH. Appraisal of the Glasgow assessment and management of alcohol guideline: a comprehensive alcohol management protocol for use in general hospitals. QJM 2012;105:649–56.

142. Ng SK, Hauser WA, Brust JC, et al. Alcohol consumption and withdrawal in new-onset seizures. N Engl J Med 1988;319:666–73.

143. Sampliner R, Iber F. Diphenylhydantoin control of alcohol withdrawal seizures. JAMA 1974;230:1430–2.

144. Alldredge BK, Lowenstein DH, Simon RP. Placebo-controlled trial of intravenous diphenylhydantoin for short-term treatment of alcohol withdrawal seizures. Am J Med 1989;87:645–8.

145. Rathlev NK, D'Onofrio G, Fish SS, et al. The lack of efficacy of phenytoin in the prevention of recurrent-alcohol related seizures. Ann Emerg Med 1994;23:513–8.

146. Sellers EM, Naranjo CA, Harrison M, et al. Diazepam loading: simplified treatment of alcohol withdrawal. Clin Pharmacol Ther 1983;34:822–6.

147. **D'Onofrio G, Rathlev NK, Ulrich AS, et al. Lorazepam for the prevention of recurrent seizures related to alcohol. N Engl J Med 1999;340:915–9.** *After alcohol withdrawal seizure, 186 patients were randomized to 2 mg lorazepam intravenously or placebo. In the next 6 hours, those who received lorazepam had a lower rate of recurrent seizure (3% vs. 24%).*

148. **Mayo-Smith MF, Beecher LH, Fischer TL, et al. Management of alcohol withdrawal delirium. An evidence based practice guideline. Arch Intern Med 2004;164:1405–12.** *In this meta-analysis of nine prospective controlled trials, neuroleptics, when used in the setting of alcohol withdrawal delirium, carried a relative risk of death of 6.6 compared to that of benzodiazepines. There were no deaths in any study when benzodiazepines were used.*

149. DeCarolis DD, Rice KL, Willenbring ML, Cassaro S. Symptom-driven lorazepam protocol of severe alcohol withdrawal delirium in the intensive care unit. Pharmacotherapy 2007;27:510–8.

150. Ely EW, Truman B, Shintani A, et al. Monitoring sedation status over time in ICU patients: reliability and validity of the Richmond Agitation-Sedation Scale (RASS). JAMA 2003;289:2983–91.

151. Bertholet N, Daeppen JB, Wietlisbach V, et al. Reduction of alcohol consumption by brief alcohol intervention in primary care: systematic review and meta-analysis. Arch Intern Med 2005;165:986–95.

152. Saitz R. Alcohol screening and brief intervention in primary care: absence of evidence for efficacy in people with dependence or very heavy drinking. Drug Alcohol Rev 2010;29:631–40.

153. Saitz R, Palfai TP, Cheng DM, et al. Brief intervention for medical inpatients with unhealthy alcohol use—a randomized controlled trial. Ann Intern Med 2007;146:167–76.

154. Walitzer KS, Dermen KH, Barrick C. Facilitating involvement in Alcoholics Anonymous during out-patient treatment: a randomized clinical trial. Addiction 2009:104:391–401.

155. **Hoffmann NG, Harrison PA, Belille CA. Alcoholics Anonymous after treatment: attendance and abstinence. Int J Addict 1983;18:311–8.** *In this cohort study of 900 alcoholics who completed inpatient detoxification found that at 6 months, 73% of those who attended AA at least once/week were abstinent, compared to 33% of those who attended less than once/week.*

156. Witbrodt J, Mertens J, Kaskutas LA, et al. Do 12-step meeting attendance trajectories over 9 years predict abstinence? J Subst Abuse Treat 2012;43:30–43.

157. Gossop M, Harris J, Best D, et al. Is attendance at Alcoholics Anonymous meetings after inpatient treatment related to improved outcomes? A 6-month follow-up study. Alcohol Alcohol 2003;38:421–6.

158. Timko C, DeBenedetti A, Billow R. Intensive referral to 12-step self-help groups and 6-month substance use disorder outcomes. Addiction 2006;101:678–88.

159. **Walsh DC, Hingson RW, Merrigan DM, et al. A randomized trial of treatment options for alcohol abusing workers. N Engl J Med 1991;325:775–82.** *Consecutive workers identified by an employee assistance program as needing treatment for alcohol abuse (n = 227) were randomized to (1) inpatient treatment, (2) AA meetings, or (3) their choice of treatment. All three groups improved, with no difference in job-related outcomes, but the inpatient group was less likely to need further inpatient treatment in follow-up—23% versus 38% of the choice group and 63% of the AA group.*

160. White A, Kavanagh D, Stallman H, et al. Online alcohol interventions: a systematic review. J Med Internet Res 2010;12:e62.

161. Gustafson DH, McTavish FM, Chih MY, et al. Smartphone application to support recovery from alcoholism: a randomized clinical trial. JAMA Psychiatry 2014;71:566–72.

162. Gajecki M1, Berman AH, Sinadinovic K, et al. Mobile phone brief intervention applications for risky alcohol use among university students: a randomized controlled study. Addict Sci Clin Pract 2014;9:11.

163. **Jonas D, Amick HR, Feltner C, et al. Pharmacotherapy for adults with alcohol use disorders in outpatient settings: a systematic review and meta-analysis. JAMA 2014;311:1889–1900.** *This systematic review of studies assessed treatment with acamprosate (27 studies, n = 7519) and naltrexone (53 studies, n = 9140). The number needed to treat (NNT) to prevent return to any drinking for acamprosate was 12 (95% CI, 8 to 26; risk difference [RD], –0.09; 95% CI, –0.14 to –0.04) and for oral naltrexone was 20 (95% CI, 11 to 500; RD, –0.05; 95% CI, –0.10 to –0.002). For injectable naltrexone, meta-analyses found no significant association with return to any drinking (RD, –0.04; 95% CI, –0.10 to 0.03) or heavy drinking (RD, –0.01; 95% CI, –0.14 to 0.13)*

164. **Fuller RK, Roth HP. Disulfiram for the treatment of alcoholism: an evaluation of 128 men. Ann Intern Med 1979;90:901–4.** *In this trial, 128 alcoholic men were randomized to (1) disulfiram 250 mg/day, (2) disulfiram 1 mg/day, or (3) no medication. There was no significant difference in abstinence rates by intention to treat; however, abstinence rates were higher among those who took the disulfiram compared to those who did not.*

165. **Fuller RK, Branchey L, Brightwell DR, et al. Disulfiram treatment of alcoholism. A Veterans Administration cooperative study. JAMA 1986;256:1449–55.** *In this trial, 605 men were randomized to disulfiram 250 mg/day, placebo, or no medication (all received behavioral counseling); there was no difference in total abstinence or time to first drink.*

166. Jorgensen C, Pedersen B, Tonnesen H. The efficacy of disulfiram for the treatment of alcohol use disorder. Alcoholism: Clin Exp Res 2011;35:1749–1758.

167. Anton RF, O'Malley SS, Ciraulo DA, et al. Combined pharmacotherapies and behavioral interventions for alcohol dependence: the COMBINE study: a randomized controlled trial. JAMA 2006;295:2003–17.

168. **Krystal JH, Cramer JA, Krol WF, et al. Naltrexone in the treatment of alcohol dependence. N Engl J Med 2001;345:1734–9.** *In this trial, 627 veterans (97% male) were randomized to 12 months of naltrexone*

(50 mg/day), 3 months of naltrexone followed by 9 months of placebo, or 12 months of placebo. All were offered individual counseling and encouraged to attend AA. At 13 weeks, there were no differences in days to relapse, and at 52 weeks, no differences in drinking days or number of drinks/drinking day.

169. Rosner S, Hackl-Herrwerth A, Leucht S, et al. Opioid antagonists for alcohol dependence. Cochrane Database Syst Rev 2010;(12):CD001867.

170. **Garbutt JC, Kranzler HR, O'Malley SS, et al. Efficacy and tolerability of long-acting injectable naltrexone for alcohol dependence: a randomized controlled trial. JAMA. 2005;293:1617–25.** *This 6-month trial with 624 subjects compared three treatments—placebo, and depot naltrexone, 190 or 380 mg. Compared with placebo, those on 380 mg naltrexone had a 25% decrease in heavy drinking days (p = 0.02, but 0.28 for women and <0.001 for men); those on 190 mg of naltrexone had a 17% decrease (p = 0.07).*

171. Chamorro AJ, Marcos M, Mirón-Canelo JA, et al. Association of the μ-opioid receptor (OPRM1) gene polymorphism with response to naltrexone in alcohol dependence: a systematic review and meta-analysis Addict Biol 2012;17:505–12.

172. Kalk NJ, Lingford-Hughes AR. The clinical pharmacology of acamprosate. Br J Clin Pharmacol 2014;77:315–23.

173. **Tempesta E, Janiri L, Bignamini A, et al. Acamprosate and relapse prevention in the treatment of alcohol dependence: A placebo-controlled study. Alcohol Alcohol 2000;35:202–9.** *After detoxification, 330 alcoholics were randomized to acamprosate or placebo; all received counseling. At 6 months, abstinence rate was higher in the acamprosate group (58% vs. 45%), but 3 months after the end of the study (with no medication), there was no difference between the groups.*

174. **Gual A, Lehert P. Acamprosate during and after acute alcohol withdrawal: a double-blind placebo controlled study in Spain. Alcohol Alcohol 2001;36:413–8.** *After detoxification, 296 alcoholics were randomized acamprosate or placebo for 180 days; all received counseling; 110 patients dropped out from the study. By intention-to-treat analysis, mean abstinence duration was longer for the acamprosate group (93 vs. 74 days; p = 0.01). Full abstinence was achieved by 35 on acamprosate and 26 on placebo (p = 0.07).*

175. **Chick J, Howlett H, Morgan MY, et al. United Kingdom multicentre acamprosate study: a 6-month prospective study of acamprosate versus placebo in preventing relapse after withdrawal from**

alcohol. *Alcohol Alcohol 2000;35:176–87. After detoxification, 581 alcoholics were randomized to acamprosate or placebo; all received counseling. Compliance was poor with only 57% of patients taking ≥90% of pills by week 2. There was no difference in outcomes between groups, with abstinence rates of 12% for acamprosate versus 11% on placebo.*

176. Rösner S, Hackl-Herrwerth A, Leucht S, et al. Acamprosate for alcohol dependence. Cochrane Database of Syst Rev 2010;9:CD004332.

177. Mason BJ, Lehert P. Acamprosate for alcohol dependence: a sex-specific meta-analysis based on individual patient data. Alcohol Clin Exp Res 2012; 36:497–508.

178. **Johnson BA, Ait-Daoud N, Bowden CL, et al. Oral topiramate for treatment of alcohol dependence: a randomised controlled trial. Lancet 2003;361:1677–85.** *In this study, 150 alcoholics were randomized to topiramate at escalating doses of 25–300 mg/day or placebo. Those on topiramate had significantly fewer drinks/day, fewer drinks/drinking day, and more days abstinent (44% vs. 18%).*

179. Johnson BA, Rosenthal N, Capece JA, et al. Topiramate for treating alcohol dependence: a randomized clinical trial. JAMA 2007;298:1641–51.

180. Paparrigopoulos T, Tzavellas E, Karaiskos D, et al. Treatment of alcohol dependence with low-dose topiramate: an open-label controlled study. BMC Psychiatry 2011;11:41.

181. Kranzler HR, Covault J, Feinn R. Topiramate treatment for heavy drinkers: moderation by a GRIK1 polymorphism. Am J Psych 2014;171:445–52.

182. **Mason BJ, Quello S, Goodell V, et al. Gabapentin treatment for alcohol dependence: a randomized clinical trial. JAMA Intern Med 2014;174:70-7.** *This trial (n = 150) compared gabapentin dosages (of 0 [placebo], 900 mg, or 1800 mg/day). Over 12 weeks, gabapentin improved the rates of abstinence and no heavy drinking. Abstinence rate was 4% with placebo, 11% with 900 mg, and 17% with 1800 mg (p = 0.04 for linear dose effect; NNT = 8 for 1800 mg). No heavy drinking rate was 23% with placebo, 30% with 900 mg, and 45% with 1800 mg (p = 0.02 for linear dose effect; NNT = 5 for 1800 mg).*

183. Pani PP, Trogu E, Pancini M, Maremmani I. Anticonvulsants for alcohol dependence. Cochrane Database Syst Rev 2014;2:CD008544.

184. **Litten RZ, Ryan ML, Fertig JB, et al. A double-blind, placebo-controlled trial assessing the efficacy of varenicline tartrate**

for alcohol dependence. J Addict Med 2013;7:277–86. *In this study, 200 individuals with alcohol dependence received varenicline or placebo with a computerized behavioral intervention. The varenicline group had lower weekly percent heavy drinking days (adjusted mean difference 10 days), drinks/day, drinks/drinking day, and alcohol craving. The treatment effect on alcohol use was similar for smokers and nonsmokers.*

5

Sedative-Hypnotics

Background

The sedative-hypnotics are central nervous system (CNS) depressants. These agents are used therapeutically at low doses for treatment of anxiety, panic disorder, and insomnia, and at higher doses for sedation or anesthesia. Sedative-hypnotics are also used for treating status epilepticus (benzodiazepines) and for preventing seizures (barbiturates). Butalbital, an intermediate-acting barbiturate, is an ingredient in migraine medications. Table 5.1 shows a list by category of commonly used sedative-hypnotics.

TABLE 5.1 Sedative-Hypnotic Drugs

Generic	Brand Name
Benzodiazepines	
Alprazolam	Xanax
Chlordiazepoxide	Librium
Clonazepam	Klonopin
Clorazepate	Tranxene
Diazepam	Valium
Flunitrazepam	Rohypnol
Flurazepam	Dalmane
Lorazepam	Ativan
Oxazepam	Serax
Temazepam	Restoril
Triazolam	Halcion

(continued)

TABLE 5.1 (Continued)

Barbiturates	
Amobarbital	
Butabarbital	
Butalbital	Fiorinal*
Pentobarbital	Nembutol
Phenobarbital	
Secobarbital	Seconol
Others	
Carisoprodol	Soma
Chloral hydrate	
Eszopiclone	Lunesta
Gamma-hydroxybutyrate	Xyrem
Meprobamate	Miltown, Equanil
Zaleplon	Sonata
Zolpidem	Ambien

*Combination with aspirin and caffeine.

Bromides, introduced in 1826, were the first sedative-hypnotic drugs, followed by barbital, the first barbiturate, in 1903, chloral hydrate in 1932, and meprobamate in1955. Chlordiazepoxide (Librium), introduced in 1961, was the first benzodiazepine. Benzodiazepines quickly overtook barbiturates as the most prescribed sedative-hypnotic, as they were able to decrease anxiety with less sedation and less risk for respiratory depression.

All barbiturates are derived from barbituric acid. They are classified into three groups by duration of action. The short-acting barbiturates are used to induce anesthesia and are generally administered intravenously. The intermediate-acting barbiturates are prescribed as oral sedative-hypnotics and are the group most commonly abused. The long-acting barbiturates are prescribed for oral use as anticonvulsants.

Benzodiazepines can be divided into three groups: those that have active metabolites (chlordiazepoxide, diazepam, flurazepam, flunitrazepam, clorazepate); those that do not produce active metabolites (lorazepam, oxazepam); and a group that produces an active metabolite with little clinical activity (alprazolam, triazolam). A classification of benzodiazepines based on potency, onset of action, and half-life is shown in Table 5.2; roughly equivalent oral doses are also provided.

When first introduced, benzodiazepines were thought to have low risk for abuse and were not classified as scheduled drugs. Subsequently, abuse liability studies in animals and humans of benzodiazepines showed them to be drugs that may lead to abuse and addiction.[1,2] Most individuals who abuse benzodiazepines abuse other drugs as well.[3] Nonmedical use of benzodiazepines is commonly related to attempts at self-medicating anxiety or agoraphobia.[4] The indications for prescribing benzodiazepines are limited, especially as other safer medications can be prescribed for anxiety. The American Geriatric Society and the American Board of Internal Medicine Foundation Choosing Wisely Campaign recommend against the use of benzodiazepines in adults aged 65 and older.[5] There is evidence that direct patient education can reduce inappropriate benzodiazepine prescribing to older adults.[6]

Abuse liability of benzodiazepines is greatest for drugs with rapid onset of action.[7,8,9] The newer sedative-hypnotics zolpidem (Ambien and Intermezzo), eszopiclone (Lunesta), ramelteon (Rozerem), and zaleplon (Sonata) are used for insomnia and are chemically distinct from the benzodiazepines, but bind to the same receptors.[10] Other sedative-hypnotics include chloral hydrate (no longer available in the United States) used in the treatment of insomnia; meprobamate

TABLE 5.2 Comparison of Benzodiazepines

Class/Agent (Brand Name)	Equipotent Oral Dose (mg)*
Short-Acting/Low Potency	
Oxazepam (Serax)	30
Temazepam (Restoril)	60
Short-Acting/High Potency	
Alprazolam (Xanax)	1
Lorazepam (Ativan)	2
Triazolam (Halcion)	1
Long-Acting/Low Potency	
Chlordiazepoxide (Librium)	25
Clorazepate (Tranxene)	15
Diazepam (Valium)	10
Flurazepam (Dalmane)	60
Long-Acting/High Potency	
Clonazepam (Klonopin)	1
Flunitrazepam (Rohypnol)	2

*Roughly equivalent to 30 mg of phenobarbital.

(Miltown or Equanil), an anxiolytic with high abuse potential; carisoprodol (Soma), whose metabolite is meprobromate; and gamma-hydroxybutyrate (GHB). GHB is therapeutically used for the treatment of narcolepsy. Abused GHB is produced illicitly and is used recreationally at raves. Two drugs related to GHB, 1,4-butanediol (used to clean electronic equipment) and gamma-butyrolactone, are metabolized to GHB. GHB is easily manufactured in illicit laboratories as a powder that is dissolved in water and often mixed in alcoholic beverages. Flunitrazepam (Rohypnol) has gained attention for abuse as "the date rape drug."[11,12] It is not licensed in the United States but is sold illicitly. Some users grind flunitrazepam into a powder and then use it by intranasal route.

Epidemiology

Data on use of sedatives are somewhat difficult to interpret because the U.S. National Survey on Drug Use and Health (NSDUH) divides this category into two somewhat arbitrary groups: *tranquilizers* and *sedatives*. For the purposes of this chapter, we will refer to both groups as sedatives unless we are specifically referring to NSDUH data. *Tranquilizers* includes most benzodiazepines, the "muscle relaxers" cyclobenzaprine and carisoprodol, the antihistamine hydroxyzine, along with buspirone and meprobamate. *Sedatives* includes barbiturates, the benzodiazepines temazepam, flurazepam, and triazolam, as well as methaqualone, chloral hydrate, and ethchlorvynol. Additionally, not all surveys related to substance use report prevalence data specific to sedatives or tranquilizers.

The 2013 NSDUH estimated that 23.5 million Americans have used a tranquilizer nonmedically in their lifetime (9.0% of those aged 12 and older); 5.3 million (2.0%) have used one in the past year, and 1.7 million (0.6%) were current (past month) nonmedical users. For sedatives, 7.5 million (2.9%) have used these in their lifetime, 639,000 (0.2%) in the past year, and 251,000 (0.1%) in the past month.[13] The tranquilizers or sedatives most commonly taken nonmedically are alprazolam, followed by diazepam and clonazepam.

Most sedative users abuse other drugs as well; in 2010, there were 33,701 treatment admissions for combined benzodiazepine and opioid abuse.[14] For individuals with substance use disorders, and especially those on methadone maintenance, abuse of benzodiazepines is common.[15,16,17,18] Patients with alcoholism are also at greater risk for benzodiazepine abuse.[19,20,21] Childhood traumatic experiences may be a risk factor for benzodiazepine use disorder in individuals with opiate use disorder.[22] Benzodiazepine misuse appears to be particularly widespread among young adults 18–29 who report regular attendance at large dance clubs, with one survey reporting a prevalence of 25%.[23]

In 2012, tranquilizers were reported as the primary substance of abuse by 1% of drug treatment admissions and sedatives were reported as the primary substance of abuse by 0.25%.[24] Emergency room visits related to nonmedical use of alprazolam totaled 123,744 in 2011.[25] Of these visits, 81% involved nonmedical use of alprazolam along with another drug. As many clinicians have shifted benzodiazepine prescribing to clonazepam, significant abuse liability for clonazepam has been reported.[26]

Reported misuse of zolpidem has increased over the past decade. As with other sedatives, most cases occur in individuals who abuse other drugs.[27] In a survey of adolescents ages 12–17, zolpidem misuse was present in 1.4%.[28] In 2009–2010, there were 42,274 emergency room visits related to zolpidem;[29] this was twice the number seen in 2005–2006. Just over half of the visits in 2009–2010 were related to zolpidem in combination with other drugs. In 2010, 26% of the emergency room visits related to zolpidem led to admissions to an intensive care unit.

Carisoprodol misuse has only recently being recognized, leading to its reclassification as a scheduled drug in 2012. It has been removed from the market in most European countries. In a 6-month study at a university hospital in San Diego, 19 of 4245 urine samples had positive drug tests for carisoprodol.[30] All of the 19 patients had clinical complications thought related to carisoprodol, with most patients lethargic or obtunded, and several presenting with seizures.

Drug Effects

Sedative-hypnotics interact at the gamma-aminobutyric acid (GABA) receptor. GABA is an inhibitory transmitter in the central nervous system. Benzodiazepines do not directly bind to GABA receptors, but rather potentiate the actions of GABA by causing

GABA to bind more tightly to receptors, enhancing CNS inhibitory tone. Barbiturates bind to the GABA receptor complex and prolong opening of chloride channels, inhibiting excitable cells in the CNS. There is some evidence that there is a specific barbiturate receptor site, with a correlation between binding affinity and drug effect.[31] Carisoprodol and its active metabolite meprobamate also act directly at the GABA receptor complex.

Acute Effects

Sedatives cause intoxication similar to that seen with alcohol. They produce a depression of cortical function and relax social and personal inhibitions. Mood is elevated and anxiety is reduced. Barbiturates are more likely than benzodiazepines to cause motor incoordination, slurred speech, and respiratory depression. While reinforcing effects of benzodiazepines are variable, barbiturates have consistently demonstrated high abuse liability. Patients, including those with anxiety disorders, do not necessarily find the effects of benzodiazepines pleasurable or reinforcing. Used for sleep, sedative-hypnotic drugs decrease sleep latency and temporarily diminish awakenings from sleep. Effects on sleep lessen with chronic use. Additionally, REM sleep (restful sleep) is actually diminished. Benzodiazepines also cause acute amnesia after high-dose intravenous administration, an effect used therapeutically for medical procedures.

Carisoprodol has clinical effects similar to those of the benzodiazepines, but may also cause tachycardia, involuntary movements, hand tremor, and horizontal gaze nystagmus.[32] Psychomotor impairment may occur without individuals perceiving effects.[33] GHB has clinical effects 15–30 minutes after oral ingestion, producing an initial euphoria, followed by dizziness, hypersalivation, and drowsiness.[34]

Acute Toxicity and Overdose

The DSM-5 diagnostic criteria for "sedative, hypnotic, or anxiolytic intoxication" require the presence of "clinically significant maladaptive behavioral or psychological changes plus one (or more) of the following signs or symptoms after use: (1) slurred speech, (2) incoordination, (3) unsteady gait, (4) nystagmus, (5) cognitive impairment, and (6) stupor or coma.[35] The ICD-10 code depends on whether there is a comorbid use disorder and the severity of the disorder; it is F13.929 if there is no use disorder, F13.129 if a mild disorder, and F13.229 if moderate-severe.

At the extreme, overdose may lead to respiratory depression, vasomotor collapse, and death. Benzodiazepines (compared with barbiturates) cause less loss of motor coordination and rarely cause death on their own, even when taken in large doses, unless given rapidly by intravenous route (e.g., midazolam or diazepam) or in combination with alcohol or other drugs. Barbiturates carry a higher risk of overdose and fatality than benzodiazepines and other sedatives.[36] There is one case report of a near-fatal overdose of carisoprodol.[37] For benzodiazepine overdose, flumazenil, a specific benzodiazepine antagonist, should be administered—0.2 mg intravenously followed by 0.3 mg in 30 seconds and another 0.5 mg every 60 seconds for up to six doses. Flumazenil has a short duration of action, so repeated doses may need to be administered, even after a satisfactory initial response. For benzodiazepine-dependent patients, flumazenil may cause symptoms of withdrawal. Flumazenil may also be effective in the treatment of carisoprodol intoxication.[38]

Severe intoxication with GHB may produce coma and apnea.[39] Overdose is common, as the strength of street GHB can vary greatly. Agitation, myoclonus, and seizures are common. In addition, GHB overdose may result in bradycardia or hypothermia in about a third of individuals.[40,41] Intoxication with 1,4 butanediol produces more prolonged symptoms, especially sedation.[42] Treatment of GHB overdose is supportive. Bradycardia does not usually produce hemodynamic instability. Endotracheal intubation may be temporarily necessary in individuals with severely depressed mental status. Fomepizole, an alcohol dehydrogenase inhibitor approved for treatment of ethylene glycol and methanol intoxication, may be useful in 1,4 butanediol overdose.[43]

Withdrawal

Withdrawal symptoms from sedatives are similar to those with alcohol withdrawal. The DSM-5 diagnostic criteria for "sedative, hypnotic, or anxiolytic withdrawal" require the presence of two or more of the following signs or symptoms in the setting of cessation or reduction in use: (1) autonomic hyperactivity (sweating or tachycardia), (2) tremor, (3) insomnia, (4) nausea or vomiting, (5) transient visual, tactile or auditory hallucinations or illusions, (6) psychomotor agitation, (7) anxiety, and (8) grand mal seizures.[36] The ICD-10 code is F13.232 if there are perceptual disturbances and F13.239 if there are none.

The onset of withdrawal symptoms from benzodiazepines and barbiturates is related to drug half-life, with cessation of shorter-acting drugs leading to withdrawal symptoms in 24–48 hours and withdrawal from longer-acting drugs typically occurring in 48–96 hours. Most withdrawal seizures occur 24–72 hours after cessation of use. From a clinical point of view, it is important to recognize that many patients with physical dependence on sedative-hypnotics also misuse other drugs concurrently. Seizures are more likely to occur in individuals who also consume alcohol. Withdrawal symptoms may last for a few weeks or more.[44] For individuals taking a short-acting benzodiazepine only at night for insomnia, withdrawal symptoms will likely be limited to re-emergence and heightening of their insomnia. A rare but serious complication of benzodiazepine withdrawal is nonconvulsive status epilepticus. Individuals with this syndrome may be unresponsive or exhibit bizarre behavior, and it may be confused with intoxication. The diagnosis can be made with an electroencephalogram (EEG), and patients respond rapidly to the administration of benzodiazepines.[45]

Signs and symptoms of GHB withdrawal include tremor, tachycardia, anxiety, hallucinations (auditory, tactile and visual), paranoia, delusions, delirium, diaphoresis, hypertension, and nausea. There has been one reported death.[46] Withdrawal usually starts 24–48 hours after last use and may last several days.

Carisoprodol withdrawal has been reported in patients taking high doses for an extended period, with symptoms of insomnia, anxiety, headache, and irritability.[47,48,49] There are case reports of delirium and psychosis in the setting of withdrawal from carisoprodol that responded to treatment with benzodiazepines.[50,51] Withdrawal symptoms seem to peak 2–3 days after cessation of use.

Assessment

Chronic use of benzodiazepines may go undetected until confusion, irritability, slurred speech, or ataxia is recognized as signs of sedative toxicity. Physical examination may include ecchymoses from injuries. Urine drug tests will detect barbiturates and most benzodiazepines, with the exception of flunitrazepam and clonazepam, which may not be detected by all testing assays. Other sedative-hypnotics are not detected by routine urine drug tests, but may be detected by more extensive testing.

The DSM-5 criteria for "sedative, hypnotic, or anxiolytic use disorder" are the same as those for other substances; see Chapter 1 for more details.[36] The ICD-10 code for a mild disorder is F13.10 and for moderate-severe, F13.20.

Medical Complications

Virtually all of the literature on medical complications of sedative-hypnotic use is specific to benzodiazepines. The most serious complications are cognitive impairment and accidental injury.

Cognitive Impairment

Memory impairment may occur in some individuals using benzodiazepines chronically.[52,53] This effect appears more prevalent in the elderly[54] and in individuals using high-potency, short half-life benzodiazepines.[55] One study showed sustained cognitive impairment 6 months after patients were withdrawn from long-term benzodiazepine use.[56] Moreover, a 2014 case-control study found that older benzodiazepine users were at increased risk of Alzheimer's dementia.[57] Elderly patients who discontinue chronic benzodiazepine use may see improvement in memory and cognitive functioning.[58,59] Because alcohol is known to produce brain atrophy, several studies have examined whether chronic benzodiazepines use also leads to pathological changes. While some studies show an effect,[60,61] other studies do not.[62,63]

Accidental Injury

Benzodiazepine use may increase the risk of accidental injury.[64] Several epidemiological studies have shown that benzodiazepines and other sedative-hypnotics increase the risk of falls[65,66,67,68,69] and hip fractures in the elderly.[70,71,72,73] One study found an increased risk of incurring an accidental injury within 6 months of receiving a prescription for a benzodiazepine.[74] Additionally, in a study of older adults, an elevated rate of automobile accidents was found in benzodiazepine users.[75]

Treatment

There are limited data on the treatment of individuals with a sedative use disorder and most of the literature is on the treatment of withdrawal. It is reasonable to try psychosocial modalities used for other substances, including self-help groups and counseling. There is no evidence to support any long-term pharmacological treatments for these individuals.

Medically supervised withdrawal (detoxification) from benzodiazepines in patients receiving them therapeutically can be managed by tapering the prescribed benzodiazepine[76] or by switching to a benzodiazepine with a longer half-life and tapering it over several weeks.[77] Typically, the dose can be reduced 50% within a few days, the next 25% over a week or two, and the last 25% over a few weeks. The final 25% is most often the most difficult stage for patients.[78]

Inpatient treatment is often required for high-dose users and can be managed similarly to alcohol withdrawal with symptom-triggered benzodiazepines, using a withdrawal scale to guide administration. A 20-item withdrawal scale, the Clinical Institute Withdrawal Assessment–Benzodiazepines (CIWA-B), has been developed to measure withdrawal symptoms,[79] but there are limited data on its use. In our experience, given the similarity between alcohol and sedative withdrawal, the CIWA-Ar can be used and is simpler to implement.

Phenobarbital can also be used for benzodiazepine withdrawal; it has a long half-life (80–100 hours) and provides the pharmacokinetic umbrella to prevent withdrawal symptoms, including seizures. For patients misusing benzodiazepines, self-report of daily use may not be reliable. Table 5.2, presented earlier in this chapter, shows milligram equivalents between the benzodiazepines, with conversions doses for treating benzodiazepine withdrawal with phenobarbital.

We have had success treating benzodiazepine withdrawal in hundreds of patients using phenobarbital according to the fixed schedule shown in Box 5.1.[80] Doses are withheld for sedation or unsteady gait. It should be noted that this protocol was generally used in individuals who were not medically ill and there was limited

---

BOX 5.1 Phenobarbital Dosing Protocol for Treatment of Benzodiazepine Withdrawal

Phenobarbital 200 mg orally, then
Phenobarbital 100 mg orally every 4 hours times five doses, then
Phenobarbital 60 mg orally every 4 hours times four doses, then
Phenobarbital 60 mg orally every 8 hours for three doses.
Note—Hold dose if patient is sedated.

experience with older patients. Phenobarbital can also be used for treating barbiturate withdrawal, with evidence of successful treatment in patients withdrawing from butalbital containing headache medications.[81]

A gradual taper of carbamazepine also seems to be modestly effective and may be preferable to barbiturates if withdrawal is done in an outpatient setting.[82] There are also reports on the use of topiramate (a single case successfully treated)[83] and captodiamine[84] (not available in the United States, but potentially useful once further studies are performed) in the treatment of benzodiazepine withdrawal. Other drugs (propranolol,[85] clonidine, oxcarbamazepine,[86] and buspirone) have been used anecdotally as adjuncts in the treatment of sedative-hypnotic withdrawal, but there is insufficient evidence to support their use. Ondansetron[87] and paroxetine[88] have not been found to be useful. Studies combining cognitive-behavioral therapy with a gradual taper for benzodiazepine dependence failed to show a benefit over taper alone.[89,90]

GHB withdrawal can be managed similar to alcohol withdrawal using benzodiazepines as outlined in Chapter 4. There is also one report of using diazepam in the treatment of zolpidem withdrawal in an individual taking over 400 mg/day.[91]

A number of studies have looked at interventions to reduce benzodiazepine use among patients who are prescribed them but do not necessarily have a substance use disorder. In one trial, a mailed educational booklet describing the risks of benzodiazepine use and providing a tapering protocol was effective at reducing benzodiazepine use among a cohort of older adults.[7] In a systematic review of supervised withdrawal to reduce benzodiazepine use among the elderly, prescribing interventions were not effective used alone, but they were effective when combined with psychotherapy, education, or other interventions.[92]

For patients prescribed benzodiazepines and those taking them nonmedically, treatment for benzodiazepine dependence improves quality of life.[93,94] However, following successful cessation of benzodiazepine use, individuals continue to have high rates of morbidity, including high rates of depression and suicide.[95,96,97] Comorbid mental illness warrants ongoing psychiatric care.

Notes

1. Ator NA, Griffiths RR. Self-administration of barbiturates and benzodiazepines: a review. Pharmacol Biochem Behav 1987;27:391–8.

2. DuPont RL. Abuse of benzodiazepines: the problems and the solutions. Am J Drug Alcohol Abuse 1988;14:S1–S69.

3. Busto UE, Romach MK, Sellers EM. Multiple drug use and psychiatric comorbidity in patients admitted to the hospital with severe benzodiazepine dependence. J Clin Psychopharmacol 1996;16:51–7.

4. Becker WC, Fiellin DA, Desai RA. Non-medical use, abuse and dependence on sedatives and tranquilizers among U.S. adults: Psychiatric and socio-demographic correlates. Drug Alcohol Depend 2007;90:280–7.

5. The American Geriatrics Society 2012 Beers Criteria Update Expert Panel. American Geriatrics Society Updated Beers Criteria for potentially inappropriate medication use in older adults. J Am Geriatr Soc 2012; 60:616–31.

6. Tannenbaum C, Martin P, Tamblyn R, Benedetti A. Reduction of inappropriate benzodiazepine prescriptions among older adults through direct patient education: the EMPOWER cluster randomized trial. JAMA Intern Med 2014;174:890–8.

7. Bergman U, Griffiths RR. Relative abuse of diazepam and oxazepam: Prescription forgeries and theft/loss reports in Sweden. Drug Alcohol Depend 1986;16:293–301.

8. Griffiths RR, McLeod DR, Bigelow GE, et al. Relative abuse liability of diazepam and oxazepam: behavioral and subjective dose effects. Psychopharmacology 1984;84:147–54.

9. Griffiths RR, Wolf B. Relative abuse liability of different benzodiazepines in drug abusers. J Clin Psychopharmacol 1990;10:237–43.

10. Hajak G, Muller WE, Wittchen HU, et al. Abuse and dependence potential for the non-benzodiazepine hypnotics zolpidem and zopiclone: a review of case reports and epidemiologic data. Addiction 2002;98:1371–8.

11. Druid H, Holmgren P, Ahlner J. Flunitrazepam: an evaluation of use, abuse and toxicity. Forens Sci Int 2001;122:136–41.

12. Woods JH, Winger G. Abuse liability of flunitrazepam. J Clin Psychopharmacol 1997;17:1S–57S.

13. Substance Abuse and Mental Health Services Administration. *Results from the 2013 National Survey on Drug Use and Health: Summary of National Findings.* NSDUH Series H-46, HHS Publication No. (SMA) 14-4863. Rockville, MD: Substance Abuse and Mental Health Services Administration; 2014.

14. Substance Abuse and Mental Health Services Administration, Center for Behavioral Health Statistics and Quality. *The TEDS Report: Admissions Reporting Benzodiazepine and Narcotic Pain Reliever Abuse at Treatment Entry.* Rockville, MD; December 13, 2012.

15. Barnas C, Rossmann M, Roessler H, et al. Benzodiazepines and other psychotropic drugs abused by patients in a methadone maintenance program: familiarity and preference. J Clin Psychopharmacol 1992;12:397–402.

16. Iguchi MY, Handelsman L, Bickel WK, Griffiths RR. Benzodiazepine and sedative use/abuse by methadone maintenance clients. Drug Alcohol Depend 1993;32:257–66.

17. Darke S, Swift W, Hall W, Ross M. Drug use, HIV risk-taking and psychosocial correlates of benzodiazepine use among methadone maintenance clients. Drug Alcohol Depend 1993;34:67–70.

18. Chen KW, Berger CC, Forde DP, et al. Benzodiazepine use and misuse among patients in a methadone program. BMC Psychiatry 2011;11:90.

19. Ciraulo DA, Sands BF, Shader RI. Critical review of liability for benzodiazepine abuse among alcoholics. Am J Psychiatry 1988;145:1501–6.

20. Ciraulo DA, Barnhill JG, Greenblatt DJ, et al. Abuse liability and clinical pharmacokinetics of alprazolam in alcoholic men. J Clin Psychiatry 1988;49:333–7.

21. Ross HE. Benzodiazepine use and anxiolytic abuse and dependence in treated alcoholics. Addiction 1993;88:209–18.

22. Vogel M, Dursteler-MacFarland KM, Walter M et al. Prolonged use of benzodiazepines is associated with childhood trauma in opioid-maintained patients. Drug Alcohol Depend 2011;119:93–8.

23. Kurtz SP, Surratt HK, Levi-Minzi MA, Mooss A. Benzodiazepine dependence among multidrug users in the club scene. Drug Alcohol Depend 2011;119:99–105.

24. Substance Abuse and Mental Health Services Administration, Center for Behavioral Health Statistics and Quality. *Treatment Episode Data Set (TEDS): 2002–2012. National Admissions to Substance Abuse Treatment Services.* BHSIS Series S-71, HHS Publication No. (SMA) 14-4850. Rockville, MD: Substance Abuse and Mental Health Services Administration; 2014.

25. Substance Abuse and Mental Health Services Administration, Center for Behavioral Health Statistics and Quality. *The DAWN Report: Emergency Department Visits Involving Nonmedical Use of the Anti-anxiety Medication Alprazolam.* Rockville, MD; May 22, 2014.

26. Frauger E, Pauly V, Pradel V. Evidence of clonazepam abuse liability: results of the tools developed by the French Centers for Evaluation and Information on Pharmacodependence (CEIP) network. Fundem Clin Pharmacol 2010;25:633–41.

27. Hajak G, Muller WE, Wittchen HU, et al. Abuse and dependence potential for the non-benzodiazepine hypnotics zolpidem and zopiclone; a review of case reports and epidemiologic data. Addiction 2003;98:1371–8.

28. Ford JA, McCutcheon J. The misuse of Ambien among adolescents: prevalence and correlates in a national sample. Addictive Behav 2012;37:1389–94.

29. Substance Abuse and Mental Health Services Administration, Center for Behavioral Health Statistics and Quality. *Emergency Department Visits for Adverse Reactions Involving the Insomnia Medication Zolpidem.* Rockville, MD; May 1, 2013.

30. Bailey DN, Briggs JR. Carisoprodol—an unrecognized drug of abuse. Am J Clin Pathol 2002;117:396–400.

31. Olsen RW, Yang JS, Ransom RW. GABA-stimulated 36Cl—flux in brain slices as an assay for modulation by CNS depressant drugs. Adv Biochem Psychopharmacol 1988;45:125–33.

32. Bramness JG, Skurtveit S, Morland J. Impairment due to intake of carisoprodol. Drug Alcohol Depend 2004;74:311–8.

33. Zacny JP, Paice JA, Coalson DW. Characterizing the subjective and psychomotor effects of carisprodol in healthy volunteers. Pharmacol Biochem Behav 2011;100:139–43.

34. Oliveto A, Brooks Gentry W, Pruzinsky R. Behavioral effects of gamma-hydroxybutyrate (GHB) in humans. Behav Pharmacol 2010; 21:332–42.

35. American Psychiatric Association. (2013). *Diagnostic and Statistical Manual of Mental Disorders*, Fifth Edition. Arlington, VA: American Psychiatric Publishing.

36. Buckley NA, McManus PR. Changes in fatalities due to overdose of anxiolytic and sedative drugs in the UK (1983–1999). Drug Saf 2004;27:135–41.

37. Siddiqi M, Jennings CA. A near-fatal overdose of carisoprodol (soma): a case report. J Toxicol Clin Toxicol 2004;42:239–40.

38. Roberge RJ, Lin E, Krenzelok EP. Flumazenil reversal of carisoprodol (soma) intoxication. J Emerg Med 2000;18:61–4.

39. Mason PE, Kerns WP. Gamma hydroxybutyric acid (GHB) intoxication. Acad Emerg Med 2002;9:730–9.

40. Chin RL, Sporer KA, Cullison B, et al. Clinical course of gamma-hydroxybutyrate overdose. Ann Emerg Med 1998;31:716–22.

41. Li J, Stokes SA, Woeckener A. A tale of novel intoxication: seven cases of gamma-hydroxybutyric acid overdose. Ann Emerg Med 1998;31:723–8.

42. Mycyk MB, Wilemon C, Aks SE. Two cases of withdrawal from 1,4-butanediol use. Ann Emerg Med 2001;38:345–6.

43. Tancredi, DN, Shannon MW. Case 30-2003: a 21-year-old man with sudden alteration of mental status. N Engl J Med 2003;349:1267–75.

44. Busto U, Sellers EM, Naranjo CA, et al. Withdrawal reaction after long-term therapeutic use of benzodiazepines. N Engl J Med 1986;315:854–9.

45. Olnes MJ, Golding A, Kaplan PW. Nonconvulsive status epilepticus resulting from benzodiazepine withdrawal. Ann Intern Med 2003;139:956–8.

46. McDonough M, Kennedy N, Glasper A, Bearn J. Clinical features and management of gamma-hydroxybutyrate (GHB) withdrawal; a review. Drug Alcohol Depend 2004;75:3–9.

47. Reeves RR, Parker JD. Somatic dysfunction during carisoprodol cessation: evidence for a carisoprodol withdrawal syndrome. J Am Osteopath Assoc 2003;103:75–80.

48. Reeves RR, Beddingfield JJ, Mack JE. Carisoprodol withdrawal syndrome. Pharmacotherapy 2004;12:1804–6.

49. Reeves RR, Hammer JS, Pendarvis RO. Is the frequency of carisoprodol withdrawal syndrome increasing? Pharmacotherapy 2007;27:1462–6.

50. Ni K, Cary M, Zarkowski P. Carisoprolol withdrawal induced delirium: a case study. Neuropsychiatr Dis Treat 2007;3:679–82.

51. Eleid MF, Krahn LE, Argwal N, Goodman BP. Carisoprodol withdrawal after Internet purchase. Neurologist 2010;16:262–4.

52. Golombok S, Moodley P, Lader M. Cognitive impairment in long-term benzodiazepine users. Psychol Med 1988;18:365–74.

53. Curran HV. Benzodiazepines, memory and mood: a review. Psychopharmacology 1991;105:1–8.

54. Billioti de Gage S, Begaud B, Bazin F, et al. Benzodiazepine use and risk of dementia: prospective population-based study. BMJ 2012;345:e6231.

55. Foy A, O'Connell D, Henry D, et al. Benzodiazepine use as a cause of cognitive impairment in elderly hospital inpatients. J Gerontol Med Sci 1995;50A:M99–M106.

56. Tata PR, Rollings J, Collins M, et al. Lack of cognitive recovery following withdrawal from long-term benzodiazepine use. Psychol Med 1994;24:203–13.

57. Billoti de Gage S, Moride Y, Ducruet T, et al. Benzodiazepine use and risk of Alzheimer's disease: case-control study. BMJ 2014;349:g5205.

58. Salzman C, Fisher J, Nobel K, et al. Cognitive improvement following benzodiazepine discontinuation in elderly nursing home residents. Int J Gen Psychiatry 1992;7:89–93.

59. Larson EB, Kukull WA, Buchner D, Reifler BV. Adverse drug reactions associated with global cognitive impairment in elderly persons. Ann Intern Med 1987;107:169–73.

60. Lader MH, Ron M, Petursson H. Computed axial brain tomography in long-term benzodiazepine users. Psychol Med 1984;14:203–6.

61. Moodley P, Golombok S, Shrine PH, Lader M. Computed axial brain tomograms in long-term benzodiazepine users. Psychiatr Res 1993;48:135–44.

62. Perera KMH, Powell T, Jenner FA. Computerized axial tomographic studies following long-term use of benzodiazepines. Psychol Med 1987;17:775–7.

63. Poser W, Poser S, Roscher D, Argyrakis A. Do benzodiazepines cause cerebral atrophy? Lancet 1983;8326:715.

64. Oster G, Huse DM, Adams SF, et al. Benzodiazepine tranquilizers and the risk of accidental injury. Am J Pub Health 1990;12:1467–70.

In this study, 4,554 persons who had been prescribed a benzodiazepine were compared with 13,662 who had been prescribed a drug other than a benzodiazepine. Accident-related care was two-fold more likely for those who had been prescribed benzodiazepines, with the probability of an accident-related medical encounter higher during months in which a prescription for a benzodiazepine had recently been filled. Those who had filled three or more prescriptions for a benzodiazepine in the 6 months following initiation of therapy had a significantly higher risk of an accident-related medical event than those who had filled only one prescription.

65. Lichtenstein MJ, Griffin MR, Cornell JE, et al. Risk factors for hip fractures occurring in the hospital. Am J Epidemiol 1994;140:830–8.

66. Myers AH, Baker SP, Van Natta ML, et al. Risk factors associated with falls and injuries among elderly institutionalized persons. Am J Epidemiol 1991;133:1179–90.

67. Khong TP, de Vries F, Goldenberg JS, et al. Potential impact of benzodiazepine use on the rate of hip fractures in five large European countries and the United States. Calcif Tissue Int 2012;91:24–31.

68. Sorock GS, Shimkin EE. Benzodiazepine sedatives and the risk of falling in a community-dwelling elderly cohort. Arch Intern Med 1988;148:2441–4.

69. Bartlett G, Abrahamowicz M, Grad R, et al. Association between risk factors for injurious fall and new benzodiazepine prescribing in elderly persons. BMC Fam Pract 2009;10:1.

70. **Wagner AK, Zhang F, Soumerai SB. Benzodiazepine use and hip fractures in the elderly. Arch Intern Med 2004;164:1567–72.** *This was an analysis of 125,203 New Jersey Medicaid health care claims over 42 months in which there were 2312 hip fractures. Hip fracture rate was significantly higher among patients with exposure to any benzodiazepine than among patients with no benzodiazepine exposure (incidence rate ratio [IRR] 1.24), for a short half-life, high-potency benzodiazepine (IRR, 1.27), during the first 2 weeks after starting a benzodiazepine (IRR, 2.05), during the second 2 weeks after starting a benzodiazepine (IRR, 1.88), and for continued use (IRR, 1.18).*

71. Cummings SR, Nevitt MC, Browner WS, et al. Risk factors for hip fracture in white women. N Engl J Med 1995;332:767–73.

72. Herings RMC, Stricker BH, de Boer A, et al. Benzodiazepines and the risk of falling leading to femur fractures. Dosage more important than elimination half-life. Arch Intern Med 1995;155:1801–7.

73. Ray WA, Griffin MR, Downey W. Benzodiazepines of long and short elimination half-life and the risk of hip fracture. JAMA 1989;262:3303-7.

74. Oster G, Huse DM, Adams SF, et al. Benzodiazepine tranquilizers and the risk of accidental injury. Am J Public Health 1990;80:1467-70.

75. Ray WA, Fought RL, Decker MD. Psychoactive drugs and the risk of injurious motor vehicle crashes in elderly drivers. Am J Epidemiol 1992;136:873-83.

76. Oude Voshaar RC, Gorgels WJ, Mol AJ, et al. Tapering off long-term benzodiazepine use with or without group cognitive-behavioural therapy: three-condition, randomized controlled trial. Br J Psychiatry 2003;182:498-504.

77. Sullivan JT, Sellers EM. Detoxification for triazolam physical dependence. J Clin Psychopharmacol 1992;12:124-7.

78. Schweizer E, Rickels K, Case WG, Greenblatt DJ. Long-term therapeutic use of benzodiazepines. II. Effects of gradual taper. Arch Gen Psychiatry 1990;47:908-15.

79. Busto UE, Sykora K, Sellers EM. A clinical scale to assess benzodiazepine withdrawal. J Clin Psychopharmacol 1989;9:412-6.

80. **Sharfstein-Kawasaki S, Jacapraro JS, Rastegar DA. Safety and effectiveness of a fixed-dose phenobarbital protocol for inpatient benzodiazepine detoxification. J Subst Abuse Treat 2012; 43:331-4.** *This study involved 310 inpatients treated with a 3-day fixed dose phenobarbital taper for benzodiazepine dependence. There were no seizures, falls, or delirium, and only three patients requiring readmission within 30 days for withdrawal symptoms.*

81. **Loder E, Biondi D. Oral phenobarbital loading: a safe and effective method of withdrawing patients with headache from butalbital compounds. Headache 2003;43:904-9.** *In this study, 19 patients who stopped butalbital (8–20 tablets/day) were treated with phenobarbital doses of 120 mg/hour until sedated (range of 8–13 doses). There were no adverse effects and all patients underwent successful withdrawal.*

82. Denizs C, Fatseas M, Lavie E, Auriacombe M. Pharmacological interventions for benzodiazepine mono-dependence management in outpatient settings. Cochrane Database Syst Rev 2006;19:CD005194.

83. Chesaux M, Monnat M, Zullino DF. Topiramate in benzodiazepine withdrawal. Hum Psychopharmacol 2003;18:375-7.

84. Mercier-Guyon C, Chabannes JP, Saviuc P. The role of captodiamine in the withdrawal from long-term benzodiazepine treatment. Curr Med Res Opin 2004;9:1347–55.

85. Cantopher T, Olivieri S, Cleave N, Edwards JG. Chronic benzo-diazepine dependence—a comparative study of abrupt withdrawal under propranolol cover versus gradual withdrawal. Br J Psychiatry 1990;156:406–11.

86. Croissant B, Grosshans M, Diehl A, Mann K. Oxcarbazepine in rapid benzodiazepine detoxification. Am J Drug Alcohol Abuse 2008;34:534–50.

87. Romach MK, Kaplan HL, Busto UE, et al. A controlled trial of ondansetron, a 5-HT3 anagonist, in benxodiazepine discontinuation. J Clin Psychopharmacol 1998;18:121–31.

88. Zitman FG, Couvee JE. Chronic benzodiazepine use in general prac-tice patients with depression: an evaluation of controlled treatment and taper-off. Report on behalf of the Dutch chronic benzodiazepine working group. Br J Psychiatry 2001;178:317–24.

89. Vorma H, Naukkarinen H, Sarna S, Kuoppasalmi K. Treatment of outpatients with complicated benzodiazepine dependence: comparison of two approaches. Addiction 2002;97:851–9.

90. Voshaar RC, Gorgels WJ, Mol AJ, et al. Tapering off long-term benzodiazepine use with or without group cognitive behav-ioural therapy: three-condition, randomised trial. Br J Psychiatry 2003;182:498–504.

91. Rappa LR, Larose-Pierre M, Payne DR, et al. Detoxification from high-dose zolpidem using diazepam. Ann Pharmacother 2004;38:590–4.

92. Gould RL, Coulson MC, Patel N, et al. Interventions for reducing benzodiazepine use in older people: meta-analysis of randomised con-trolled trials. Br J Psychiatry 2014;204:98–107.

93. Vorma H, Naukkarinen H, Sarna S, Kuoppasalmi K. Symptom severity and quality of life after benzodiazepine withdrawal treat-ment in participants with complicated dependence. Addict Behav 2004;29:1059–65.

94. Lugoboni F, Mirijello A, Faccini M, et al. Quality of life in a cohort of high-dose benzodiazepine dependent patients. Drug Alcohol Depend 2014;142:105–9.

95. Ashton H. Benzodiazepine withdrawal: outcome in 50 patients. Br J Addict 1987;82:665–71.

96. Allgulander C, Borg S, Vikander B. A 4–6-year follow-up of 50 patients with primary dependence on sedative and hypnotic drugs. Am J Psychiatry 1984;141:1580–2.

97. Rickels K, Case WG, Schweizer E, et al. Long-term benzodiazepine users 3 years after participation in a discontinuation program. Am J Psychiatry 1991;148:757–61.

6

Opioids

Background

Opioids have been used for centuries for their analgesic effect and for the control of dysenteries, as well as for their pleasurable effects. Opium, which is produced from the juice of the opium poppy, is the original opioid. *Opioids* are the family of compounds related to opium, while *opiates* are those found in opium: morphine, thebaine, and codeine. Morphine, the main active ingredient of opium, was first purified in 1805. Diacetylmorphine was later synthesized from morphine in 1874 and was initially marketed by Bayer, under the brand name "Heroin." A number of opioids are derived from thebaine, including oxycodone, hydrocodone, and hydromorphone. Methadone is a synthetic opioid developed in Germany in 1937 as an analgesic, and has subsequently found use as a treatment for opioid dependence. Buprenorphine is a partial opioid agonist and antagonist derived from thebaine, which was developed in the 1970s as a safer analgesic. But it is increasingly used for treatment of opioid dependence because of its partial agonist properties.

Epidemiology

According to the 2013 National Survey on Drug Use and Health (NSDUH),[1] approximately 4.8 million Americans reported using heroin at some time in their lives (1.8% of those aged 12 or older); 681,000 (0.3%) had used heroin in the past year and 289,000 (0.1%) in the past month. The number of past-year heroin users increased from 373,000 in 2007 to 681,000 in 2013. The nonmedical use of prescription opioids rose steadily during the 1990s but gradually declined afterward. An estimated 628,000 Americans used these agents for the first time in 1990; this figure rose to 2.4 million in 2001 and fell to 1.5 million in 2013. Nevertheless, such use remains a significant problem: in 2013, 35.5 million (14%) people reported lifetime nonmedical use of prescription pain relievers (primarily opioids); 11.1 million (4.2%) had used them in the past year and 4.5 million (1.7%) in the past month.

With increased attention on the problems associated with prescription opioids, the trend of increasing prescribing and misuse of prescription opioids from the early 1990s to 2010 appears to have abated, and the rates have plateaued or decreased between 2011 and 2013.[2] However, with the decline in prescription opioid misuse, there has been an increase in heroin use as prescription opioid users are transitioning to heroin. With this transition, there has been a shift in the demographics of heroin users from primarily urban non-white men to white men and women living outside of large urban areas, most of whom were introduced to opioids through prescription drugs.[3]

Opioid use disorder is an important medical problem. According to the 2013 NSDUH, the number of Americans with heroin dependence or abuse was estimated to be 517,000—this is more than twice the number in 2002 (214,000). The number of Americans with prescription pain reliever abuse or dependence was estimated to be 1.9 million. In 2011, it was estimated that over 250,000 emergency department visits in the United States were related to heroin use; for prescription opioids, the number was 488,000.[4]

Drug Effects

Opioids exert their effect by mimicking the effect of endorphins (endogenous opioid peptides). They bind to three distinct opioid receptors: mu (μ), delta (δ), and kappa (κ) receptors.[5] Stimulation of all three receptors is thought to have an analgesic effect. Stimulation of the mu receptor is also associated with euphoria, respiratory depression, suppression of cough, decreased gastrointestinal motility, and miosis. It is also thought to be the receptor that is most responsible for the rewarding effects of opioids. Kappa receptors are also associated with sedation, dysphoria, and miosis. Experienced users develop tolerance to the sedative effects and respiratory depression, but not to the constipating and miotic effects of opioids.

Acute Effects

Users of opioids administer them through a variety of routes: oral, intranasal, smoking, and by intravenous, intramuscular, or subcutaneous injection. For heroin users, the drug peaks in the serum within a minute of intravenous use, 3–5 minutes of intranasal or intramuscular use, and 5–10 minutes of subcutaneous use. Drug users prefer heroin (over morphine) because its greater lipid solubility allows for better penetration of the blood-brain barrier. Users experience euphoria, sedation, analgesia, and a sense of well-being.

A list of selected opioid analgesics and their relative potency is provided in Table 6.1. It should be noted that the relative doses are rough estimates of comparative potency and are generally derived from studies of single-dose efficacy for treatment of acute pain. Comparative dosing may be quite different for patients who are on chronic opioid treatment; this is particularly important when considering conversion to (or from) methadone. While a single dose of methadone has roughly equivalent efficacy (1:1 dose ratio) to that of morphine in reducing acute pain, for patients on chronic opioids, the morphine-to-methadone ratio may be closer to 10:1, and even as high as 20:1 among those receiving high doses of morphine (over 1,000 mg/day).[6] This issue is further complicated by high rates of variability between patients and potential drug interactions (see Chapter 14).

Acute Toxicity and Overdose

The typical presentation of opioid overdose is the triad of depressed level of consciousness, decreased respiration, and miotic (constricted) pupils. The DSM-5 criteria for opioid intoxication requires the presence of "clinically significant problematic behavioral or psychological changes" along with pupillary constriction (or dilation due to anoxia from severe overdose), and one (or more) of the following signs or symptoms: (1) drowsiness or coma, (2) slurred speech, and (3) impairment of attention or memory.[7] The ICD-10 code for opioid intoxication depends on whether there is a perceptual disturbance

TABLE 6.1 Characteristics and Dosing of Selected Opioid Analgesics

Generic Name	Trade Names*	Equianalgesic Parenteral Dose[†]	Equianalgesic Oral Dose[†]	Starting Oral Dose[‡]
Morphine	MSIR, Avinza[1], Kadian[1], MSContin[1], OramorphSR[1]	10 mg	30 mg	15–30 mg q 3–4 h
Buprenorphine	Bunavail[2], Buprenex, Butrans, Suboxone[2], Zubsolv[2]	0.4 mg	4 mg (sublingual)	2–4 mg (sublingual)
Butorphanol	Stadol	2 mg	—	—
Codeine	Tylenol #3*, Tylenol#4*	75 mg	200 mg	30–60 mg q 3–4 h
Diacetylmorphine	Heroin	6 mg	30 mg	—
Dihydrocodeine	PanlorDC*, PanlorSS*, SynalgosDC*	—	160 mg	16–32 mg q 4h
Fentanyl	Duragesic, Sublimaze, Ionsys, Actiq, Fentora, Onsolis	0.1 mg (100 mcg)	100 mcg (buccal)	100 mcg (buccal)

(continued)

TABLE 6.1 (Continued)

Generic Name	Trade Names*	Equianalgesic Parenteral Dose[†]	Equianalgesic Oral Dose[†]	Starting Oral Dose[‡]
Hydrocodone	Anexia*, Lortab*, Lorcet*, Maxidone*, Norco*, Vicodin*, Zydone*, Vicoprofen*, Reprexain* Zohydro[1]	—	30 mg	5–10 mg q 3–4 h
Hydromorphone	Dilaudid, Exalgo[1]	1.5 mg	7.5 mg	4–6 mg q 3–4 h
Levorphanol	Levo-Dromoran	2 mg	4 mg	4 mg q 6–8 h
Meperidine	Demerol	75 mg	300 mg	50–100 mg q 3–4 h
Methadone	Dolophine, Methadose	10 mg	20 mg (acute) 10 mg (chronic)[3]	10–20 mg q 6–8 h

Oxycodone	OxyIR, Oxyfast, Endocet*, Percocet*, Roxicet*, Tylox*, Percodan*, Combunox*, Oxycontin[1], Xartemis XR*[1], Targiniq ER[1,2]	—	20 mg	5–10 mg q 3–4 h
Oxymorphone	Numorphan, Opana, Opana ER[1]	1 mg	10 mg	5–10 mg q 4–6 h
Pentazocine	Talwin, Talwin NX[2], Talacen*	60 mg	50 mg	50 mg q 4–6 h
Tapentadol	Nucynta	—	100 mg	50–100 mg q 4–6 h
Tramadol	Ultram, Ultracet*	—	100 mg	50–100 mg q 4–6 h

*Combinations with acetaminophen, aspirin, or ibuprofen.

†Doses approximately equivalent to 10 mg of parenteral morphine.

‡For adults ≥50 kg; frequency is for non-sustained-release formulations.

[1]Sustained-release formulations.

[2]Combined with naloxone.

[3]The conversion ratio of morphine and methadone varies by dose; see text for more information.

or a comorbid use disorder, as well as the severity of the disorder. Death does not generally occur immediately after use; most individuals are thought to expire hours after their overdose.

Overdose is a common and serious complication of opioid use. In one study of injection heroin users in San Francisco, 48% had reported having at least one overdose and 33% reported having two or more in the past.[8] In an Australian cohort of heroin users, 68% had experienced at least one overdose, and 24% reported five or more lifetime overdoses. Those who had overdosed recently were more likely to have used benzodiazepines, opioids other than heroin, and stimulants.[9] In a cohort of 1,075 opioid-dependent individuals seeking treatment in the UK in the mid-1990s who were followed for 4 years, 68% of the deaths were due to overdose, and the risk of overdose was increased with the concurrent use of other substances, especially alcohol, benzodiazepines, and amphetamines.[10] In recent years in the United States, the majority of opioid overdose deaths have been due to prescription opioids: in 2008, there were 36,450 fatal overdoses; in 20,044, one or more prescription drugs were involved and prescription opioids were involved in 14,800 (74%) of these.[11]

The risk of overdose is also heightened by recent abstinence,[12] such as occurs after detoxification[13,14] or release from prison,[15] because tolerance is reduced. Overdose deaths may also occur after sudden changes in the purity of heroin sold on the market or the addition of more potent opioids, such as fentanyl.[16] The risk factors for prescription opioid overdose include mental health problems, high prescribed dosage, concurrent use of benzodiazepines, and receiving medication from multiple prescribers;[17] this topic is covered further in Chapter 13.

The standard treatment for opioid overdose is naloxone, which can be given intravenously (usually 0.4 mg) or subcutaneously (0.8 mg); both appear to be equally effective.[18] A higher dose (1–2 mg) can be tried if the initial dose is not effective. Higher doses may be required to treat overdoses with propoxyphene, pentazocine, and buprenorphine. Intranasal or intramuscular administration of naloxone is also effective, though generally given at higher doses (1–2 mg).[19] Naloxone can also be given via endotracheal tube in an intubated patient. Naloxone is not effective orally, since it is highly metabolized by the liver when given by this route. Animal studies[20] and case reports[21] suggest that the partial agonist buprenorphine can also reverse the effects of a full-agonist overdose.

Naloxone is relatively short-acting (45–90 minutes); therefore, it is possible that the overdose victim may have recurrent toxicity and require further treatment, even after a satisfactory initial response. For this reason, it is standard practice to take overdose victims to a hospital after resuscitation in the field; 2–3 hours of observation after an overdose is usually sufficient.[22]

There are a number of clinical signs that may help in identifying overdose victims who can be discharged an hour after receiving naloxone. In one study of 573 presumed opioid overdose victims, the presence of the following six clinical factors was used to identify those who could be safely discharged an hour after naloxone: (1) patient can mobilize as usual, (2) room air O_2 saturation >92%, (3) respiratory rate between 10 and 20 breaths/minute, (4) temperature between 35.0 and 37.5°C, (5) heart rate between 50 and 100 beats/minute, and (6) Glasgow coma scale of 15.[23] Among heroin users who refuse transport to the hospital, the risk of recurrent toxicity appears to be fairly low,[24,25] but this may not be the case for those who overdose on long-acting opioids.[26] Overdose may also be complicated by noncardiogenic pulmonary edema; this is generally clinically apparent within 2 hours after an overdose and should be considered in anyone with a cough or hypoxia after overdose. Overdose victims may also develop rhabdomyolysis or compartment syndrome.

Addiction treatment is probably the most effective way to prevent overdose deaths. Several studies have found that methadone maintenance treatment is associated with a lower risk of overdose.[27] Furthermore, the introduction of buprenorphine for treatment of opioid addiction has been associated with a reduction in overdose deaths.[28,29] The establishment of supervised injecting facilities has also been associated with a reduction in overdose deaths.[30]

Distribution of naloxone with overdose education has been shown to reduce overdose fatalities.[31] Naloxone has been distributed in kits that include a syringe with naloxone and a nasal adaptor. A device that administers naloxone by means of a hand-held auto-injector has been approved by the U.S. Food and Drug Administration (FDA) and is marketed under the brand name Evzio.

Withdrawal

The opioid withdrawal syndrome typically begins within 12 hours of discontinuation of regular use of short-acting opioids, such as heroin; this may be delayed in users of longer-acting preparations, such as methadone. The DSM-5 diagnostic criteria for opioid withdrawal require the presence of three (or more) of the following signs or symptoms in the setting of cessation or reduction in opioid use: (1) dysphoric mood, (2) nausea and vomiting, (3) muscle aches, (4) lacrimation or rhinorrhea, (5) pupillary dilation, piloerection, or sweating, (6) diarrhea, (7) yawning, (8) fever, and (9) insomnia.[7] The ICD-10 code for opioid withdrawal is F11.23. The symptoms can be very unpleasant but are generally not life-threatening. However, patients who have coexisting medical conditions may experience serious complications. Withdrawal symptoms generally resolve within a week of abstinence but may be prolonged to 2 weeks or more in patients withdrawing from longer-acting opioids. Table 6.2 provides the 11-item Clinical Opiate Withdrawal Scale (COWS), which can be used to assess the severity of withdrawal and response to treatment.

Assessment

The DSM-5 diagnostic criteria for opioid use disorders are the same as other substances; see Chapter 1 for details.[7] The ICD-10 code for a mild disorder is F11.10, and F11.20 for moderate-severe. Anyone who uses opioids on a regular basis for an extended period of time will develop physical dependence; that is, they will develop

TABLE 6.2 Clinical Opiate Withdrawal Scale (COWS)

Resting pulse rate *after resting for 1 minute*
0 <80 beats/minute
1 81–100 bpm
2 101–120 bpm
4 >120 bpm

Sweating *over past ½ hour, not accounted for by room temperature or patient activity*
0 no report of chills or flushing
1 subjective report of chills or flushing
2 flushed or observable moistness on face
3 beads of sweat on brow or face
4 sweat streaming off face

Restlessness *observation during assessment*
0 able to sit still
1 patient reports difficulty sitting still, but able to do so
3 frequent shifting or extraneous movements of legs or arms
5 unable to sit still for more than a few seconds

GI upset *over last ½ hour*
0 no GI symptoms
1 stomach cramps
2 nausea or loose stool
3 vomiting or diarrhea
5 multiple episodes of diarrhea or vomiting

Tremor *observation of outstretched hands*
0 no tremor
1 tremor can be felt, but not observed
2 slight tremor observable
4 gross tremor or muscle twitching

Yawning *observation during assessment*
0 no yawning
1 yawning once or twice during assessment
2 yawning three or more times during assessment
4 yawning several times/minute

(continued)

TABLE 6.2 (Continued)

Pupil size
0 pupils pinned or normal in size for room light
1 pupils possibly larger than normal for room light
2 pupils moderately dilated
4 pupils are so dilated that only rim of iris is visible

Bone or joint aches *if patient was having pain previously, only additional component attributable to opiate withdrawal*
0 not present
1 mild diffuse discomfort
2 patient reports severe diffuse aching of joints or muscles
4 patient rubbing joints or muscles and is unable to sit still because of discomfort

Runny nose or tearing *not accounted for by cold symptoms or allergies*
0 not present
1 nasal stuffiness or unusually moist eyes
2 nose rubbing or tearing
4 nose constantly running or tears streaming down cheeks

Anxiety or irritability
0 none
1 patient reports increasing irritability or anxiousness
2 patient is obviously irritable or anxious
4 patient is so irritable or anxious that participation in assessment is difficult

Gooseflesh skin
0 skin is smooth
3 piloerection of skin can be felt or hairs standing up on arms
5 prominent piloerection

Total Score _____
5–12 mild
13–24 moderate
25–36 moderately severe
>36 severe withdrawal

Adapted from Wesson DR, Ling W. The Clinical Opiate Withdrawal Scale (COWS). J Psychoactive Drugs 2003;35:253-9.

tolerance to the drug effects and withdrawal symptoms if the substance is abruptly discontinued. This is also true for patients who take prescribed opioids for chronic pain. It may be difficult for these patients to distinguish physical dependence from addiction (meaning a pattern of use that is harmful rather than therapeutic). While tolerance and withdrawal are 2 of the 11 DSM-5 criteria for a substance use disorder, the DSM-5 specifies that these are not sufficient to make a diagnosis of a substance use disorder for individuals who are prescribed opioids and that they must meet at least one other criterion. This topic is covered further in Chapter 13.

Physical Exam

A number of findings on examination should raise the consideration of opioid dependence, including constricted pupils, drowsiness, or frequent "nodding." Patients may exhibit signs of withdrawal from opioids (covered earlier in this section). Intranasal users may have nasal septal erosion or perforation (especially those who use cocaine as well). Injection drug users often have needle marks or track marks in the antecubital fossae or forearms; however, some inject in other locations, including veins in the neck, legs, groin, or axilla, or subcutaneously into the upper arm, thigh, or buttock.

Laboratory Testing

Opioid use may be detected through urine drug testing, though its utility as screening test in unselected populations is limited. It is important to be aware of the test's performance characteristics. Many standard urine immunoassays for drugs of abuse will detect opioids that are structurally similar to morphine (such as codeine or heroin), but not other opioids (such as oxycodone, methadone, meperidine, or buprenorphine). There are specific assays for methadone, oxycodone, and buprenorphine; these are useful for monitoring individuals on methadone or buprenorphine maintenance and those prescribed oxycodone for pain. It is also important to keep in mind that the main metabolite of heroin is morphine and that standard immunoassays for opiates will not differentiate between those who are using heroin and those using prescription opiates. Detection of 6-acetyl-morphine (6-AM), which is a heroin-specific metabolite, can be used to differentiate between heroin and other opiates.[32] Urine drug testing is covered further in Chapter 2.

In addition, since many injection drug users are infected with hepatitis C,[33] the presence of antibodies to this virus or an elevated serum alanine immunotransferase (ALT) may also be clues to a history of injection drug use.

Medical Complications

As discussed earlier, the most serious complication of opioid use is overdose. In a cohort of U.S. adults surveyed in 1991, heroin was the only illicit drug associated with increased 15-year mortality.[34] Other than overdose, opioids are associated with relatively few medical complications, even with long-term use. Most of the medical complications that users acquire are due to the use of needles to administer the drug; complications of injection drug use are reviewed further in Chapter 14.

Pulmonary Complications

Pulmonary complications with opioid use are not common. Although respiratory depression can be an acute effect of opioid use, most chronic users develop tolerance to this side effect. However, opioid users have been noted to sometimes develop acute noncardiogenic pulmonary edema, generally in the setting of overdose. In one series of 1,278 heroin overdoses treated at one hospital, 27 (2.1%) developed pulmonary edema and 9 required mechanical ventilation; most recovered within 24 hours.[35] Finally, inhalation of heroin may trigger an attack in asthmatic patients,[36] and there is a case report of hypersensitivity pneumonitis associated with intranasal heroin use.[37]

Cardiovascular Complications

The synthetic opioids methadone and levacetylmethadol (LAAM) are associated with a dose-dependent prolongation of the QT interval.[38] This has been attributed to blockade of the cardiac potassium ion channel, resulting in prolongation of cardiac repolarization, and may lead to syncope and sudden cardiac death. Of note, buprenorphine, another opioid used for addiction treatment, does not appear to cause QT prolongation.[39] This topic is covered further in Chapter 14, in the section "Care of Patients on Opioid Agonist Treatment."

Gastrointestinal Complications

Opioids slow gastrointestinal transit; one of their first therapeutic uses was to treat diarrheal illnesses. Constipation is a common problem for chronic opioid users. Use of bulking (e.g., fiber) and osmotic agents (e.g., polyethylene glycol) generally helps alleviate this. Methylnaltrexone, a mu-opioid receptor antagonist that is given subcutaneously and has restricted ability to cross the blood-brain barrier, has been shown to be effective at relieving constipation for patients on methadone maintenance[40] and for patients with advanced illness on chronic opioids[41] without causing opioid withdrawal. Two oral peripherally acting mu-opioid receptor antagonists, alvimopan (brand name Entereg)[42] and naloxegol (brand name Movantik),[43] have also been shown to be effective for opioid-associated constipation without antagonizing central opioid effects and analgesia.

Renal Complications

Opioids seem to have little, if any, deleterious effect on the kidneys.[44] However, in the 1970s and 80s, an association was observed between injection heroin use and nephrotic syndrome, sometimes leading to end-stage renal disease; this was referred to as "heroin nephropathy." These patients were generally African-American men, and pathological evaluation revealed sclerosing glomerulo-nephritis.[45] The etiology of this condition has never been clearly established and may have been due to impurities or adulterants; unrecognized hepatitis C or HIV infection may also played a role.[46] It appears that heroin nephropathy has declined (or disappeared) since then.[47] In a postmortem study of 129 illicit drug users in Germany, heroin use was not associated with histopathological alterations in the kidney.[48]

Endocrine Complications

Experimental and clinical studies have shown that opioids can produce hypogonadotropic hypogonadism; in practice, this is generally seen in individuals on methadone maintenance or high doses of opioids for chronic pain. This topic is covered further in Chapter 14, in the section "Care of Patients on Opioid Agonist Treatment." There is also an association between tramadol and hypoglycemia.[49]

Neuromuscular Complications

Patients receiving meperidine (Demerol), especially those with renal failure, are at risk for neurotoxicity due to accumulation of the drug and its active metabolite, normeperidine.[50] Symptoms include agitation, tremor, myoclonus, and seizures.[51] Use of tramadol, an analgesic with opioid agonist activity, has also been associated with seizures.[52]

Treatment

Screening and counseling outpatients who use heroin appears to be modestly effective at reducing subsequent drug use.[53] Beyond simple counseling, the treatment options for an opioid-dependent individual can be roughly categorized as (1) medically supervised withdrawal (detoxification), which is generally followed by psychosocial treatment; (2) psychosocial treatment; and (3) medication-assisted treatment with the use of an opioid agonist (methadone or buprenorphine) or an opioid antagonist (naltrexone).

There are a number of agents that are effective at reducing the symptoms of withdrawal. However, most studies of detoxification focus on short-term outcomes (i.e., completion of detoxification), and there is less evidence supporting their long-term effectiveness. Aftercare in the form of self-help groups, outpatient treatment, or residential programs may help addicts maintain abstinence. Maintenance treatment with an opioid agonist appears to be most effective at reducing illicit opioid use.

Medically Supervised Withdrawal

Opioid withdrawal is unpleasant but not life-threatening. Medically supervised withdrawal, or detoxification, is a palliative procedure to minimize the symptoms and help individuals take the first step toward recovery and abstinence. Unfortunately, long-term abstinence after detoxification is the exception rather than the rule.[54,55] Most controlled trials of detoxification are limited by a focus on short-term outcomes (completion of detoxification) and the data on longer-term outcomes are primarily from observational studies. Nevertheless, some studies suggest a modest reduction in drug use in the months following detoxification.[56,57] However, studies consistently show maintenance treatment to be more effective than a supervised taper.[58,59]

Administration of any opioid will relieve the symptoms of withdrawal but will not necessarily help reduce dependence. A number of agents and protocols have been used to help ameliorate the symptoms of withdrawal and have been studied for use in detoxification. Withdrawal scales may be helpful to assess and monitor patients during detoxification, as discussed earlier in this chapter. Most research on detoxification has been done on heroin users; these procedures may not be as effective for those dependent on long-acting opioids such as methadone. We address this specific issue at the end of this section.

Treatment Setting

One of the first decisions that must be made is the optimal treatment setting. The ASAM has developed patient placement criteria to help guide this decision;[60] an overview of placement criteria is provided in Chapter 3. Often, this decision is limited by availability, health insurance, and other practical considerations. Many opioid-dependent individuals can be safely withdrawn from the drug in an ambulatory setting, and this process can be coordinated in a primary care office. Other options include intensive outpatient treatment, residential treatment, and inpatient hospitalization. Indications for treatment at a more intensive level of care include concurrent dependence on other substances (particularly alcohol or benzodiazepines), previous unsuccessful attempts at detoxification, unstable social situation, or a concurrent medical or psychiatric condition that requires more intensive care. There is some evidence that those who receive inpatient treatment are more likely to complete detoxification[61] and some have argued that this makes it cost-effective;[62] however, evidence supporting the longer-term superiority of inpatient treatment is lacking.[63]

Agents Used for Treatment of Opioid Withdrawal

Buprenorphine

Buprenorphine is a long-acting partial opioid agonist, which was first proposed as a treatment for opioid dependence in 1978[64] and is currently the only FDA-approved medication for the treatment of opioid dependence that is accessible to office-based physicians. The partial opioid-agonist properties give buprenorphine some advantages over other opioids: it has a ceiling effect[65] and a lower risk of overdose than other opioids. Furthermore, cessation of buprenorphine is associated with fewer withdrawal symptoms than cessation from full agonists.[66] A number of studies have shown it to be effective for treating withdrawal symptoms.[67] A 2009 Cochrane review concluded that "buprenorphine is more effective than clonidine" and "may offer some advantages over methadone, at least in inpatient settings, in terms of quicker resolution of withdrawal symptoms and possibly slightly higher rates of completion of withdrawal."[68] Studies have also demonstrated the feasibility and effectiveness of using buprenorphine in primary care settings.[69] The U.S. Substance Abuse and Mental Health Service Administration (SAHMSA) has issued treatment guidelines for use of buprenorphine for detoxification and maintenance treatment; these can obtained via the Internet (www.samhsa.gov).[70]

The optimal buprenorphine regimen for treatment of withdrawal has not been established. A symptom-triggered dose-titration study of buprenorphine for heroin withdrawal found that the median dose was 4 mg on day 1, 6 mg on day 2, 4 mg on day 3, and 2 mg on day 4; most individuals (72%) required no further medication on the fifth day.[71] A small study comparing a 5-day low-dose buprenorphine regimen (2-4-8-4-2 mg/day) with a high-dose regimen (8-8-8-4-2 mg/day) found that the high-dose regimen was more effective at relieving withdrawal symptoms without any reported adverse effects.[72] For our inpatient 3-day withdrawal protocol, we have used 4 mg on admission and 4 mg at night on day 1 (8 mg total), 4 mg in morning and 4 mg at night on day 2 (8 mg total), 4 mg in morning and 2 mg at night on day 3 (6 mg total), and a 2 mg dose on the morning of discharge. This has been effective for most patients,[73] although some require an additional 2 mg after the initial 4 mg dose on admission.

In the outpatient setting, patients can be titrated up to a target dose of 12 to 16 mg/day over 2–3 days and then gradually tapered over 1–4 weeks (or longer). The higher initial doses with the extended detoxification are closer to usual maintenance doses of buprenorphine (discussed later in this chapter). While the optimal tapering schedule has not been determined, a study comparing a 7-day taper with a 28-day taper for subjects who had initially received 4 weeks of buprenorphine found no significant differences in withdrawal, craving, or abstinence from other drugs.[74] It should be pointed out that even with extended tapering schedules, most individuals are not able to maintain abstinence.[75] Table 6.3 gives suggested protocols for 3- to 10-day inpatient treatment of withdrawal using buprenorphine in the sublingual formulation.

TABLE 6.3 Inpatient Protocols for Opioid Detoxification with Buprenorphine: Suggested Doses (mg of Sublingual Buprenorphine)

Day	10-Day (Fixed Dose)	7-Day (Fixed Dose)	3-Day (Fixed Dose)	5-Day (Flexible Dose)
1	8 mg	8 mg	12 mg	4 mg at onset of withdrawal, additional 2–4 mg as needed
2	6 mg	8 mg	8 mg	4 mg morning, 2–4 mg evening dose as needed
3	4 mg	4 mg	8 mg	4 mg morning, 2 mg evening dose as needed
4	4 mg	4 mg		2 mg morning, 2 mg evening dose as needed
5	4 mg	2 mg		2 mg as needed
6	2 mg	2 mg		
7	2 mg	0 mg		
8	2 mg			
9	2 mg			
10	0 mg			

Adapted from Johnson RE, et al. Drug Alcohol Depend 2003;70:S59–S77, and Lintzeris N, et al. Drug Alcohol Depend 2003;70:287–94.

There have been no studies that compare fixed-dose opioid withdrawal regimens with symptom-triggered dosing. Fixed-dose protocols (with "rescue dosing" as needed) are simpler and minimize negotiations (or haggling) over dosing. Furthermore, it may be better to treat in anticipation of withdrawal symptoms, rather than wait for symptoms to appear.

Both inpatient and outpatient protocols can be supplemented with symptomatic medication (analgesics, antiemetics, antidiarrheal agents). Providing other treatment modalities, such as behavioral therapy, may offer additional benefits.[76]

Methadone

Methadone has been used for decades for treatment of opioid addiction, both for treatment of withdrawal and as a maintenance treatment. A variety of protocols have been utilized with different doses of methadone and lengths of treatment. The starting dose is typically 20–30 mg/day, and duration of treatment varies from a week to a month (or longer). One study comparing a 10-day with 21-day inpatient methadone taper reported higher and earlier peak withdrawal symptoms with the 10-day protocol; however, completion rates were similar.[77] A 2013 Cochrane review of methadone taper for opioid withdrawal reported that "programs vary widely with regard to the assessment of outcomes measures, impairing the application of meta-analysis." Nevertheless, they concluded that "slow tapering with temporary substitution of long-acting opioids can reduce withdrawal severity."[78] As a practical consideration, in the United States, the use of methadone (and other opioids) for addiction treatment on an outpatient basis is limited to licensed treatment programs, so it cannot be used for office-based treatment in other settings.

Clonidine

Clonidine is a centrally acting alpha 2-adrenergic receptor agonist that was originally developed for treatment of hypertension. In 1978, it was first reported that this drug also helped reduce the symptoms of opioid withdrawal.[79] Clonidine seems to be associated with fewer withdrawal symptoms in the later phases of detoxification than methadone,[80] but long-term outcomes (i.e., abstinence from opioids on follow-up) are no better.[81] A 2014 Cochrane review of the use of alpha 2-adrenergic agonists for opioid withdrawal detected no significant difference in efficacy between these agents and the traditional methadone taper.[82] Some treatment programs use a combination of methadone or buprenorphine taper with clonidine.

For opioid detoxification using clonidine, patients are typically given 0.1 to 0.2 mg every 4–6 hours tapered over 5–12 days, with a maximal daily dosage of 1.0 mg/day. Often, treatment programs supplement this with analgesics, antiemetics, and antidiarrheal/antispasmodic medications to further ameliorate the symptoms of withdrawal.

Side effects of clonidine include dry mouth, sedation, and orthostatic hypotension. Abrupt withdrawal of the medication may be complicated by rebound hyperadrenergic symptoms, including hypertension, sweating, agitation, flushing, and headache.[83] Clonidine is frequently misused by opioid-dependent individuals to potentiate opioid effects.[84] There have even been reports of clonidine abuse in the absence of concurrent opioid use.[85] Use of the transdermal clonidine patch may be less subject to misuse, but we have observed overdoses among opioid-dependent individuals after deliberately chewing these patches.[86]

Tramadol
Tramadol is a centrally acting synthetic analgesic with opioid activity. A pharmacological study found that doses of 200 or 400 mg were modestly effective at suppressing opioid withdrawal symptoms; lower doses (50 and 100 mg) were no more effective than placebo.[87] However, a clinical trial found that buprenorphine is more effective at treating opioid withdrawal symptoms and there is a substantial risk of seizures with tramadol.[88]

Special Considerations

Rapid and Ultra-Rapid Detoxification
The withdrawal process can be accelerated by the addition of an opioid antagonist such as naloxone or naltrexone; some have postulated that combining these with a medication that ameliorates withdrawal symptoms (such as clonidine) may improve success rates

("rapid detoxification"). However, a randomized controlled trial of this approach found no better treatment retention, though more patients were "successfully detoxified."[89] The addition of naltrexone to buprenorphine can also help shorten the duration of withdrawal, although it increases the intensity of these symptoms.[90]

Some have tried speeding the process further by heavily sedating or anesthetizing patients while administering an opioid antagonist—this practice is sometimes referred to as "ultra-rapid detoxification" or "anesthesia-assisted rapid opioid detoxification (AAROD)." While there have been reports of favorable success rates and safety with this strategy,[91,92] a randomized controlled trial found no benefit with its use and reinforced concerns about its safety.[93] Moreover, a 2012 investigation of a New York City clinic found that of 75 patients treated with AAROD, 7 required hospitalization within 72 hours and 2 of them died.[94] A 2010 Cochrane systematic review concluded that "this form of treatment should not be pursued."[95]

Withdrawal from Long-Acting Opioids

As noted earlier in this section, research on treatment of withdrawal has generally been done on heroin users and less is known about the optimal strategy for users of long-acting opioids. One study of heroin and methadone users who were treated with a 10-day methadone taper found more severe withdrawal symptoms among the methadone users, but no significant difference in onset or duration of withdrawal.[96] In our experience, the withdrawal syndrome from long-acting opioids is generally delayed and prolonged compared with that of users of short-acting opioids. Therefore, treatment will generally need to start later after the last use and continue for a longer period of time. Furthermore, the partial-agonist properties of buprenorphine and its high affinity for opioid receptors may initially precipitate withdrawal symptoms in patients on high doses of long-acting opioids.

We have found that the shorter withdrawal protocols generally do not work as well with users of long-acting opioids and a better strategy may be to slowly taper the dose of the long-acting opioid rather than attempt withdrawal over a few days. If withdrawal is attempted, it is probably best to try to begin at 36 to 48 hours after the last dose (especially if using buprenorphine) and be prepared to extend treatment beyond what is generally needed (a few weeks of withdrawal symptoms is not unusual). The use of buprenorphine is not recommended for those using 60 mg or more of methadone/day (or its equivalent in other long-acting opioids). However, a study of subjects receiving 100 mg/day of methadone found that some experienced no withdrawal symptoms, and the remainder had less withdrawal when given lower, repeated doses of buprenorphine rather than a single, higher dose.[97] This finding suggests that a strategy of low, repeated doses of buprenorphine (e.g., 2 mg) may be safe and effective. Another option may be to switch to a short-acting opioid as a bridge to treatment with buprenorphine.

Psychosocial Treatment

There are a number of psychosocial treatment options; often these are employed after withdrawal from opioids in the form of aftercare. Withdrawal alone is rarely effective, and although there is a paucity of experimental data to support this, some observational studies suggest that aftercare is beneficial. In one study of opioid-dependent individuals who participated in a variety of drug treatments, those who received detoxification alone did not do as well as those in therapeutic communities or outpatient drug-free programs; in fact, they fared no better than those who received "intake-only" (i.e., no treatment).[98] Psychosocial treatment options include brief interventions, self-help groups such as Narcotics Anonymous (NA), outpatient counseling, or residential treatment.

Brief Interventions

The data on the effectiveness of brief interventions for opioid use are mixed. One trial of a single-session motivational intervention for cocaine or heroin use reported effectiveness,[99] while other trials of drug users (including opioids) have failed to show a benefit.[100,101] Brief interventions are discussed further in Chapter 2.

Self-Help Groups

Self-help groups are probably the most commonly used treatment modality. Many of these groups, such as Narcotics Anonymous (www.na.org), are based on the 12-step philosophy of Alcoholics Anonymous and offer meetings throughout North America. There is relatively little experimental data on their effectiveness: observational studies indicate that participation in these groups is associated with better outcomes,[102] and one randomized trial in a cohort who used a variety of substances, including heroin, reported that an intensive referral to self-help groups was somewhat more effective than a passive referral, particularly for those with less previous experience with these groups.[103]

Outpatient Counseling

Outpatient programs take on a variety of forms and use a wide range of strategies. There are some data to support the effectiveness of certain types of programs. One common approach is counseling combined with self-help groups. A randomized controlled trial of a weekly 3-hour recovery training and self-help group reported significant reduction in opioid use and improvements in employment and (self-reported) criminal activity after 1 year.[104]

Another approach is to offer incentives for drug abstinence ("contingency management"). This approach appears to lead to more drug abstinence while the incentives are offered, but this effect dissipates thereafter. One example is a study that reported modestly improved short-term (one month) outcomes with abstinent-contingent reinforcement in the form of access to financial assistance, in addition to individual counseling, as well as job and social skills training.[105] In a follow-up of this study, offering abstinent-contingent incentives for a longer period of time (3 months vs. 1 month) was associated with high abstinence rates among a select group of opioid-dependent subjects over that period of time.[106] A 2005 Cochrane systematic review of psychosocial treatments for opioid abuse and dependence concluded that these "are not adequately proved treatment modalities."[107]

Residential Treatment

Residential treatment programs differ widely in approach, setting, and length of treatment. Some halfway houses are little more than a place to stay, while other programs, such as "therapeutic communities," offer more intensive treatment. There are limited data on their effectiveness, mostly in the form of observational studies, which are limited by selection bias and incomplete follow-up of subjects. In one study, heroin addicts who participated in one of three therapeutic communities had better outcomes than those who did not, but this was limited by nonrandom assignment and the likelihood of selection bias.[108]

Another study that prospectively studied a select group of individuals with a variety of drug abuse problems and randomly assigned them to a day program or a residential program did report significantly better outcomes with residential treatment on some measures, but concluded that the outcomes were not significantly better overall.[109] With these limitations in mind, it is clear that some opioid-dependent individuals are able to maintain sobriety for extended periods of time in these programs, but they are in the minority.[110,111]

Medication-Assisted Treatment

There are currently three available pharmacotherapies for opioid use disorders: the full agonist methadone, the partial agonist buprenorphine, and the antagonist naltrexone. The evidence suggests that agonist treatments are the most effective ones. While some view agonist treatment as substituting one drug for another, the goal is to reduce the medical and societal harm associated with addiction by substituting illicit drug use with the supervised provision of another opioid. Some have also proposed harm reduction through the provision of heroin to those who fail other treatments.[112]

Methadone

Methadone has been used for decades as maintenance treatment for opioid dependence, and studies have shown that this reduces illicit opioid use[113] and is more effective than detoxification followed by psychosocial treatment.[114] Higher doses of methadone appear to be more effective,[115] and the incorporation of abstinence reinforcement (such as rewards for negative urine drug tests) appears to be effective as well.[116] A 2009 Cochrane review of methadone maintenance that included 11 studies with 1,969 participants concluded that it is effective in reducing illicit opioid abuse and retaining users in treatment.[117] Another review concluded that doses of 60–100 mg/day are more effective than lower doses.[118]

A detailed discussion of methadone treatment protocols and regulations is beyond the scope of this handbook. Guidelines have been developed by Center for Substance Abuse Treatment (CSAT) and are available as a treatment improvement protocol.[119] Patients are typically started at 20–30 mg daily and the dose is gradually titrated up to usual doses of 60–120 mg/day. Patients are initially given supervised doses daily but can earn "take-home" doses once they are stabilized.

Methadone programs typically provide varying levels of psychosocial services. There have been a number of studies of outcomes at different levels of services. The provision of methadone alone with limited services has been shown to reduce drug use[120,121] and to be more effective than detoxification.[122] "Standard" services, which include counseling and reinforcement, may lead to better outcomes over medication alone; the addition of onsite medical/psychiatric care and family and employment counseling ("enhanced" services) has been reported to be associated with further improvements, at least during the first 6 months of enrollment.[123] On the other hand, "standard" services appear to be most cost-effective[124] and a 2011 Cochrane systematic review concluded that the addition of psychosocial services to standard agonist maintenance treatments does not offer additional benefits.[125]

The effectiveness of methadone as a treatment for opioid dependence is limited by its restricted availability. Despite evidence that supports the use of this treatment in the primary care setting,[126] only licensed programs can dispense methadone for the treatment of opioid dependence in the United States (though physicians can prescribe it for treatment of chronic pain).

Buprenorphine

Buprenorphine is a long-acting partial opioid agonist with a high affinity for opioid receptors and has been shown to be effective for treating opioid withdrawal and as a maintenance treatment. Sublingual and buccal formulations have been approved for use as maintenance treatment in the United States and are accessible to physicians who undergo the necessary training and licensing. Studies show buprenorphine to be as effective as methadone when dispensed on a three-times-a-week basis by a treatment program;[127] it can also be dispensed twice weekly.[128] When given three times a week, a double dose (two times the daily dose) can be given on Monday and Wednesday, and a triple dose on Friday; for twice-weekly treatment, a quadruple dose can be given on Monday and triple on Friday.

Physicians who wish to prescribe buprenorphine are required to undergo 8 hours of training and obtain a special license from the Drug Enforcement Administration (DEA). Courses are regularly offered throughout the United States and the necessary training can be done on the Internet using Web-based training modules; information on both of these is available on the SAMHSA website (www.samhsa.gov). Current federal law limits each licensed physician to treating 30 individuals at a time during the first year; this can be increased to 100 afterwards.

Buprenorphine maintenance has been shown to be safe and effective when used in office-based settings,[129] including when it is integrated into primary care.[130] A 2014 Cochrane review concluded that buprenorphine is "an effective intervention for use in the maintenance treatment of heroin dependence."[131] As noted earlier, SAMHSA has issued treatment recommendations for the use of buprenorphine that can be obtained free of charge via the Internet (www.samhsa.gov).[70]

Buprenorphine has some advantages over methadone. It is less likely to cause overdose, even in individuals who have not built up tolerance to opioids. Withdrawal symptoms from buprenorphine are less severe than methadone. Moreover, when given in repeated doses over time, buprenorphine appears to have minimal effect on cognitive and psychomotor performance.[132] For pregnant women, buprenorphine has the advantage of causing less intense neonatal abstinence syndrome.[133] One disadvantage of buprenorphine is its higher cost; however, the prescription cost of buprenorphine is fairly comparable to that of a typical methadone program. Studies suggest that methadone is somewhat more effective than buprenorphine,[134] but office-based buprenorphine attracts many individuals who would not enter or do not have access to methadone programs.

Buprenorphine is available in the United States in a number of formulations. The one most commonly used is a sublingual formulation that is a combination of buprenorphine and naloxone in a 4:1 ratio; the naloxone is not active orally and is added to discourage injection or intranasal use. It is generally recommended that patients be prescribed the formulation combined with naloxone, unless they have a sensitivity to naloxone or are pregnant. To streamline the discussion in this section, we will refer to "buprenorphine" instead of "buprenorphine/naloxone" and to the buprenorphine dose alone, rather than the combination (e.g., "2 mg" instead of "2/0.5 mg").

Sublingual tablet formulations are available with and without naloxone in 2 and 8 mg formulations and must be used sublingually because this route bypasses hepatic metabolism. There are also sublingual strips (brand name Suboxone), which are only available in combination with naloxone and in dosages of 2, 4, 8, and 12 mg of buprenorphine. There are also two buccal formulations of buprenorphine/naloxone available—a tablet (brand name Zubsolv) and a film (brand name Bunavail). The buprenorphine dosages for the buccal formulations are different than the sublingual formulations; 5.4 mg of the buccal tablet and 4.2 mg of the buccal film are roughly equivalent to 8 mg of the sublingual tablet or film.

Buprenorphine Induction

Earlier guidelines recommended observed induction in the office setting, but a number of studies have shown that induction can be done safely and effectively at home.[135] In our experience, most patients can be started on buprenorphine at home; this is particularly true for those who have experience with taking the medication previously. The main risks during induction are precipitated withdrawal and incomplete suppression of withdrawal symptoms or craving, neither of which are dangerous. The risk of precipitated withdrawal can be minimized by having the patient wait until they are experiencing withdrawal symptoms before taking the first dose and starting with a low dose of buprenorphine (e.g., 2–4 mg of a sublingual tablet). Studies suggest that individuals taking 8–16 mg daily of the sublingual formulation should not have significant withdrawal or craving, though higher doses may be more effective for some in the long term. It is important to make sure that the patient knows how to take the medication properly in order to get the full effect; we find that this is often the problem when patients feel that the dose is inadequate. We generally prescribe a 1-week supply of medication initially and provide enough to take up to 16 mg daily of the sublingual formulation. The optimal regimen for induction has not been established; in one observational study, 89% of those prescribed 16 mg or more daily during induction successfully transitioned to maintenance treatment without relapse, compared to 68% of those prescribed 8 mg, 61% prescribed 4 mg, and 49% prescribed 2 mg.[136] Box 6.1 gives some suggestions for treatment induction. It should be noted that splitting the tablets or cutting the film version is officially not recommended, but in practice many patients can and do split them.

Patients who are dependent on methadone or other long-acting opioids may have a difficult transition, especially if they are taking high doses. As noted earlier, because of its high affinity for opioid receptors and its partial agonist effect, buprenorphine can cause "precipitated withdrawal" in patients who have been taking long-acting opioids, particularly methadone. It is generally recommended that the dose be tapered down to the equivalent of 30 mg/day of methadone, and the transfer of patients on doses over 60 mg/day is not recommended. However, as noted earlier, a study of subjects on 100 mg/day of methadone suggested that giving low, repeated doses of buprenorphine (e.g., 2 mg) may be an effective

BOX 6.1 Suggested Instructions for Buprenorphine Induction for an Individual Using Short-Acting Opioids with Sublingual* Buprenorphine Tablet or Film

Day 1

- Begin the first dose at least 4 hours after last opioid use, preferably when having some withdrawal symptoms. Make sure the tablet or film dissolves completely and do not drink or eat anything for at least 30 minutes afterward.
- Take 4 mg of buprenorphine (two 2 mg tab/films or one half of an 8 mg tab/film).
- Wait 1–3 hours, take another 4 mg of buprenorphine if still having withdrawal symptoms.
- Wait another 1–3 hours and take a third dose of 4 mg of buprenorphine if still having withdrawal symptoms.
- Do not take more than 12 mg in the first 24 hours.

Day 2

- **If day 1 total was 4 mg** and there were no withdrawal symptoms: take 4 mg in the morning. If having withdrawal symptoms in the morning, take 8 mg. Take another 4 mg later in the day if having withdrawal symptoms.
- **If day 1 total was 8–12 mg** and there were no withdrawal symptoms in the morning, take 8 mg again. If having withdrawal symptoms, take 12 mg. Take another 4 mg later in the day if having withdrawal symptoms. Do not take more than 16 mg total for the day.

Day 3

- If you felt well on day 2, repeat the same dose.
- If tired, groggy, or oversedated on day 2, take 2–4 mg less.

- If the day 2 dose was 4–12 mg and you are having withdrawal symptoms in the morning, take 12 mg in the morning. Take another 4 mg in the evening if still having withdrawal symptoms. Do not take more than 16 mg total for the day.

Day 4–7

- Take the dose used on day 3; you can take it once daily or split it into two doses. Do not take more than 16 mg per day without speaking to the physician first.

---

*For buccal formulations: 5.7 mg tablet (Zubsolv) and 4.2 mg film (Bunavail) are roughly equivalent to 8 mg sublingual tablet or film.

strategy to prevent precipitated withdrawal during this transition.[97] Table 6.4 provides some advice on buprenorphine induction for individuals who are taking long-acting opioids.

It is generally recommended that patients be evaluated at least weekly during the initial treatment phase to determine if they are having any adverse effects and are handling the medication responsibly. Having the patient sign an agreement at the onset of treatment can be helpful to clarify and document the responsibilities and expectations; Figure 6.1 provides an example of one such agreement. Once the patient is stabilized and provides urine samples that are free of illicit opioids, less frequent visits (biweekly or monthly) may be sufficient. Of note, buprenorphine is not detected in many currently available commercial urine drug tests, although there are specific assays available for its detection.

For those who have urine drug tests positive for other substances, a variety of strategies can be used. Many opioid-dependent individuals also use cocaine. Continued use while on buprenorphine is generally not grounds for discontinuing treatment,[137] but physicians should counsel patients on their use and may wish to provide incentives to patients for abstinence (such as increasing the interval between visits). Those who are using sedatives or alcohol in combination with buprenorphine should be warned of the risks of combining these and should receive treatment for their other substance use disorders. In some cases, it may be best to discontinue treatment with buprenorphine if the individual continues

TABLE 6.4 Buprenorphine Induction from Long-Acting Opioids (Methadone, Sustained-Release Oxycodone/Morphine)

Step 1:

- If patient is on an opioid maintenance program or prescribed long-acting opioids, treatment should be coordinated with the program or prescriber.

- Patients should be warned that they may experience discomfort or dysphoria for up to 2 weeks with the transition.

Step 2:

- If possible, taper to a dose of 30 mg/day of methadone (or its equivalent). Splitting the dose may help.

- If not possible, transfers can be done with a dose of 30–60 mg/day of methadone (or its equivalent), at the lowest dose that is tolerable to the patient.

- For patients who cannot be tapered below 60 mg of methadone/day, *transfer is not generally recommended.* There have been reports of patients being transferred to a short-acting opioid followed by transition to buprenorphine. (This may be allowable for only 3 days by federal regulations.)

- **Normal transfer** (methadone dose ≤30 mg/day): at least 24 hours should pass from the last dose of long-acting opioid before giving the first dose of buprenorphine.

- **High-dose transfer** (methadone dose 30–60 mg/day): the first dose of buprenorphine should be given at least 48–96 hours after the last dose of long-acting opioid, or until the patient experiences maximal withdrawal discomfort. Earlier dosing is highly likely to precipitate withdrawal.

(continued)

TABLE 6.4 (Continued)

• Recommended dosing schedule is given below:			
Long-Acting Opioid Dose (mg of methadone/day)	**≤10 mg**	**10–40 mg**	**40–60 mg**
1st day buprenorphine target dose	2–4 mg	4–8 mg	4–8 mg
Optional dose review 2–4 hours after 1st dose	Dose review not required	Dose review not required	Dose review required: give 2–4 mg additional if needed
2nd day buprenorphine target dose	4 mg	8 mg (4–8 mg)	8 mg (6–10 mg)
3rd day buprenorphine target dose	6 mg (6–8 mg)	12 mg (8–12 mg)	12 mg (10–16 mg)

Adapted from *Dosing Guide for Suboxone and Subutex*. Distributed by Reckitt Benckiser Pharmaceuticals, Inc.

to abuse alcohol or sedatives and does not comply with treatment. For those who continue to use other opioids or are diverting the buprenorphine, referral to more intensive treatment with closer monitoring (e.g., a methadone maintenance program) is generally appropriate.

Buprenorphine Dosing

There is some controversy over the optimal dosing of buprenorphine. In our experience, most patients can be maintained on a dose of 8–16 mg/day of sublingual buprenorphine. Dosages over 24 mg/day should be used with caution and dosages over 32 mg/day

Patient Responsibilities

____ The patient will agree to store the medication properly. The medication can be harmful to others. The pills should be stored in a safe, secure place, out of reach of children, preferably a lock box. If anyone other than the patient ingests the medication, the patient must call the poison control center or 911 immediately.

____ The patient is responsible for the safekeeping of the prescription and medication. Lost or stolen prescriptions or medications will not be replaced.

____ The patient will agree to take the medication only as prescribed. The patient must not change or adjust the dose without prior approval of the treating physician. If the patient wishes to have a dose change, the patient must contact their physician first.

____ The patient will agree to inform us if prescribed any other medication by another practitioner. Failure to inform the clinic of receiving prescriptions for controlled substances may result in termination of treatment.

____ The patient will agree to comply with pill counts or urine tests when requested. The patient must be prepared to provide a urine sample for testing at each visit and to show their pill bottle for a pill count whenever requested.

____ The patient will agree to notify the physician in case of relapse or other drug use. The use of other drugs while on buprenorphine maintenance can be life-threatening and an appropriate treatment plan needs to be developed as soon as possible. The physician should be informed of drug use before a urine test shows it.

____ The patient will agree to follow clinic procedures and rules. This includes the hours, phone numbers, procedure for making appointments, fees, and appropriate behavior.

Patient Name _____

Patient Signature_____ Date _____

Provider Name _____

Provider Signature _____ Date _____

FIGURE 6.1 *Sample Buprenorphine Treatment Agreement.*

are generally not recommended.[138] A study found that doses over 8 mg/day provided minimal additional benefit in terms of withdrawal suppression and opioid blockade.[139] A study analyzing the impact of an insurance process that required progressively more frequent authorizations for doses over 16 mg/day found that this reduced the number of individuals on doses over 24 mg/day and there was a temporary increase in relapse rates, but no long-term increase.[140] On the other hand, a 2010 systematic review[141] and a clinical trial published in 2013 found that higher sublingual buprenorphine doses (up to 32 mg/day) were associated with better treatment outcomes.[142]

The main concern with prescribing higher doses of buprenorphine is that it will lead to diversion; there is no evidence of harm to those who take higher doses. Diversion is a common phenomenon;[143] however, at least in the United States, it appears that most individuals who take diverted buprenorphine are already opioid dependent and take it to avoid withdrawal.[144,145] While it is generally thought that buprenorphine has less misuse potential than other opioids, it is clear that it may be misused, and there are countries with high rates of intravenous buprenorphine use, primarily the pure form (without naloxone).[146] While no studies on interventions have been shown to reduce diversion, experts recommend a number of strategies, including random call backs/pill counts, testing urine for buprenorphine, limiting the quantity of medication dispensed, and using prescription-monitoring programs. Those who are prescribed the film-strip version can be asked to return the wrappers, which have serial numbers. Increasing the availability of treatment may also lead to less demand for diverted medication.[147] Buprenorphine delivered through a long-acting depot injection formulation[148] or implants[149,150] are promising treatment options on the horizon that may help reduce diversion.

Buprenorphine and Adjunctive Counseling

It is generally recommended that maintenance treatment with buprenorphine be part of a broader treatment plan and that patients participate in other psychosocial treatment modalities.[70] This can be in the form of attending self-help groups or receiving office-based counseling; the optimal approach probably depends on the patient's background and their stage in treatment. It should be noted that the addition of psychosocial treatments to standard medical management has not been shown to be beneficial in clinical trials[75,151,152]

TABLE 6.5 Summary of Opioid Use Disorder Treatment Studies

Intervention	Studies	Outcomes
Brief advice	RCTs	May be effective for reducing opioid use; data are mixed
Self-help groups	Observational	Participation associated with better outcomes
Drug counseling	RCT	Effective (in one study)
Contingency management	RCTs Meta-analysis	Effective (while incentives are offered)
Residential treatment	Observational RCT	Participation associated with better outcomes. Better than outpatient treatment in some measures (in one RCT)
Medically Supervised Withdrawal		
Methadone taper	RCTs Meta-analysis	Effective at reducing severity of withdrawal
Clonidine	RCTs Meta-analysis	Effective, but no more than methadone for withdrawal symptoms
Buprenorphine	RCTs Meta-analysis	Effective—more so than clonidine, but not methadone—for symptoms
Medication-Assisted Treatment		
Methadone	RCTs Meta-analysis	Effective, more so than detoxification. Higher doses more effective
Buprenorphine	RCTs Meta-analysis	Effective, but less so than methadone Effective in office-based setting

(continued)

TABLE 6.5 (Continued)

Intervention	Studies	Outcomes
Medication-Assisted Treatment		
Naltrexone	RCTs Meta-analysis	Effective for selected patients; long-acting injectable more effective; limited comparison with methadone or buprenorphine

See text for references and more details.
RCT: randomized controlled trial.

and in a 2011 systematic review.[125] This does not mean that no one would benefit from these services, but patients should not be forced to participate, particularly those who are doing well with medical management alone.

Naltrexone

Naltrexone, a long-acting orally active opioid antagonist, blocks the effects of opioids and has been an attractive theoretical option for relapse prevention. Unfortunately, its effectiveness is limited by low rates of patient acceptance[153] and adherence to the drug.[154] Unlike methadone and buprenorphine, individuals must be abstinent from opioids before initiating treatment. A report of a 12-week trial published in 2013 indicated that a 4-week buprenorphine taper followed by oral naltrexone therapy was effective, with 50% of the subjects remaining in treatment and abstinent from opioids, but this protocol was not compared with continuation of the buprenorphine.[155] There are few data on the effectiveness of naltrexone in comparison with methadone and buprenorphine. In one study performed in Malaysia, buprenorphine was more effective than oral naltrexone and naltrexone was not significantly better than placebo.[156]

The use of naltrexone in combination with behavioral treatments, such as contingency management, may be more effective.[157] It may also be beneficial in a subset of highly motivated individuals, such as healthcare professionals,[158] business executives,[159] or parolees.[160] A 2011 Cochrane systematic review of the efficacy of oral naltrexone for opioid dependence concluded that the available studies do not allow "an adequate evaluation."[161]

Long-acting implantable[162,163] or injectable forms of opioid antagonists may prove to be more effective. Two studies have reported positive results with extended-release injectable naltrexone when compared with placebo,[164,165] but there are no trials comparing it with buprenorphine or methadone. A 2008 Cochrane systematic review concluded that there is "insufficient evidence to evaluate the effectiveness" of the long-acting injectable formulation.[166] Similarly, a 2014 systematic review concluded that naltrexone implant use should be "limited to clinical trials."[167]

A summary of studies on treatment of opioid use disorder is given in Table 6.5

Notes

1. Substance Abuse and Mental Health Services Administration. *Results from the 2013 National Survey on Drug Use and Health: National Findings.* NSDUH Series H-48, HHS Publication No. (SMA) 14-4863. Rockville, MD: Substance Abuse and Mental Health Services Administration; 2014.

2. Dart RC, Surratt HL, Cicero TJ, et al. Trends in opioid analgesic abuse and mortality in the United States. N Engl J Med 2015;372:241–8.

3. Cicero TJ, Ellis MS, Surratt HL, Kurtz SP. The changing face of heroin use in the United States: a retrospective analysis of the past 50 years. JAMA Psychiatry 2014;71:821–5.

4. Substance Abuse and Mental Health Services Administration, Center for Behavioral Health Statistics and Quality. *The DAWN Report: Highlights of the 2011 Drug Abuse Warning Network (DAWN) Findings on Drug-Related Emergency Department Visits.* Rockville, MD; 2011.

5. Borg L, Buonora BS, Butelman ER, et al. The pharmacology of opioids. In Ries RK, Fiellin DA, Miller SC, Saitz R, eds. *The ASAM Principles of Addiction Medicine*, 5th ed. Philadelphia: Wolters Kluwer; 2014:135–50.

6. Lawlor PG, Turner KS, Hanson J, Bruera ED. Dose ratio between morphine and methadone in patients with cancer pain: a retrospective study. Cancer 1998;82:1167–73.

7. American Psychiatric Association. (2013). *Diagnostic and Statistical Manual of Mental Disorders*, Fifth Edition. Arlington, VA: American Psychiatric Publishing.

8. Seal KH, Kral AH, Gee L, et al. Predictors and prevention of nonfatal overdose among street-recruited injection heroin users in the San Francisco Bay area, 1998–1999. Am J Public Health 2001;91:1842–6.

9. Darke S, Marel C, Mills KL, et al. Patterns and correlates of non-fatal heroin overdose at 11-year follow-up: findings from the Australian Treatment Outcome Study. Drug Alcohol Depend 2014;144:148–52.

10. Gossop M, Stewart D, Treacy S, Marsden J. A prospective study of mortality among drug misusers during a 4-year period after seeking treatment. Addiction 2002;97:39–47.

11. Centers for Disease Control and Prevention (CDC). Vital signs: overdoses of prescription pain relievers—United States, 1999–2008. MMWR Morbid Mortal Wkly Rep 2011;60:1487–92.

12. Tagliaro F, DeBattisti Z, Smith FP, Marigo M. Death from heroin overdose: findings from hair analysis. Lancet 1998;351:1923–5.

13. Strang J, McCambridge J, Best D, et al. Loss of tolerance and overdose mortality after inpatient opiate detoxification: follow up study. BMJ 2003;326:959–60.

14. Ravndal E, Amundsen EJ. Mortality among drug users after discharge from inpatient treatment: an 8-year prospective study. Drug Alcohol Depend 2010;108:65–9.

15. Binswanger IA, Blatchford PJ, Yamashita S, et al. Trends in overdose deaths after release from state prison, 1999–2009. Drug Alcohol Depend 2014;140:e14.

16. Algren DA, Monteilh CP, Punja M, et al. Fentanyl-associated fatalities among illicit drug users in Wayne County, Michigan (July 2005–May 2006). J Med Toxicol 2013;9:106–15.

17. Paulozzi LJ. Prescription drug overdoses: a review. J Safety Res 2012;43:283–9.

18. Wanger K, Brough L, Macmillan I, et al. Intravenous vs. subcutaneous naloxone for out-of-hospital management of presumed opioid overdose. Acad Emerg Med 1998;5:293–9.

19. Kerr D, Kelly AM, Dietze P, et al. Randomized controlled trial comparing the effectiveness and safety of intranasal and intramuscular naloxone for the treatment of suspected heroin overdose. Addiction 2009;104:2067–74.

20. Zamani N, Hassanian-Moghaddam H, Bayat AH, et al. Reversal of overdose syndrome in morphine-dependent rats using buprenorphine. Toxicol Lett 2015;232:590–4.

21. Welsh C, Sherman SG, Tobin KE. A case of heroin overdose reversed by sublingually administered buprenorphine/naloxone (Suboxone). Addiction 2008;103:1226–28.

22. Sporer KA. Acute heroin overdose. Ann Intern Med 1999;130:584–90.

23. Christenson J, Etherington J, Grafstein E, et al. Early discharge of patients with presumed opioid overdose: development of a clinical prediction rule. Acad Emerg Med 2000;7:1110–8.

24. Vilke GM, Sloane C, Smith AM, Chan TC. Assessment for deaths in out-of-hospital heroin overdose patients treated with naloxone who refuse treatment. Acad Emerg Med 2003;10:893–6.

25. Wampler DA, Molina DK, McManus J, et al. No deaths associated with patient refusal of transport after naloxone-reversed opioid overdose. Prehosp Emerg Care 2011;15:320–4.

26. Watson WA, Steele MT, Muelleman RL, Rush MD. Opioid toxicity recurrence after initial response to naloxone. J Toxicol Clin Toxicol 1998;36:11–17.

27. Caplehorn JR, Dalton MS, Haldar F, et al. Methadone maintenance and addicts' risk of fatal heroin overdose. Subst Use Misuse 1996;31:177–96.

28. Lepere B, Gourarier L, Sanchez M, et al. [Reduction in the number of lethal heroin overdoses in France since 1994. Focus on substitution treatments] Ann Med Interne (Paris) 2001;152(Suppl3):IS5–IS12.

29. Schwartz RP, Gryczynski J, O'Grady KE, et al. Opioid agonist treatments and opioid overdose deaths in Baltimore, Maryland. Am J Pub Health 2013;103:917–22.

30. Marshall BD, Milloy MJ, Wood E, et al. Reduction in overdose mortality after the opening of North America's first medically supervised

safer injecting facility: a retrospective population-based study. Lancet 2011;377:1429–37.

31. Walley AY, Xuan Z, Hackman HH, et al. Opioid overdose rates and implantation of overdose education and nasal naloxone distribution in Massachusetts: interrupted time series analysis. BMJ 2013;346:f174.

32. Smith ML, Shimomura ET, Summers J, et al. Detection times and analytical performance of commercial urine opiate immunoassays following heroin administration. J Anal Toxicol 2000;24:522–9.

33. Fingerhood MI, Jasinski DR, Sullivan JT. Prevalence of hepatitis C in a chemically dependent population. Arch Intern Med 1993;153:2025–30.

34. Muhuri PK, Gfroerer JC. Mortality associated with illegal drug use among adults in the United States. Am J Drug Alcohol Abuse 2011;37:155–64.

35. Sporer KA, Dorn E. Heroin-related noncardiogenic pulmonary edema: a case series. Chest 2001;120:1628–32.

36. Cygan J, Trunsky M, Corbridge T. Inhaled heroin-induced status asthmaticus. Five cases and a review of the literature. Chest 2000;117:272–5.

37. Karne S, D'Ambrosio C, Einarsson O, O'Connor PG. Hypersensitivity pneumonitis induced by intranasal heroin use. Am J Med 1999;107:392–5.

38. Martell BA, Arnsten JH, Ray B, Gourevitch MN. The impact of methadone on cardiac conduction in opiate users. Ann Intern Med 2003;139:154–5.

39. Wedam EF, Bigelow GE, Johnson RE, et al. QT-interval effects of methadone, levomethadyl and buprenorphine in a randomized trial. Arch Intern Med 2007;167:2469–75.

40. Yuan SC, Foss JF. Oral methylnaltrexone for opioid-induced constipation. JAMA 2000;284:1383–4.

41. Thomas J, Karver S, Cooney GA, et al. Methylnaltrexone for opioid-induced constipation in advanced illness. N Engl J Med 2008; 358:2332–43.

42. Paulson DM, Kennedy DT, Donovick RA, et al. Alvimopan: an oral, peripherally acting, mu-opioid receptor antagonist for the treatment of opioid-induced bowel dysfunction—a 21-day treatment-randomized clinical trial. J Pain 2005;6:184–92.

43. Chey WD, Webster L, Sostek M, et al. Naloxegol for opioid-induced constipation in patients with noncancer pain. N Engl J Med 2014;370:2387-96.

44. Arruda JA, Kurtzman NA, Pillay VK. Prevalence of renal disease in asymptomatic heroin addicts. Arch Intern Med 1975;135:535-7.

45. Cunningham EE, Brentjens JR, Zielezny MA, et al. Heroin nephropathy. A clinicopathologic and epidemiologic study. Am J Med 1980;68:47-53.

46. Jaffe JA, Kimmel PL. Chronic nephropathies of cocaine and heroin abuse: a critical review. Clin J Am Soc Nephrol 2006;1:655-67.

47. Friedman EA Tao TK. Disappearance of uremia due to heroin-associated nephropathy. Am J Kidney Dis 1995;25:689-93.

48. Buettner M, Toennes SW, Suettner S, et al. Nephropathy in illicit drug abusers: a postmortem analysis. Am J Kidney Dis 2014;63:945-53.

49. Fournier JP, Azoulay L, Yin H, et al. Tramadol use and the risk of hospitalization for hypoglycemia in patients with noncancer pain. JAMA Intern Med 2015;175:186-93.

50. Szeto HH, Inturrisi CE, Houde R, et al. Accumulation of normeperidine, an active metabolite of meperidine, in patients with renal failure or cancer. Ann Intern Med 1977;86:738-41.

51. Hershey LA. Meperidine and central neurotoxicity. Ann Intern Med 1983;98:548-9.

52. Labate A, Newton MR, Vernon GM, Berkovic SF. Tramadol and new-onset seizures. Med J Australia 2005;182:42-43.

53. **Bernstein J, Bernstein E, Tassiopoulos K, et al. Brief motivational intervention at a clinic visit reduces cocaine and heroin use. Drug Alcohol Depend 2005;77:49–59.** *Patients at walk-in clinics at were screened for heroin or cocaine use and randomized to (1) a brief intervention (by a trained counselor)—motivational interview, active referrals, and written handout with a list of treatment resources, followed by a phone call 10 days later, or (2) handout only. A total of 23,669 were screened, 1,232 (5%) were eligible, 1,175 enrolled, and 778 were used in the final analysis. At 6-month follow-up, the intervention group was more likely to be abstinent from heroin alone (40% vs. 31%), cocaine alone (22% vs. 17%), and both drugs (17% vs. 13%).*

54. Gossop M, Green L, Phillips G, Bradley B. What happens to opiate addicts immediately after treatment: a prospective follow up study. BMJ 1987;294:1377-80.

55. Davison JW, Sweeney ML, Bush KR, et al. Outpatient treatment engagement and abstinence rates following inpatient opioid detoxification. J Addict Dis 2006;25:27–35. *Of 112 male veterans who received detoxification followed by abstinence-oriented outpatient care, 78% completed detox, but only 22% remained in aftercare at 90 days and <3% had toxicology-verified abstinence. At 1-year follow-up, 20% were readmitted for detox and 4.5% had died.*

56. Broers B, Giner F, Dumont P, Mino A. Inpatient opiate detoxification in Geneva: follow-up at 1 and 6 months. Drug Alcohol Depend 2000;58:85–92. *Of 73 admitted for inpatient detox (most with methadone, average 15 days), 73% completed it and at 6 months, 22/60 interviewed were abstinent, 11 had at least one overdose.*

57. Chutuape MA, Jasinski DR, Fingerhood MI, Stitzer ML. One-, three-, and six-month outcomes after brief inpatient opioid detoxification. Am J Drug Alcohol Abuse 2001;27:19–44. *After undergoing inpatient 3-day detoxification, 116 heroin users who agreed to participate in the study were followed for 6 months. Compared to baseline, they (1) used less heroin, cocaine, and alcohol, (2) engaged in less criminal activity, (3) were more likely to be employed, and (4) were more likely to have a regular place to live. Approximately a third were not using heroin at 6 months, another third using intermittently, and the rest using regularly.*

58. Sees KL, Delucchi KL, Masson C, et al. Methadone maintenance vs. 180-day psychosocially enriched detoxification for treatment of opioid dependence. JAMA 2000;283:1303–10. *Subjects (n = 179) were randomized to methadone maintenance or methadone-assisted detox and followed for 12 months. Those on maintenance had better treatment retention, a lower rate of drug-related HIV risk behaviors, and fewer legal problems. Heroin use decreased in both arms, more so among those on maintenance. There was no difference in employment, family functioning, or alcohol use.*

59. Fiellin DA, Schottenfeld RS, Cutter CJ, et al. Primary care-based buprenorphine taper vs, maintenance therapy for prescription opioid dependence: a randomized clinical trial. JAMA Intern Med 2014;174:1947–54. *Subjects with prescription opioid dependence in a primary care practice (n = 113) received 2-week buprenorphine induction then randomly received either a stable dosage for 4 weeks followed by a gradual taper over 3 weeks or a stable dose for 14 weeks. Those assigned to taper had lower mean percentage of opioid negative urine samples (33% vs. 53%), achieved fewer mean maximum consecutive weeks of opioid abstinence (2.7 vs. 5.2), and were less likely to complete the trial (11% vs. 66%).*

60. Mee-Lee D, Shulman GD, Fishman MJ, Gastfriend DR, Miller MM, eds. The *ASAM Criteria: Treatment Criteria for Addictive, Substance-Related, and Co-Occurring Conditions*, 3rd ed. Carson City, NV: Change Companies; 2013.

61. Gossop M, Johns A, Green L. Opiate withdrawal: inpatient versus outpatient programmes and preferred versus random assignment to treatment. BMJ 1986;293:103–4.

62. Gossop M, Strang J. Price, cost and value of opiate detoxification. Br J Psychiatry 2000;177:262–6.

63. Day E, Ison J, Strang J. Inpatient versus other settings for detoxification for opioid dependence. Cochrane Database Syst Rev 2005;2:CD004580.

64. Jasinski DR, Pevnick JS, Griffith JD. Human pharmacology and abuse potential of the analgesic buprenorphine: a potential agent for treating narcotic addiction. Arch Gen Psychiatry 1978;35:501–16.

65. Walsh SL, Preston KL, Stitzer ML, et al. Clinical pharmacology of buprenorphine: ceiling effects at high doses. Clin Pharmacol Ther 1994;55:569–80.

66. Tompkins DA, Smith MT, Mizer MZ, et al. A double-blind, within subject comparison of spontaneous opioid withdrawal from buprenorphine versus morphine. J Pharmacol Exp Ther 2014;348:217–26.

67. **Lintzeris N, Bell J, Bammer G, et al. A randomized controlled trial of buprenorphine in the management of short-term ambulatory heroin withdrawal. Addiction 2002;97:1395–404.** *Heroin users (n = 114) were randomized to detox with 8 days of clonidine or 5 days of buprenorphine. Those on buprenorphine had better treatment retention at days 8 (86% vs. 57%) and 35 (62% vs. 39%). They also had less severe withdrawal symptoms.*

68. Gowing L, Ali R, White JM. Buprenorphine for the management of opioid withdrawal. Cochrane Database Syst Rev 2009;3:CD002025.

69. **Gibson AE, Doran CM, Bell JR, et al. A comparison of buprenorphine treatment in clinic and primary care settings: a randomised trial. Med J Aust 2003;179:38–42.** *Heroin-dependent subjects (n = 115) were randomized to 5-day outpatient detox at a drug treatment center or a general practice. There were no significant differences in detox completion (~75%) or participation in post-detox treatment (~56%). At 3-month follow-up, self-reported heroin use in both arms was about the same, but lower than before detox.*

70. Center for Substance Abuse Treatment. *Clinical Guidelines for the Use of Buprenorphine in the Treatment of Opioid Addiction.* Treatment improvement protocol (TIP) Series 40. DHHS Publication No. (SMA) 04-3939. Rockville, MD: Substance Abuse and Mental Health Services Administration; 2004.

71. Lintzeris N, Bammer G, Rushworth L, et al. Buprenorphine dosing regimen for inpatient heroin withdrawal: a symptom-triggered dose titration study. Drug Alcohol Depend 2003;70:287–94.

72. **Oreskovich MR, Saxon AJ, Ellis MLK, et al. A double-blind, double-dummy, randomized, prospective pilot study of the partial Mu opiate agonist, buprenorphine, for acute detoxification from heroin. Drug Alcohol Depend 2005;77:71–9.** *Heroin-dependent adults (n = 30) with moderate-severe withdrawal symptoms (COWS ≥13) were randomized to inpatient detox with (1) low-dose buprenorphine, (2) high-dose buprenorphine, or (3) clonidine. Both buprenorphine regimens were better at suppressing withdrawal than clonidine; the high dose was somewhat better than the low dose in some measures.*

73. Soeffing JM, Rastegar DA. Treatment completion on an inpatient detoxification unit: impact of a change to sublingual buprenorphine-naloxone. J Subst Abuse Treat 2007;33:401–4.

74. Ling W, Hillhouse M, Domier C, et al. Buprenorphine tapering schedule and illicit opioid use. Addiction 2009;104:256–65.

75. Weiss RD, Potter JS, Fiellin DA, et al. Adjunctive counseling during brief and extended buprenorphine-naloxone treatment for prescription opioid dependence: a 2-phase randomized controlled trial. Arch Gen Psychiatry 2011;68:1238–46.

76. Amato L, Minozzi S, Davoli M, Vecchi S. Psychosocial and pharmacological treatments versus pharmacological treatments for opioid detoxification. Cochrane Database Syst Rev 2011;9:CD005031.

77. Gossop M, Griffiths P, Bradley B, Strang J. Opiate withdrawal symptoms in response to 10-day and 21-day methadone withdrawal programmes. Br J Psychiatry 1989;154:360–3.

78. Amato L, Davoli M, Minozzi S, et al. Methadone at tapered doses for the management of opioid withdrawal. Cochrane Database Syst Rev 2013;2:CD:003409.

79. Gold MS, Redmond DE, Kleber HD. Clonidine in opiate withdrawal. Lancet 1978;311:929–30.

80. Washton AM, Resnick RB. Clonidine versus methadone for opiate detoxification. Lancet 1980;316:1297.

81. Kleber HD, Riordan CE, Rounsaville B, et al. Clonidine in outpatient detoxification from methadone maintenance. Arch Gen Psychiatry 1985;42:391–4.

82. Gowing L, Farrell M, Ali R, White JM. Alpha-2-adrenergic agonists for the management of opioid withdrawal. Cochrane Database Syst Rev 2014;3:CD002024.

83. Reid JL, Dargie HJ, Davies DS, et al. Clonidine withdrawal in hypertension. Changes in blood-pressure and plasma and urinary noradrenaline. Lancet 1977;309:1171–4.

84. Dennison SJ. Clonidine abuse among opiate addicts. Psychiatr Q 2001;72:191–5.

85. Markowitz JS, Myrick H, Hiott W. Clonidine dependence. J Clin Psychopharmacol 1997;17:137–38.

86. Rapko DA, Rastegar DA. Intentional clonidine patch ingestion by 3 adults in a detoxification unit. Arch Intern Med 2003;163:367–8.

87. Lofwall MR, Walsh SL, Bigelow GE, Strain EC. Modest opioid withdrawal suppression efficacy of oral tramadol in humans. Psychopharmacology (Berl). 2007;194(3):381–93.

88. Chawla JM, Pal H, Lai R, et al. Comparison of efficacy between buprenorphine and tramadol in the detoxification of opioid (heroin)-dependent subjects. J Opioid Manag 2013;9:35–41.

89. O'Connor PG, Carroll KM, Shi JM, et al. Three methods of opioid detoxification in a primary care setting: a randomized trial. Ann Intern Med 1997;127:526–30.

90. Umbricht A, Montoya ID, Hoover DR, et al. Naltrexone shortened opioid detoxification with buprenorphine. Drug Alcohol Depend 1999;56:181–90.

91. Seoane A, Carrasco G, Cabré L, et al. Efficacy and safety of two methods of rapid intravenous detoxification in heroin addicts previously treated without success. Br J Psychiatry 1994;171:340–5.

92. Hensel M, Kox WJ. Safety, efficacy, and long-term results of a modified version of rapid opiate detoxification under general anaesthesia: a prospective study in methadone, heroin, codeine and morphine addicts. Acta Anaesthesiol Scand 2000;44:326–33.

93. Collins ED, Kleber HD, Whittington RA, Heitler NE. Anesthesia-assisted vs. buprenophine or clonidine-assisted heroin detoxification and naltrexone induction: a randomized controlled trial. JAMA 2005;294:903–13.

94. Centers for Disease Control and Prevention. Deaths and severe adverse events associated with anesthesia-assisted rapid detoxification—New York City, 2012. MMWR Morbid Mortal Wkly Rep 2013;62:777–80.

95. Gowing L, Ali R, White JM. Opioid antagonists under heavy sedation or anaesthesia for opioid withdrawal. Cochrane Database Syst Rev 2010;20:CD002022.

96. Gossop M, Strang J. A comparison of the withdrawal responses of heroin and methadone addicts during detoxification. Br J Psychiatry 1991;158:697–9.

97. Rosado J, Walsh SL, Bigelow GE, Strain EC. Sublingual buprenorphine/naloxone precipitated withdrawal in subjects maintained on 100 mg of daily methadone. Drug Alcohol Depend 2007;90:261–9.

98. Bracy SA, Simpson DD. Status of opioid addicts 5 years after admission to drug abuse treatment. Am J Drug Alcohol Abuse 1982;9:115–27.

99. Bernstein J, Bernstein E, Tassiopoulos K, et al. Brief motivational intervention at a clinic visit reduces cocaine and heroin use. Drug Alcohol Depend 2005;77:49–59.

100. Saitz R, Palfai TPA, Cheng DM, et al. Screening and brief intervention for drug use in primary care-The ASPIRE randomized clinical trial. JAMA 2014;312:502–13.

101. Roy-Byrne P, Bumgardner K, Krupski A, et al. Brief interventions for problem drug in safety-net primary care settings—a randomized clinical trial. JAMA 2014;312:492–501.

102. Christo G, Franey C. Drug users' spiritual beliefs, locus of control and the disease concept in relation to Narcotics Anonymous attendance and six-month outcomes. Drug Alcohol Depend 1995;38:51–6.

103. **Timko C, DeBenedetti A, Billow R. Intensive referral to 12-step self-help groups and 6-month substance use disorder outcomes. Addiction 2006;101:678–88.** *Veterans in an outpatient treatment program (n = 345) were randomized to an intensive referral (three individual meetings with a counselor arranging for self-help group participation) or standard referral (a list of self-help groups). Among the 281 (81%) who completed 6-month follow-up, there was no difference in self-help group*

participation or number of meetings attended, but those assigned to the intensive referral had somewhat greater improvement in ASI scores and were more likely to be abstinent from drugs (78% vs. 70%), but not alcohol. Among those with less previous self-help group experience, intensive referral was associated with attendance at more meetings and greater improvement in ASI scores.

104. **McAuliffe WE. A randomized controlled trial of recovery training and self-help for opioid addicts in New England and Hong Kong. J Psychoactive Drugs 1990;22:197–209.** *In this study, 168 volunteers who completed drug treatment (detox, therapeutic community, halfway house, etc.) were randomized to weekly 3-hour sessions that included recovery training led by a drug counselor and a peer-led self-help group; they also participated in recreational activities and community service. The control arm received no treatment. Among those who had follow-up interviews, opioid abstinence and "rare use" was significantly higher in the treatment arm during the first 6 months (47% vs. 29%) and second 6 months (36% vs. 19%).*

105. **Gruber K, Chutuape MA, Stitzer ML. Reinforcement-based intensive outpatient treatment for inner city opiate abusers: a short-term evaluation. Drug Alcohol Depend 2000;57:211–23.** *In this study, 28 of 52 opioid-dependent subjects (of 91 initially recruited) who completed inpatient 3-day detoxification were randomized to a 3-month program that included (during the first month) counseling, social skills training, employment and housing assistance, recreational activities, and abstinent-contingent rewards. During the next 2 months they had counseling only. Only 5 completed the program; participants were more likely to be abstinent from heroin/cocaine at 30 days (50% vs. 21%), but not at 3-month follow-up.*

106. **Katz EC, Gruber K, Chutuape MA, Stitzer ML. Reinforcement-based outpatient treatment for opiate and cocaine abusers. J Subst Abuse Treat 2001;20:93–8.** *In this study, 37 recently detoxified opioid-dependent subjects in a program like the one in reference 105 (Gruber et al.) were given abstinence-contingent rewards over 3 months instead of 1 month; 16 (43%) completed the program; 92% of their urine samples were opioid/cocaine free, versus 56% of the dropouts' urine samples.*

107. Mayet S, Farrell M, Ferri M, et al. Psychosocial treatment for opiate abuse and dependence. Cochrane Database Syst Rev 2005;1:CD004330.

108. **Bale RN, Zarcone VP, Van Stone WW, et al. Three therapeutic communities. A prospective controlled study of narcotic**

addiction treatment: process and two-year follow-up results. Arch Gen Psychiatry 1984;41:185–91. *In this study, 181 opioid-dependent subjects who spent at least a week in one of three therapeutic communities were compared with 166 who only completed detox. After 2 years, those who participated in two of the three programs were more likely to be working or attending school and less likely to have been convicted of a crime. Most of the drug and alcohol use outcome measures were not significantly better.*

109. Guydish J, Sorensen JL, Chan M, et al. A randomized trial comparing day and residential drug abuse treatment: 18-month outcomes. J Consult Clin Psychology 1999;67:428–34. *In this study, 534 drug abusers were randomized to day or residential treatment in a therapeutic community; 261 (49%) completed 2 weeks and 188 (35%) completed all the follow-up interviews over 18 months. Overall, both groups improved. Those assigned residential treatment had better outcomes in terms of psychiatric symptoms and social problem severity, but not other measures, including addiction severity and employment.*

110. Keen J, Oliver P, Rowse G, Mathers. Residential rehabilitation for drug users: a review of 13 months' intake to a therapeutic community. Fam Pract 2001;18:545–8. *Of 138 drug users admitted to a residential treatment program in the UK, 17(13%) completed the one-year program and remained abstinent.*

111. Gossop M, Marsden J, Stewart D, Kidd T. The national treatment outcome research study (NTORS): 4- to 5-year follow-up results. Addiction 2003;98:291–303. *Drug misusers (418 of 650 eligible) who were treated in a variety of settings, including residential treatment, were followed for 4–5 years. The 142 in residential treatment reported significant declines in criminal activity, and almost half of the heroin users reported being abstinent in the previous 90 days at their follow-up interview.*

112. Strang J, Metrebian N, Lintzeris N, et al. Supervised injectable heroin or injectable methadone versus optimised oral methadone as treatment for chronic heroin addicts in England after persistent failure in orthodox treatment (RIOTT): a randomised trial. Lancet 2010;375:1885–95.

113. Newman RG, Whitehill WB. Double-blind comparison of methadone maintenance treatments of narcotic addicts in Hong Kong. Lancet 1979;314:485–8. *In this study, 100 subjects were stabilized on 60 mg of methadone over 2 weeks and then randomized to (1) methadone taper (1 mg/day) followed by placebo or (2) methadone maintenance*

(30–130 mg/day). Retention rates were better on maintenance, both at 32 weeks (76% vs. 10%) and 3 years (56% vs. 2%).

114. Sees KL, Delucchi KL, Masson C, et al. Methadone maintenance vs. 180-day psychosocially enriched detoxification for treatment of opioid dependence. JAMA 2000;283:1303–10.

115. **Strain EC, Bigelow GE, Liebson IA, Stitzer ML. Moderate- vs. high-dose methadone in the treatment of opioid dependence. JAMA 1999;281:1000–5.** *In this study, 179 subjects were randomized to low-dose (40–50 mg/day) or high-dose (80–100 mg/day) methadone. At week 30, the high-dose group had lower rates of illicit opioid use (53% vs. 62%) and were more likely to have completed the 40-week program (33% vs. 20%), but this difference was not statistically significant.*

116. **Preston KL, Umbricht A, Epstein DH. Methadone dose increase and abstinence reinforcement for treatment of continued heroin use during methadone maintenance. Arch Gen Psychiatry 2000;57:395–404.** *Subjects on methadone (n = 120) who had ≥3 positive urine drug tests (opiates or cocaine) over 5 weeks were randomized to (1) methadone dose increase (from 50 to 70 mg/day), (2) vouchers as a reward for negative drug tests, (3) both dose increase and vouchers, or (4) neither (control). Dose increase and vouchers were equally effective at reducing use over 8 weeks, but the combination was not significantly better.*

117. Mattick RP, Breen C, Kimber J, Davoli M. Methadone maintenance therapy versus no opioid replacement therapy for opioid dependence. Cochrane Data Syst Rev 2009;3:CD002209.

118. Faggiano F, Vigna-Taglianti F, Versino E, Lemma P. Methadone maintenance at different dosages for opioid dependence. Cochrane Database Syst Rev 2003;3:CD002208.

119. Center for Substance Abuse Treatment. Medication-Assisted Treatment for Opioid Addiction in Opioid Treatment Programs. Treatment Improvement Protocol (TIP) Series 43. HHS Publication No. (SMA) 12-4214. Rockville, MD: Substance Abuse and Mental Health Services Administration; 2005.

120. Yancovitz SR, DesJarlais DC, Peyser NP, et al. A randomized trial of an interim methadone maintenance clinic. Am J Public Health 1991;81:1185–91.

121. Schwartz RP, Kelly SM, O'Grady KE, et al. Interim methadone treatment compared to standard methadone treatment: 4-month findings. J Subst Abuse Treat 2011;41:21–9.

122. Gruber VA, Delucchi KL, Kielstein A, Batki SL. A randomized trial of 6-month methadone maintenance with standard or minimal counseling versus 21-day detoxification. Drug Alcohol Depend 2008;94:199–206.

123. McLellan AT, Arndt IO, Metzger DS, et al. The effects of psychosocial services in substance abuse treatment. JAMA 1993;269:1953–9. *Opioid-dependent subjects (n = 92) were randomized to (1) "minimum methadone services" (MMS): methadone alone without additional services; (2) "standard methadone services" (SMS): methadone plus counseling and reinforcement; or (3) "enhanced methadone services" (EMS): SMS plus onsite medical/psychiatric care, employment counseling, and family therapy. "Treatment failure" was defined as eight consecutive opiate/cocaine-positive urine tests or three "emergency situations" requiring immediate health care, and was higher over 24 weeks among MMS subjects (69%) than SMS (41%) or EMS (19%) subjects—most were due to cocaine use.*

124. **Kraft MK, Rothbard AB, Hadley TR, et al. Are supplementary services provided during methadone maintenance really cost-effective? Am J Psychiatry 1997;154:1214–9.** *This study calculated the cost-effectiveness of the three levels of services from the previous reference. The annual cost per abstinent client was $16,485 at the minimum level, $9,804 at the standard level, and $11,818 at the enhanced level.*

125. Amato L, Minozzi S, Davoli M, Vecchi S. Psychosocial combined with agonist maintenance treatment versus agonist maintenance treatments alone for treatment of opioid dependence. Cochrane Database Syst Rev 2011;10:CD004147.

126. **Fiellin DA, O'Connor PG, Chawarski M, et al. Methadone maintenance in primary care. JAMA 2001;286:1724–31.** *Opioid-dependent subjects (n = 47) on methadone for a year without evidence of illicit drug use were randomized to receive methadone at a primary care office or to continue their program. Illicit drug use over 6 months was the same in both groups (40–50%); subjects were more satisfied with office-based treatment.*

127. **Johnson RE, Chutuape MA, Strain EC, et al. A comparison of levomethadyl acetate, buprenorphine, and methadone for opioid dependence. N Engl J Med 2000;343:1290–7.** *Opioid dependent subjects (n = 55) were randomized to (1) levomethadyl acetate (3 times/week), (2) methadone (daily), (3) buprenorphine (3 times/week), or (4) low-dose methadone (essentially a control group). The three active treatments were roughly equivalent and better than low-dose methadone in terms of retention and abstinence (26–36% vs. 8%).*

128. Marsch LA, Bickel WK, Badger GJ, Jacobs EA. Buprenorphine treatment for opioid dependence: the relative efficacy of daily, twice and thrice weekly dosing. Drug Alcohol Depend 2005;77:195–204. *Opioid-dependent subjects (n = 134) were randomized to daily, thrice-weekly, or twice-weekly buprenorphine (dosage: 4–12 mg/day, mean ~7.5 mg). Of all subjects, 69% completed 24 weeks; drug use and addiction severity index improved equally in all three arms.*

129. Fudala PJ, Bridge TP, Herbert S, et al. Office-based treatment of opiate addiction with a sublingual-tablet formulation of buprenorphine and naloxone. N Engl J Med 2003;349:949–58. *Opioid-dependent subjects (n = 326) were randomized to (1) placebo, (2) buprenorphine, or (3) buprenorphine-naloxone. The trial had two parts: (1) 4-week placebo-controlled trial (16 mg/day), followed by (2) 48–52 weeks open-label efficacy trial. During the first phase, those in either buprenorphine arm had more opiate-negative urine drug tests (~20% vs. 6%) and improved self-rated health and well-being, but cocaine use in all arms was the same (~40%). Buprenorphine appeared to be safe and effective during the efficacy phase.*

130. Soeffing JM, Martin LD, Fingerhood MI, et al. Buprenorphine maintenance treatment in a primary care setting: outcomes at 1 year. J Subst Abuse Treat 2009;37:426–30.

131. Mattick RP, Breen C, Kimber J, Davoli M. Buprenorphine maintenance versus placebo or methadone maintenance for opioid dependence. Cochrane Database Syst Rev 2014;2:CD002207.

132. Mintzer MZ, Correia CJ, Strain EC. A dose-effect study of repeated administration of buprenorphine/naloxone on performance in opioid-dependent volunteers. Drug Alcohol Depend 2004;74:205–9.

133. Jones HE, Kaltenbach K, Heil SH, et al. Neonatal abstinence syndrome after methadone or buprenorphine exposure. N Engl J Med 2010;363:2320–31.

134. Fingerhood MI, King VL, Brooner RK, Rastegar DA. A comparison of characteristics and outcomes of opioid-dependent patients initiating office-based buprenorphine or methadone maintenance. Subst Abus 2014;35:122–6.

135. Lee JD, Vocci F, Fiellin DA. Unobserved "home" induction onto buprenorphine. J Addict Med 2014;8:299–308.

136. Leonardi C, Hanna N, Laurenzi P, et al. Multi-centre observational study of buprenorphine use in 32 Italian drug addiction centres. Drug Alcohol Depend 2008;94:125–32.

137. Cunningham CO, Giovanniello A, Kunins HV, et al. Buprenorphine treatment outcomes among opioid-dependent cocaine users and non-users. Am J Addict 2013;22:352–7.

138. Anonymous. Medical advisory and best-practices update. Richmond: Reckitt Benckiser Pharmaceuticals; 2006.

139. Correia CJ, Walsh SL, Bigelow GE, Strain EC. Effects associated with double-blind omission of buprenorphine/naloxone over a 98-h period. Psychopharmacology 2006;189:297–306.

140. Clark RE, Baxter JD, Barton BA, et al. The impact of prior authorization on buprenorphine dose, relapse rates, and cost for Massachusetts Medicaid beneficiaries with opioid dependence. Health Serv Res 2014;49:1964–79.

141. Fareed A, Vayalapaiil S, Casarella J, Drexler K. Effect of buprenorphine dose on treatment outcome. J Addict Dis 2012;31:8–18.

142. **Hser YI, Saxon AJ, Huang D, et al. Treatment retention among patients randomized to buprenorphine/naloxone compared to methadone in a multi-site trial. Addiction 2013;109:79–87.** *This trial randomized 1,269 opioid-dependent adults to buprenorphine (BUP) or methadone (MET). Both were directly administered; 24-week treatment completion was better with MET than with BUP (74% vs. 46%). There was a linear relationship between treatment retention and BUP dose up to 32 mg/ day. Subjects were not randomly assigned to their dose, and the paper does not explain how the dose was determined.*

143. Johanson CE, Arfken CL, di Menza S, Schuster CR. Diversion and abuse of buprenorphine: findings from national surveys of treatment patients and physicians. Drug Alcohol Depend 2012;120:190–5.

144. Genberg BL, Gillespie M, Schuster CR, et al. Prevalence and correlates of street-obtained buprenorphine use among current and former injectors in Baltimore, Maryland. Addict Behav 2013;38:2868–73.

145. Cicero TJ, Ellis MS, Surratt HL, Kurtz SP. Factors contributing to the rise of buprenorphine misuse: 2008–2013. Drug Alcohol Depend 2014;142:98–104.

146. Lofwall MR, Walsh SL. A review of buprenorphine diversion and misuse: the current evidence base and experiences from around the world. J Addict Med 2014;8:315–26.

147. Fox AD, Chamberlain A, Sohler NL, et al. Illicit buprenorphine use, interest in and access to buprenorphine treatment among syringe exchange participants. J Subst Abuse Treat 2015;48:112–16.

148. Sigmon SC, Wong CJ, Chausmer AL, et al. Evaluation of an injection depot formulation of buprenorphine: placebo comparison. Addiction 2004;99:1439–49.

149. Lin W, Casadonte P, Bigelow G, et al. Buprenorphine implants for treatment of opioid dependence: a randomized controlled trial. JAMA 2010;304:1576–83.

150. **Rosenthal RN, Ling W, Casadonte P, et al. Buprenorphine implants for treatment of opioid dependence: randomized comparison to placebo and sublingual buprenorphine/naloxone. Addiction 2013;108:2141–9.** *This study compared an 80 mg implant with 12–16 mg/day of sublingual buprenorphine. There was no significant difference in the percentage of urine tests negative for opioids. However, 22% of those randomized to an implant required additional implants, and 39% required sublingual "rescue medication" in addition to the implant.*

151. Fiellin DA, Pantalon MV, Chawarski MC, et al. Counseling plus buprenorphine-naloxone maintenance therapy for opioid dependence. N Engl J Med 2006;355:365–74.

152. Ling W, Hillhouse M, Ang A, et al. Comparison of behavioral treatment conditions in buprenorphine maintenance. Addiction 2013;108:1788–98.

153. Fram DH, Marmo J, Holden R. Naltrexone treatment—the problem of patient acceptance. J Subst Abuse Treat 1989;6:119–22.

154. San L, Pomarol G, Peri JM, et al. Follow-up after six month maintenance period on naltrexone versus placebo in heroin addicts. Br J Addict 1991;86:983–90.

155. **Sigmon SC, Dunn KE, Saulsgiver K, et al. A randomized, double-blind evaluation of buprenorphine taper duration in primary prescription opioid abusers. JAMA Psychiatry 2013;70:1347–54.** *This 12-week study compared three buprenorphine taper durations for 70 adults with prescription opioid dependence, followed by naltrexone: 1, 2, and 4 weeks. The 4-week taper was the most effective, with 50% in treatment and opioid abstinent compared to 17% with 2 weeks and 21% with 1 week.*

156. Schottenfeld RS, Chawarski MC, Mazlan M. Maintenance treatment with buprenorphine and naltrexone for heroin dependence in Malaysia: a randomised, double-blind, placebo-controlled trial. Lancet. 2008;371:2192–200.

157. Carroll KM, Ball SA, Nich C, et al. Targeting behavioral therapies to enhance naltrexone treatment of opioid dependence. Efficacy of

contingency management and significant other involvement. Arch Gen Psychiatry 2001;58:755–61.

158. Ling W, Wesson DR. Naltrexone treatment for addicted health care professionals: a collaborative private practice experience. J Clin Psychiatry 1984;45:46–8.

159. Washton AM, Gold MS, Potash AC. Naltrexone in addicted physicians and business executives. NIDA Res Monogr 1984;55:185–90.

160. **Cornish JW, Metzger D, Woody GE, et al. Naltrexone pharmacotherapy for opioid dependent federal probationers. J Subst Abuse Treat 1997;14:529–34.** *Volunteer probationers (51 of 300 eligible) were randomized to naltrexone or control; all received counseling. Over 6 months, those assigned to naltrexone had better treatment retention (52% vs. 33%); they were less likely to be reincarcerated (26% vs. 56%) or to have opiate-positive urine tests (8% vs. 30%).*

161. Minozzi S, Amato L, Vecchi S, et al. Oral naltrexone maintenance treatment for opioid dependence. Cochrane Database Syst Rev 2011;4:CD001333.

162. Hulse GK, Morris N, Arnold-Reed D, Tait RJ. Improving clinical outcomes in treating heroin dependence: a randomized, controlled trial of oral or implant naltrexone. Arch Gen Psychiatry 2009;66:1108–15.

163. Krupitsky E, Zvartau E, Blokhina E, et al. Randomized trial of long-acting sustained-release naltrexone implant vs. oral naltrexone or placebo for preventing relapse to opioid dependence. Arch Gen Psychiatry 2012;69:973–81.

164. **Comer SD, Sullivan MA, Yu E, et al. Injectable, sustained-release naltrexone for the treatment of opioid dependence. Arch Gen Psychiatry 2006;63:210–8.** *Heroin-dependent subjects (n = 60) were randomized to placebo or one of two doses of naltrexone (192 and 384 mg) and followed for 8 weeks. All received inpatient detoxification followed by 3 days of oral naltrexone, and only those who were "willing and able to tolerate" the drug were included. Those who received naltrexone had better treatment retention and were more likely to give opioid-negative urines.*

165. **Krupitsky E, Nunes EV, Ling W, et al. Injectable extended-release naltrexone for opioid dependence: a double-blind, placebo-controlled, multicenter randomised trial. Lancet 2011;377:1506–13.** *Opioid-dependent adults who were abstinent from opioids for at least 7 days (n = 250) received monthly XR-NTX or placebo; all were offered biweekly individual counseling. Completion of the 24-week*

study was higher with XR-NTX (53% vs. 38%), as was total confirmed abstinence (36% vs. 23%).

166. Lobmaier P, Kornør H, Kunøe N, Bjørndal A. Sustained-release naltrexone for opioid dependence. Cochrane Database of Syst Rev 2008;2:CD006140.

167. Larney S, Gowing L, Mattick RP, et al. A systematic review and meta-analysis of naltrexone implants for the treatment of opioid dependence. Drug Alcohol Rev 2014;33:115–28.

Tobacco and Nicotine

Background

Tobacco (*Nicotiana tabacum*) is a broad-leafed plant indigenous to the Americas that was used by natives and introduced to Europeans when they colonized the Western Hemisphere. Tobacco is now cultivated and used throughout the world. The leaves are most commonly dried and cured and smoked in the form of cigarettes or cigars. The leaves can also be chewed, or sniffed in the powdered form (snuff).

The psychoactive and habit-forming substance in tobacco is nicotine. Nicotine is an organic alkaloid that is found naturally in tobacco and in other plants in the *Solanaceae* (nightshade) family; this includes eggplant, tomato, potato, paprika, and peppers.

Epidemiology

According to the 2013 National Survey on Drug Use and Health (NSDUH),[1] 66.9 million Americans (26% of the population age 12 or older) reported current (past month) use of a tobacco product. Most of them (55.8 million; 21%) were current cigarette smokers, 12.4 million smoked cigars (4.7%), 8.8 million used smokeless tobacco (3.4%), and 2.3 million smoked tobacco in pipes (0.9%). Of the 55.8 million who were current cigarette smokers, 33.2 million (60%) were daily smokers.

Current tobacco use is highest among young adults aged 18–25 (37%) and is more prevalent among males (31%) than females (20%). Cigarette smoking rates decline with increasing level of education and are higher among unemployed than employed individuals.

The number of Americans who smoked for the first time declined from 3.3 million in 1997 to 1.9 million in 2002, but the rate has been relatively stable since then (2.1 million in 2013). About half of new cigarette smokers in 2013 initiated smoking prior to age 18.

Drug Effects

Acute Effects

Nicotine is the psychoactive component of tobacco and is responsible for its habit-forming effects. It can be absorbed through the lungs when smoked, and through the oral or nasal mucosa when chewed or sniffed. Nicotine is poorly absorbed from tobacco when ingested. The amount of nicotine absorbed from a cigarette will vary depending on a number of factors, including puff volume, number and intensity of puffs, as well as depth of inhalation. Nicotine has a half-life of about 2 hours in experienced users and is primarily metabolized by the liver into cotinine, which has a much longer half-life. Nicotine acts on selective acetylcholine receptors that are generally referred to as nicotine receptors and have a mild stimulating effect, leading to increased alertness, improved attention, and decreased appetite.[2]

Acute Toxicity and Overdose

While smoking is an important cause of morbidity and mortality worldwide, the risk of acute toxicity or overdose from tobacco is minimal, especially among regular users who have developed tolerance. There are reports of acute toxicity among children who have ingested tobacco or were exposed to nicotine patches. The nicotine liquid used in electronic cigarettes may pose a higher risk of toxicity.[3] Symptoms include nausea, vomiting, diarrhea, weakness, and dizziness.[4] There is no specific antidote to nicotine poisoning. Unlike most other substances, DSM-5 does not include "intoxication" for tobacco, but does provide for "unspecified tobacco-related disorder" (ICD-10 code: F17.209).[5]

Withdrawal

Regular users of tobacco experience a number of signs and symptoms with cessation. The DSM-5 criteria for tobacco withdrawal require the presence of four or more of the following signs or symptoms following cessation or reduction in regular tobacco use: (1) irritability, frustration, or anger, (2) anxiety, (3) difficulty concentrating, (4) increased appetite, (5) restlessness, (6) depressed mood, and (7) insomnia.[5] Tobacco users may also experience craving and slowing of heart rate.[6] The ICD-10 code for tobacco withdrawal is F17.203.

These symptoms are most intense during the first 4 days of abstinence and then decline gradually over a month. However, increased appetite and weight gain seem to persist beyond the first month—for as long as 6 months (or longer);[7] this is probably not a withdrawal symptom per se, but rather a consequence of withdrawing the appetite-suppressant effect of nicotine. The mean weight gain experienced after smoking cessation is about 3 kilograms[8] and is understandably a barrier to smoking cessation for some individuals.

Assessment

The simplest way to assess tobacco use is to ask the patient; this should be a routine part of the assessment of almost any patient. The DSM-5 criteria for "tobacco use disorder" are the same as for other substances; this is covered further in Chapter 1.[5] The ICD-10 code for this disorder is Z72.0 if mild and F17.200 if moderate-severe.

There are a number of biomarkers associated with smoking that may be used in studies to confirm smoking cessation, but they have limited clinical utility. Smokers have higher exhaled carbon monoxide concentrations when compared with healthy nonsmokers;[9] however, exhaled carbon monoxide is also increased with obstructive lung disease,[10] passive exposure to cigarette smoke,[11] and carbon monoxide poisoning. Serum carboxyhemoglobin levels are also elevated with smoking; in fact, this may falsely elevate smokers' pulse oximetry readings, as these devices cannot distinguish between oxyhemoglobin and carboxyhemoglobin.[12]

Cotinine is a metabolite of nicotine that can be detected in the serum, saliva, and urine of tobacco users and appears to be the best method to distinguish smokers from nonsmokers;[13] however, cotinine can also be detected in persons who are exposed to secondhand smoke.[14] Furthermore, cotinine does not differentiate between those using tobacco and those using nicotine replacement products; detection of the tobacco alkaloids anabasine and nornicotine in the urine is a more specific marker for tobacco use.[15] Smoking is also associated with higher serum thiocyanate levels due to trace amounts of cyanide in tobacco;[16] however, this test has a lower sensitivity than testing cotinine levels.[13]

Medical Complications

Smoking is one of the most significant preventable causes of death and disability. In 2000, an estimated 4.83 million premature deaths worldwide were attributable to smoking; the leading smoking-related causes of death were cardiovascular disease (1.69 million deaths), chronic obstructive pulmonary disease (COPD) (0.97 million), and lung cancer (0.85 million).[17] In the United States, roughly 40% of the deaths attributable to smoking are from cancer, 40% from cardiovascular disease, and 20% from respiratory disease.[18] The observed increase in mortality associated with smoking rises with the amount of cigarettes smoked and declines with cessation of smoking.[19] It remains a significant risk factor for mortality even among older individuals and decreases with cessation.[20]

An analysis of data from the Nurse's Health Study offers further insight into the health impact of smoking.[21] In this study, compared to those who never smoked, current smokers had an increased risk of mortality (adjusted hazard ratio [HR]: 2.8), as did former smokers (HR: 1.2). There was also a graded relationship between the number of cigarettes smoked and mortality among current smokers; compared to never smokers, those who smoked 1–14 cigarettes/day had an HR of 2.0, while those who smoked ≥35/day had an HR of 4.4. Those who started smoking at an earlier age (≤17) had an increased risk of mortality, particularly from lung cancer and COPD. The overall mortality for former smokers declined significantly within the first 5 years after quitting and decreased to the level of never smokers after 20 years. The risk of mortality from vascular disease declined more rapidly than that from other causes; the risk of lung cancer declined more slowly and was still significantly higher than that for never smokers 30 years after quitting.

Cigarettes harm not only smokers but also those around them. Exposure to "secondhand smoke" (sometimes referred to as "passive smoking") has been associated with an increased risk of cardiovascular disease,[22] respiratory illness,[23] COPD,[24] cognitive impairment,[25] and cancer (particularly lung cancer).[26] It is also associated with a reduced health-related quality of life,[27] particularly for individuals with heart failure.[28] While childhood exposure to tobacco smoke is associated with an increased risk of lung cancer in adulthood,[29] the cardiovascular risk appears to be associated with recent exposure, rather than lifetime cumulative exposure.[30] Childhood exposure to tobacco smoke is also associated with early-onset asthma among children with a genetic susceptibility.[31]

Establishment of smoke-free public and workplaces has been associated with reductions in cardiovascular disease[32,33] and improved health of employees, especially those with asthma.[34] The benefit appears to extend beyond those with occupational exposure, most notably children with asthma.[35]

Smoking cessation interventions have been shown to substantially reduce the subsequent mortality of smokers.[36] Furthermore, there is some evidence that these interventions are more effective when delivered to those with a serious complication from smoking.[37] This reinforces the importance of recognizing these connections and intervening to help smokers quit their habit.

Smoking is also a significant contributor to chronic illness. It has been estimated that in the United States, 6.9 million adults have at least one smoking-attributable medical condition, the most common (by far) being chronic obstructive lung disease, followed by coronary artery disease, diabetes mellitus, stroke, and cancer.[38] Specific medical conditions associated with smoking are summarized in Box 7.1 and covered briefly in the following section.

Cutaneous Complications

Smoking is associated with premature aging of the skin and increased facial wrinkling. These changes are similar to those seen with excessive sun exposure and are greatly increased by

BOX 7.1 Medical Complications Associated with Tobacco Use

Cutaneous

Premature aging and wrinkling of facial skin
Cutaneous squamous cell carcinoma

Head and Neck

Cataracts
Macular degeneration
Periodontal disease
Squamous cell carcinoma of the head and neck
Oropharyngeal cancer

Pulmonary

Chronic obstructive pulmonary disease (emphysema)
Lung cancer
Respiratory infections (tuberculosis, pneumonia, influenza)

Cardiovascular

Coronary artery disease
Peripheral vascular disease
Thromboangiitis obliterans
Aortic aneurysms

Gastrointestinal

Esophageal cancer
Pancreatic cancer
Stomach cancer
Colorectal cancer
Anal cancer
Peptic ulcer disease
Gastroesophageal reflux

Renal

Renal carcinoma
Chronic kidney disease
Renovascular disease

Genitourinary

Bladder cancer
Cervical cancer
Erectile dysfunction

Neuromuscular

Stroke
Rheumatoid arthritis

the combination of smoking and sun exposure.[39] Smoking is also associated with an increased risk of cutaneous squamous cell carcinoma, but not basal cell carcinoma or melanoma.[40] Furthermore, smoking has been found to be associated with an increased risk of psoriasis.[41]

Head and Neck Complications

Individuals who smoke tobacco are at higher risk for periodontal disease and tooth loss; those who chew tobacco can develop gingival recession and tooth abrasion.[42] The most serious head and neck complications associated with tobacco use are malignancies. Tobacco smoking is associated with an increased risk of squamous cell carcinoma of the head and neck. In one study, when compared with those who never smoked, those who ever smoked had a four-fold higher risk and active smokers had a 6.5 times higher risk; this is further increased with concomitant alcohol use—heavy drinkers who smoked had a 22-fold higher risk than that of nonsmokers who did not drink or drank moderately.[43] Furthermore, among smokers who do develop head and neck cancer, continued smoking is associated with poorer therapeutic outcomes.[44] The increased risk of oropharyngeal squamous cell cancers in smokers may be at least partly due to human papilloma virus (HPV) infection; one cross-sectional study found an association between tobacco use and oral HPV-16 prevalence.[45]

Some studies have found an association between chewing tobacco and oral and pharyngeal cancers.[46] However, in a Swedish study, no such association was found; this may be due to differences in the preparation of chewing tobacco used in Sweden (also known as "snus").[43]

Smokers also experience higher rates of ocular complications, including cataracts[47] and macular degeneration.[48]

Pulmonary Complications

Chronic Obstructive Pulmonary Disease

Smoking is the main risk factor for COPD, which is one of the most important causes of morbidity and mortality attributable to smoking.[49] The prevalence of COPD among smokers in published studies varies depending on the length of exposure and the definition of COPD. In a 25-year prospective cohort study, approximately a quarter of continuous smokers developed moderate to severe COPD;[50] in another study, about a half of elderly (76–77 years old) smokers were found to have COPD.[51] Pipe and cigar smoking are also associated with obstructive lung disease.[52] For those who have reversible airway obstruction (i.e., asthma), smoking increases the severity of the illness[53] and impairs their response to anti-inflammatory therapy.[54]

Smoking invariably causes airway inflammation, but those who go on to develop COPD seem to have a more pronounced response, which leads to lung destruction and airway obstruction.[55] There are probably a number of genetic factors that account for the variability of the effect of smoking on lung function. The best known of these is alpha-1 antitrypsin deficiency, which, in its homozygous form, leads to severe COPD at a young age in smokers;[56] heterozygotes appear to have a slightly increased risk of developing COPD.[57] There are other genetic variants associated with a reduced risk of COPD among smokers.[58]

Quitting smoking will slow the decline in lung function, though this benefit may be partly offset by the deleterious effects of weight gain on lung function.[59] Nevertheless, in a cohort study of persons with severe COPD, recent smoking (i.e., smoking after enrollment) was the strongest predictor of mortality, indicating that smoking cessation will improve survival, even among those with severe disease.[60]

Lung Cancer

Numerous studies have shown a strong association between smoking and all types of lung cancer; this risk increases with duration and number of cigarettes smoked.[61] Moreover, active smoking at the time of diagnosis of lung cancer is associated with shortened survival.[62] Smokers who develop chronic lung disease appear to be at particularly high risk for lung cancer.[63] Carriers of the alpha-1 antitrypsin deficiency gene (heterozygotes) have also been found to be at increased risk for lung cancer.[64] Women smokers appear to be at higher risk for lung cancer than their male counterparts but have a better chance of survival.[65] The risk of lung cancer appears to be highest for users of unfiltered high-tar brands, but there does not seem to be much difference between other types of cigarettes.[66] There is some evidence that cutting down on smoking reduces the risk of lung cancer, albeit to a lesser extent than quitting.[67]

Respiratory Infections

Smoking is associated with an increased risk of respiratory infections. Smoking increases the risk of acquiring influenza and the severity of the illness among those who acquire it.[68] In a population-based case-control study in Spain, the risk of pneumonia among smokers was double that of nonsmokers; this accounted for an estimated

32% of cases.[69] A case-control study in North America found that smoking was the strongest independent risk factor for invasive pneumococcal disease among immunocompetent adults.[70] Smoking is also associated with an increased risk of tuberculosis.[71]

Cardiovascular Complications

Coronary Artery Disease

Coronary heart disease is the leading cause of death attributable to smoking. Smoking is one of the major risk factors for heart disease,[72] and the risk increases in a dose-dependent fashion with the number of cigarettes smoked.[73] There are a number of physiological effects that probably account for this association, including endothelial impairment[74] and adverse effects on lipid profiles.[75] Among smokers who suffer a myocardial infarction, continuing to smoke increases their risk for recurrent events; for those who quit, their risk declines to a rate similar to nonsmokers about 3–5 years after quitting.[76] Moreover, current smokers who have coronary artery disease are at increased risk of sudden cardiac death, while those who quit smoking have a risk comparable to those who never smoked.[77] As noted earlier, the implementation of smoke-free legislation has been associated with a decline in admissions for acute coronary syndrome, even among those who were not smokers.[33]

Use of smokeless tobacco is also associated with an increased cardiovascular risk,[78] but it appears to be lower than with cigarette smoking.[79] Nonetheless, in an observational study of snus users who suffered a myocardial infarction, those who quit using snus had a subsequent mortality risk that was half that of those who did not quit.[80]

Peripheral Vascular Disease

Peripheral vascular disease is also strongly associated with smoking in a dose-dependent fashion;[81] in fact, it appears to be the strongest risk factor for this condition.[82] There is also a strong association between smoking and thromboangiitis obliterans (Buerger's disease), and the most effective way to prevent limb loss in this devastating disease is to quit smoking.[83]

Aortic Aneurysm

Smoking is strongly associated with aortic aneurysms; in fact, the increased relative risk is even greater than that seen with smoking and coronary artery disease.[84]

Retroperitoneal Fibrosis

Retroperitoneal fibrosis is a rare condition characterized by development of fibrous and inflammatory tissue that spreads from the abdominal aorta and iliac arteries to the surrounding retroperitoneum and may cause obstruction of the ureters. It is associated with smoking, and there appears to be a multiplicative effect on the risk when smoking is combined with asbestos exposure.[85]

Gastrointestinal Complications

Smoking is associated with a number of malignancies of the gastrointestinal tract. The association is strongest for esophageal carcinoma (squamous[86] and adenocarcinoma[87]) and pancreatic cancer.[88] Cigarette smoking has also been associated with colorectal cancer incidence and mortality[89] and may account for approximately 12% of colorectal cancer deaths.[90] Use of cigarettes and other tobacco products also appears to be associated with stomach cancers.[91] Moreover, smoking is associated with a four-fold increased risk of anal carcinoma among men and women.[92]

Smokers are also at increased risk for peptic ulcer disease; there appears to be a synergistic effect with concomitant *Helicobacter pylori* infection that greatly increases this risk.[93] Smoking is also associated with an increased risk of gastroesophageal reflux disease.[94] Smokers are likewise at increased risk of developing Crohn's disease. On the other hand, active smoking is associated with a *reduced* risk of ulcerative colitis,[95] and nicotine may be beneficial for the prevention and treatment of this condition.[96]

Smokers have been found to be at increased risk for acute and chronic pancreatitis in cohort[97] and case-control studies,[98] even when alcohol use is taken into account. In these studies, there appeared to be a dose–response relationship; however, in the cohort study, both current and former smokers were at increased risk for pancreatitis (particularly acute pancreatitis), suggesting the presence of an unmeasured confounder.

Renal Complications

A number of studies suggest that smoking is associated with an accelerated decline in renal function, especially among diabetics[99] and the elderly.[100] Given the association between smoking and vascular disease elsewhere in the body, it is not surprising that smoking is also associated with renovascular disease.[101] Smokers are also at increased risk for renal cell carcinoma.[102]

Genitourinary Complications

Smoking increases the risk of erectile dysfunction among men,[103] presumably due to its effects on endothelial function.[104] It is also associated with an increased risk of bladder cancer.[105] Smoking does not appear to be a risk factor for prostate cancer,[106] but smoking at the time of prostate cancer diagnosis is associated with an increased risk of recurrence and prostate cancer mortality.[107]

Furthermore, smoking is associated with an increased risk of cervical cancer among women who are infected with oncogenic human papillomaviruses.[108] By contrast, smoking has not been found to increase the risk of ovarian cancer[21] and is associated with a *reduced* risk of endometrial cancer.[109]

Breast Cancer

Analysis of data from the Nurse's Health Study found that smoking is associated with a modest increase in risk of breast cancer (hazard ratio of 1.06); the risk increased with younger age at initiation as well as longer duration and more pack-years of smoking.[110]

Endocrine Complications

A 2007 systematic review found an association between smoking and type II diabetes. The overall relative risk compared to that of nonsmokers was 1.4, and there appeared to be a dose–response phenomenon, with heavy smokers having a higher relative risk (1.7) than lighter smokers (1.3).[111]

Neuromuscular Complications

Smokers are at increased risk for stroke[112] and have poorer outcomes if they require carotid endarterectomy.[113] The data on smoking and the risk of dementia are mixed. Earlier (case-control) studies suggested that smoking might actually reduce the risk of Alzheimer's disease,[114] whereas more recent prospective studies have found an increased risk[115,116] or no significant difference in risk.[117]

Smokers are at increased risk for developing multiple sclerosis[118] and the disease tends to progress more rapidly in smokers.[119]

Smokers also appear to be at increased risk for rheumatoid arthritis; in the Nurse's Health Study, the risk of rheumatoid arthritis was almost 50% higher among current and previous smokers than among those who never smoked.[120] Furthermore, smoking is also associated with an increase in disease activity among those with rheumatoid arthritis.[121]

Smokers have been found to have lower vitamin C levels, even when dietary intake is taken into account.[122] Severe and prolonged hypovitaminosis C can lead to scurvy, which may be manifested in joint swelling and pain, rash (petechiae, ecchymoses, and corkscrew hairs), lower extremity edema, gingival swelling, and pain.[123]

Psychiatric Complications

Smokers experience higher rates of psychological distress[124] and are at increased risk for a number of chronic psychiatric conditions.[125]

Psychiatric co-occurring disorders are covered further in Chapter 15. While tobacco users are often motivated by the positive psychoactive effects of nicotine and withdrawal can cause unpleasant psychiatric symptoms, smoking cessation is associated with an improvement in anxiety and depression.[126]

Pregnancy

Women smokers are more likely to be infertile, and those who undergo in vitro fertilization (IVF) are less likely to become pregnant.[127] Among those women who do become pregnant, smoking has been associated with a number of deleterious outcomes, including spontaneous abortion, preterm delivery, and low birth weight.[128,129] Smoking also increases the risk for placenta previa, abruptio placenta, ectopic pregnancy, and preterm premature rupture of the membrane.[130] The children of mothers who smoke are also at increased risk for sudden infant death syndrome (SIDS).[128]

Smoking by pregnant women is associated with poorer lung function in their newborn infants; the deleterious effects may persist into adulthood.[131] Providing pregnant smokers with vitamin C supplementation may improve newborn pulmonary function, at least in the short term.[132]

Treatment

Given the tremendous health burden of smoking, efforts to help smokers quit are a public health priority. The United States Preventive Services Task Force recommends that healthcare providers "ask all adults about tobacco use and provide tobacco cessation interventions for those who use tobacco products"; this is a grade A recommendation.[133] A number of studies have shown that quitting smoking improves health outcomes.[134] Although there is evidence that reducing smoking is beneficial, the goal of treatment is smoking cessation. Fortunately, a number of treatment modalities have been shown to be effective in well-designed trials, including physician advice, telephone counseling, group and individual therapy, as well as pharmacological interventions such as nicotine replacement, antidepressants (buproprion and nortriptyline), and varenicline. Unfortunately, no single intervention has yet proven to be effective for the majority of smokers. The U.S. Department of Health and Human Services has issued guidelines on treating tobacco use and dependence that were updated in 2008 and can be accessed at www.guideline.gov.[135]

While the guidelines recommend setting a "quit date" to abruptly stop, a strategy of gradually reducing smoking may be equally effective. A 2012 Cochrane review concluded that both approaches produce comparable quit rates, regardless of whether pharmacotherapy was used.[136]

Prevention

Preventing youth from initiating smoking is a public health priority. School-based programs are one way of deterring tobacco use. A 2013 Cochrane review concluded that programs that combine social competence and social influences curricula are effective (odds ratio 0.49), but programs limited to information are not effective.[137] Providing prizes or incentives to youth to prevent smoking has not been shown to be effective.[138]

Population-Based Interventions

There are a number of population-based interventions that have been found to decrease smoking rates; these include mass media campaigns, increasing the cost of cigarettes, banning smoke in public spaces, and providing financial incentives to quit. Mass media campaigns appear to be effective at changing smoking behavior in adults.[139] Increasing the cost of cigarettes through taxation appears to reduce smoking rates, particularly among adolescents.[140] Mandating smoke-free workplaces encourages smokers to cut down on cigarette use and to quit smoking.[141] A 2009 study found that providing financial incentive to employees also significantly increases smoking cessation rates.[142]

Printed Self-Help Materials

Providing smokers with printed educational materials to help them quit smoking is a simple intervention and easy to implement but, unfortunately, appears to have minimal effect. A 2014 Cochrane review of 74 trials concluded that "standard, print-based self-help materials increase quit rates compared with no intervention, but the effect is likely to be small."[143]

Counseling and Other Psychosocial Interventions

A number of studies suggest that physician advice can help individuals quit smoking. Guidelines for counseling tobacco users are summarized in Box 7.2. A 2013 Cochrane review of 42 trials concluded

---

BOX 7.2 Suggested Guidelines for Counseling Tobacco Users

1. ASK—Identify all tobacco users at every visit.
   - Expand vital signs to include tobacco use or use an alternative universal identification system.
2. ADVISE—Strongly urge all tobacco users to quit.
Advice should be:
   - *Clear*—"I think it is important for you to quit smoking now and I can help you." "Cutting down while you are ill is not enough."
   - *Strong*—"As your clinician, I need you to know that quitting smoking is the most important thing you can do to protect your health now and in the future."
   - *Personalized*—Tie tobacco use to:
     - Current health or illness
     - Social and economic costs
     - Motivation level and readiness to quit
     - Impact of tobacco use on children and others in household

3. ASSESS—Determine willingness to make a quit attempt.
   - If the patient is willing to make a quit attempt at this time, provide assistance.
   - If the patient will participate in an intensive treatment, deliver such treatment or refer to an intensive intervention.
   - If the patient clearly states that he or she is unwilling to make a quit attempt, provide motivational intervention.
   - If the patient is a member of a special population (e.g., adolescent, pregnant, ethnic minority) consider providing additional information.
4. ASSIST—Aid the patient in quitting.
   - *Set a quit date*—ideally, this should be within 2 weeks.
   - *Tell* family, friends, and coworkers about quitting and request understanding and support.
   - *Anticipate* challenges to planned quit attempt, particularly during the critical first few weeks. These include nicotine withdrawal symptoms.
   - *Remove* tobacco products from your environment. Prior to quitting, avoid smoking in places where you spend a lot of time (e.g., home, car, work).
5. ARRANGE—Schedule follow-up contact.
   - Can be done in person or by telephone
   - Preferably within the first week after quit day

Adapted from Fiore MC, Bailey WC, Cohen SJ, et al. *Treating Tobacco Use and Dependence.* Quick Reference Guide for Clinicians. Rockville, MD: U.S. Department of Health and Human Services. Public Health Service; October 2000.

that physician advice "has a small effect on smoking cessation."[144] Analysis of pooled data from 17 trials comparing brief advice with no advice found a small increase in cessation (relative risk 1.7); this translates to an absolute increase in cessation rate of 1–3%. More intensive advice appeared to be a little better than minimal advice (relative risk 1.4). Nurse-delivered counseling and education also appears to have a small but significant benefit.[145] Finally, telephone counseling has been shown to be beneficial, particularly when subjects receive multiple sessions of call-back counseling.[146]

Intensive counseling interventions provided to hospitalized patients appear to be effective if they are continued with contacts for at least 1 month after discharge. Providing nicotine replacement in addition to intensive counseling increases smoking cessation rates, and varenicline may also be effective.[147]

Group behavioral therapy is a commonly used treatment for smoking and other addictions. The approaches used in these groups vary widely, but often include components such as motivational enhancement, advice on relapse prevention, coping skills, relaxation techniques, stress management, and cognitive-behavioral therapy. A 2005 Cochrane review of this treatment modality concluded that they are "better than self-help and other less intensive interventions." However, the authors found that there is "not enough evidence to support the use of particular psychological components in a programme beyond the support and skills training normally included."[148]

Individual counseling generally uses a variety of approaches analogous to group behavioral therapy in a one-on-one setting. A number of studies have shown this approach to be effective, but it has not been shown to be any more effective than group therapy.[149]

An emerging approach is the use of Internet-based smoking cessation interventions; a 2013 Cochrane review concluded that some "can assist smoking cessation at 6 months or longer, particularly those which are interactive and tailored to individuals. However, the trials that compared Internet interventions with usual care or self help did not show consistent effects and were at risk of bias."[150]

Pharmacological Treatment

While advice to quit smoking is important and may induce some to quit, it is usually not sufficient, and smokers who wish to quit should be offered assistance in the form of pharmacotherapy. This is supported by a recent observational study of 2,325 smokers, which found that those who were offered pharmacotherapy were more likely to quit than those who were offered advice alone.[151] There are a number of medications that have been found to help smokers quit, and providing counseling and support enhances their effectiveness. A 2013 Cochrane review concluded that "providing behavioral support in person or via telephone for people using pharmacotherapy to stop smoking has a small but important effect."[152]

Nicotine Replacement

Numerous studies have shown that nicotine replacement therapy is effective for helping individuals quit smoking.[153] Overall, the provision of nicotine replacement increases smoking cessation rates by about 60%; however, since smoking cessation rates with no treatment are about 10%, this translates into an absolute increase of 6%, meaning that, on average, one additional smoker would quit out of 16 treated. Most of these studies measured outcomes 6–12 months after treatment; there are few data on longer-term outcomes.

Nicotine replacement can be given in a variety of forms, including gum, patches, nasal spray, inhaler, or sublingual tablet/lozenge. Table 7.1 gives additional information on available nicotine replacement products. The length of treatment varies in published studies, but 8–12 weeks is typical. In one trial, extending the duration of treatment from 8 to 24 weeks was associated with higher abstinence rates at week 24, but not at 52 weeks.[154] Abstinence during the first 2 weeks of treatment (particularly week 2) appears to be the best predictor of longer-term abstinence.[155]

No form of nicotine replacement therapy has been shown to be more effective than any other. However, use of higher-dose nicotine gum (4 mg) appears to be more effective for highly dependent smokers (defined by number of cigarettes smoked and time to first cigarette in the morning). Likewise, higher-dose patches may be more effective for heavy smokers; the serum nicotine levels achieved with

TABLE 7.1 Nicotine Replacement Products*

Type	Brand Names	Dosage Forms	Usual Dosage
Gum	Nicorette	2 mg, 4 mg	<25 cigs/day, use 2 mg; >25 cigs/day, use 4 mg Chew every 1–2 hours first 6 weeks, then taper
Lozenge	Commit	2 mg, 4 mg	Begin with 4 mg dose if 1st cigarette is within 30 min of waking. Dissolve lozenge in mouth every 1–2 hours for first 6 weeks, then taper
Patch	Nicoderm CQ, Nicotrol patch	7, 14, & 21 mg/24hr (Nicoderm) 5, 10, & 15 mg/24hr (Nicotrol)	If smoking >10 cigs/day, apply highest dose patch daily for 6 weeks, then next lower doses daily for 2 weeks, each sequentially
Nasal spray	Nicotrol nasal spray	10 mL bottle (10 mg/mL)	2–4 sprays per hour, up to 80/day Can taper gradually, do not use for >3 months
Inhaler	Nicotrol inhaler	10 mg cartridge (4 mg nicotine)	Puff or inhale deeply for up to 20 min, 6–16 cartridges/day for 3–6 weeks, then taper; do not use for >6 months

*Complied from manufacturer's instructions.

a 22 mg patch are significantly lower than those found in most smokers, and a 44 mg dose may be closer to what smokers are used to, especially heavy smokers (>31 cigarettes/day).[156] Combining a patch with an as-needed rapid delivery form (e.g., lozenge, spray, gum) modestly improves successful quitting rates over use of a single type.[153]

Electronic Cigarettes

Electronic cigarettes, or e-cigarettes, are battery-powered devices that deliver a nicotine vapor that is inhaled by the user. They are typically marketed as a safer alternative for smokers, one that can be used in settings where smoking cigarettes is prohibited. In one study of 300 smokers who did not intend to quit, use of e-cigarettes was associated with a significant reduction in cigarette smoking; however, there was no significant difference between those who received e-cigarettes with nicotine and those who received e-cigarettes that contained placebo.[157] In another study of 657 smokers who wanted to quit, 6-month verified abstinence was somewhat higher with an e-cigarette (7.3%) than with a nicotine patch (5.8%) or placebo e-cigarette (4.1%), but these differences were not statistically significant.[158] One observational study of smokers reported that use of e-cigarettes was not associated with quitting or cutting down on cigarette use,[159] while in a survey of smokers who attempted to quit without professional help, those who used e-cigarettes were more likely to be successful than those who tried over-the-counter nicotine replacement or no aid.[160]

There have been no adverse effects noted in the trials, but the long-term safety of e-cigarettes has not been established. There are toxic substances in the vapor, but at lower levels than found in tobacco smoke.[161]

Varenicline

Varenicline is a nicotinic acetylcholine receptor partial agonist, which works by reducing the craving for nicotine while blocking the effect of smoked nicotine. A number of studies have shown that it is effective for helping smokers quit and appears to be more effective than bupropion,[162,163] but has not been shown to be more effective than nicotine replacement therapy.[164] The usual dosage is 1 mg twice daily; in order to minimize side effects, the dose is generally titrated up from 0.5 mg daily for 3 days, then 0.5 mg twice daily for 3 days, followed by 1 mg twice daily; the manufacturer provides a "starter pack" to facilitate this. If the full dose is not tolerated, a dosage of 1 mg daily or 0.5 mg twice daily also appears to be effective. For smokers who are able to achieve abstinence on varenicline, continuation of treatment beyond 12 weeks can help them maintain abstinence.[165] For smokers who are unable to quit with the standard dose, using a higher dose of varenicline does not improve smoking cessation rates.[166]

Nausea was the most common side effect reported in studies of varenicline (about 30% of subjects), but was mild and diminished over time. Moreover, nausea infrequently led to discontinuation in these studies and was less of a problem if the dose was titrated up.[167] There have been reports of suicidal behavior associated with varenicline use, but a cohort study of 80,660 smokers who were prescribed a smoking cessation product found no increase in risk of fatal or nonfatal self-harm associated with varenicline when compared with nicotine replacement or bupropion.[168] Moreover, in a clinical trial of 525 smokers with past or stably treated current depression, varenicline was effective and was not associated with worsening depression or anxiety.[169]

Cytisine

Varenicline is derived from cytisine, an alkaloid found in a number of shrubs and small trees, and has been used for many years as a treatment for tobacco dependence, mainly in Eastern Europe. Like varenicline, it is a nicotine receptor partial agonist and has been shown to be effective for smoking cessation[164,170] and, in one study, more effective than nicotine replacement.[171] The most common side effects are nausea and sleep disorders. It is not available in the United States at this time.

Antidepressants

The antidepressants bupropion and nortriptyline have proven to be effective treatments for smoking cessation, while other antidepressants, including selective serotonin reuptake inhibitors and venlafaxine, have not been shown to be effective.[172] Bupropion is FDA approved for smoking cessation and is generally considered to be the treatment of choice because of the larger number of studies done on it. Antidepressants appear to be more effective than nicotine replacement alone, but it has not been established that the addition of nicotine replacement to antidepressants is more effective than antidepressants alone.[173] Longer-term use of antidepressants (a year or longer) may reduce relapse rates.

The dosage of nortriptyline used in the trials ranged from 50–150 mg/day (most used 75 mg), the dosage of bupropion used was 150–300 mg/day (most used 300 mg/day in two divided doses). The length of treatment ranged from 6 weeks to a year (or longer) in the studies conducted; 3 months was a typical duration. There is some evidence that continuing antidepressant therapy for up to a year after cessation helps reduce the risk of relapse, but continuing these agents beyond a year has not be shown to be helpful. Nortriptyline may cause dry mouth and sedation. Bupropion can cause insomnia and headaches, and there is a small risk of seizures.

Clonidine

Some studies have reported improved smoking cessation rates with clonidine,[174] while other studies have found no benefit.[175] A 2004 Cochrane review that included six trials concluded that "clonidine is effective in promoting smoking cessation," but did note that "there are potential sources of bias" and that "side effects limit the usefulness of clonidine for smoking cessation."[176]

Combination Treatments

There have been a few studies looking at the efficacy of combinations of pharmacotherapies. In one study, the combination of bupropion with nicotine patch was a little more effective than bupropion alone, but this difference was not statistically significant.[173] The combination of varenicline and bupropion may offer some benefits; in one study, it improved 12-week abstinence when compared to varenicline alone, but 1-year abstinence was not significantly better.[177] Combining a nicotine patch with varenicline also appears to improve smoking cessation rates over varenicline alone; while a small study failed to show a significant improvement in smoking cessation rates,[178] a subsequent larger study did show a significant improvement.[179]

Acupuncture and Related Interventions

There are a number of related interventions that have been advocated for smoking cessation, including acupuncture, acupressure, laser therapy, and electrostimulation. Some studies of auricular acupuncture have reported modestly reduced smoking rates.[180] However, a recent randomized controlled trial of acupuncture for smoking cessation failed to show a sustained effect.[181] Furthermore, a 2014 Cochrane review of 38 studies of acupuncture and related techniques for smoking cessation concluded that the evidence suggests a possible short-term effect from acupuncture, acupressure, or laser stimulation, but there is no clear evidence of a sustained benefit.[182]

Hypnosis

Some studies have reported impressive smoking cessation results with hypnosis.[183] However, a 2010 Cochrane review of 11 studies of hypnotherapy concluded that they "have not shown that hypnotherapy has a greater effect on 6-month quit rates than other interventions or no treatment."[184]

Tobacco and Other Substance Dependence

Persons who are dependent on alcohol and illicit drugs often smoke as well. Traditionally, most treatment programs focus on the alcohol or illicit drug use before addressing smoking. There are limited data to support this approach, but in a clinical trial of alcoholics who were also smokers, those who received concurrent alcoholism treatment and smoking cessation were no more likely to quit smoking and had

TABLE 7.2 Summary of Smoking Cessation Studies

Intervention	Studies	Outcomes
Self-help educational materials	RCTs Meta-analysis	Small effect (RR: 1.2)
Physician advice	RCTs Meta-analysis	Effective (RR: 1.7); more intensive advice a little more effective
Group counseling	RCTs Meta-analysis	Effective (OR: 2.2)
Individual counseling	RCTs Meta-analysis	Effective (OR: 1.6)
Telephone counseling	RCTs Meta-analysis	Effective (RR: 1.4)
Nicotine replacement	RCTs Meta-analysis	Effective (RR: 1.6)
Electronic cigarettes	RCTs	Possibly effective
Varenicline	RCTs Meta-analysis	Effective (RR: 2.3); more effective than bupropion, but not NRT
Cytisine	RCTs Meta-analysis	Effective (RR: 4.0)
Bupropion	RCTs Meta-analysis	Effective (RR: 1.6)
Nortriptyline	RCTs Meta-analysis	Effective (RR: 2.0), not significantly better than bupropion
Clonidine	RCTs Meta-analysis	Effective (RR: 1.6), but side effects are common

(*continued*)

TABLE 7.2 (Continued)

Intervention	Studies	Outcomes
Hypnosis	RCTs Meta-analysis	Not effective
Acupuncture	RCTs Meta-analysis	Not effective

See text for references and more details.

RCT: randomized controlled trial; RR: relative risk of smoking cessation with intervention compared to placebo or no intervention; OR: odds ratio—figures are from Cochrane meta-analyses.

poorer drinking outcomes compared with those who received smoking cessation 6 months after their alcohol treatment[185]

A summary of smoking cessation studies is provided in (Table 7.2).

Notes

1. Substance Abuse and Mental Health Services Administration. *Results from the 2013 National Survey on Drug Use and Health: National Findings*, NSDUH Series H-48, HHS Publication No. (SMA) 14-4863. Rockville, MD: Substance Abuse and Mental Health Services Administration; 2014.

2. Dani JA, Kosten TR, Benowitz NL. The pharmacology of nicotine and tobacco. In Ries RK, Fiellin DA, Miller SC, Saitz R, eds. *The ASAM Principles of Addiction Medicine*, 5th ed. Philadelphia: Wolters Kluwer; 2014:201–16.

3. Chatham-Stephens K, Law R, Taylor E, et al. Notes from the field: calls to poison centers for exposures to electronic cigarettes—United States, September 2010–February 2014. MMWR Morbid Mortal Wkly Rep 2014;63:292–3.

4. Woolf A, Burkhart K, Caraccio T, Litovitz T. Childhood poisoning involving transdermal nicotine patches. Pediatrics 1997;99:E4.

5. American Psychiatric Association. (2013). *Diagnostic and Statistical Manual of Mental Disorders*, Fifth Edition. Arlington, VA: American Psychiatric Publishing.

6. Hughes JR, Hatsukami D. Signs and symptoms of tobacco withdrawal. Arch Gen Psychiatry 1986;43:289–94.

7. Hughes JR, Gust SW, Skoog K, et al. Symptoms of tobacco withdrawal: a replication and extension. Arch Gen Psychiatry 1991;48:52–9.

8. Williamson DF, Madans J, Anda RF, et al. Smoking cessation and severity of weight gain in a national cohort. N Engl J Med 1991;324:739–45.

9. Middleton ET, Morice AH. Breath carbon monoxide as an indication of smoking habit. Chest 2000;117:758–63.

10. Montuschi P, Kharitonov SA, Barnes PJ. Exhaled carbon monoxide and nitric oxide in COPD. Chest 2001;120:496–501.

11. Ece A, Gurkan F, Haspolat K, et al. Passive smoking and expired carbon monoxide concentrations in healthy and asthmatic children. Allergol Immunopathol 2000;28:255–60.

12. Glass KL, Dillard TA, Phillips YY, et al. Pulse oximetry correction for smoking exposure. Mil Med 1996;161:273–6.

13. Jarvis MJ, Tunstall-Pedoe H, Feyerabend C, et al. Comparison of tests used to distinguish smokers from nonsmokers. Am J Public Health 1987;77:1435–8.

14. Repace J, Hughes E, Benowitz N. Exposure to second-hand smoke air pollution assessed from bar patrons' urinary cotinine. Nicotine Tob Res 2006;8:701–11.

15. Moyer TP, Charlson JR, Enger RJ, et al. Simultaneous analysis of nicotine, nicotine metabolites, and tobacco alkaloids in serum or urine by tandem mass spectrometry, with clinically relevant metabolic profiles. Clin Chem 2002;48:1460–71.

16. Vogt TM, Selvin S, Widdowson G, Hulley SB. Expired air carbon monoxide and serum thiocyanate as objective measures of cigarette exposure. Am J Public Health 1977;67:545–9.

17. Ezzati M, Lopez AD. Estimates of global mortality attributable to smoking in 2000. Lancet 2003;362:847–52.

18. Thun MJ, Apicella LF, Henley SJ. Smoking vs. other risk factors as the cause of smoking-attributable deaths. Confounding in the courtroom. JAMA 2000;284:706–12.

19. Vollset SE, Tverdal A, Gjessing HK. Smoking and deaths between 40 and 70 years of age in women and men. Ann Intern Med 2006;144:381–9.

20. Gellert C, Schottker B, Brenner B. Smoking and all-cause mortality in older people. Arch Intern Med 2012;172:837–44.

21. Kenfield SA, Stampfer MJ, Rosner BA, Colditz GA. Smoking and smoking cessation in relation to mortality in women. JAMA 2008;299:2037–47.

22. Barnoya J, Glantz SA. Cardiovascular effects of secondhand smoke: nearly as large as smoking. Circulation 2005;111:2684–98.

23. Janson C, Chinn S, Jarvis D, et al. Effect of passive smoking on respiratory symptoms, bronchial responsiveness, lung function, and total serum IgE in the European Community Respiratory Health Survey: a cross-sectional study. Lancet 2001;358:2103–9.

24. Yin P, Cheng KK, Lam KH, et al. Passive smoking exposure and risk of COPD among adults in China: the Guangzhou Biobank Cohort Study. Lancet 2007;370:751–7.

25. Chen R, Zhang D, Chen Y, et al. Passive smoking and risk of cognitive impairment in women who never smoke. Arch Intern Med 2012;172:271–3.

26. Wen W, Shu XO, Gao YT, et al. Environmental tobacco smoke and mortality in Chinese women who have never smoked: prospective cohort study. BMJ 2006;333:376.

27. Bridevaux PO, Cornuz J, Gaspoz JM, et al. Secondhand smoke and health-related quality of life in never smokers. Arch Intern Med 2007;167:2516–23.

28. Weeks SG, Glantz SA, De Marco T, et al. Secondhand smoke exposure and quality of life in patients with heart failure. Arch Intern Med 2011;171:1887–93.

29. Vineis P, Airoldi L, Veglia P, et al. Environmental tobacco smoke and risk of respiratory cancer and chronic obstructive pulmonary disease in former smokers and never smokers in the EPIC prospective study. BMJ 2005;330:277.

30. Stranges S, Bonner MR, Fucci F, et al. Lifetime cumulative exposure to secondhand smoke and risk of myocardial infarction in never smokers: results from the Western New York health study, 1995–2001. Arch Intern Med 2006;166:1961–7.

31. Bouzigon E, Corda E, Aschard H, et al. Effect of 17q21 variants and smoking exposure in early-onset asthma. 2008;359:1985–94.

32. Sargent RP, Shepard RM, Glantz SA. Reduced incidence of admissions for myocardial infarction associated with public smoking ban: before and after study. BMJ 2004;328:977–80.

33. Pell JP, Haw S, Cobbe S, et al. Smoke-free legislation and hospitalizations for acute coronary syndrome. N Engl J Med 2008;359:482–91.

34. Menzies D, Nair A, Williamson PA, et al. Respiratory symptoms, pulmonary function, and markers of inflammation among bar workers before and after a legislative ban on smoking in public places. JAMA 2006;296:1742–8.

35. Mackay D, Haw S, Ayers JG, et al. Smoke-free legislation and hospitalizations for childhood asthma. N Engl J Med 2010;363:1139–45.

36. **Anthonisen NR, Skeans MA, Wise RA, et al. The effects of a smoking cessation intervention on 14.5-year mortality. Ann Intern Med 2005;142:233–9.** *Smokers with asymptomatic airway obstruction (n = 5,887) were randomized to a smoking cessation program or usual care. At 5 years, those in the program were more likely to have quit smoking (22% vs. 5%); after 14.5 years, they had lower overall mortality (12% vs. 14%).*

37. Ockene J, Kristeller JL, Goldberg R, et al. Smoking cessation and severity of disease: the Coronary Artery Smoking Intervention Study. Health Psychol 1992;11:119–26.

38. Rostrib BL, Chang CM, Pechacek TF. Estimation of cigarette smoking-attributable morbidity in the United States. JAMA Intern Med 2014 174:1922–8.

39. Kadunce DP, Burr R, Gress R, et al. Cigarette smoking: risk factor for premature facial wrinkling. Ann Intern Med 1991;114:840–4.

40. DeHertog SAE, Wensveen CAH, Bastiaens MT, et al. Relation between smoking and skin cancer. J Cin Oncol 2001;19:231–8.

41. Setty AR, Curhan G, Choi HK. Smoking and the risk of psoriasis in women: Nurses' Health Study II. Am J Med 2007;120:953–9.

42. Taybos G. Oral changes associated with tobacco use. Am J Med Sci 2003;4:179–82.

43. Lewin F, Norell SE, Johansson H, et al. Smoking tobacco, oral snuff, and alcohol in the etiology of squamous cell carcinoma of the head and neck. A population-based case-referent study in Sweden. Cancer 1998;82:1367–75.

44. Browman GP, Wong G, Hodson I, et al. Influence of cigarette smoking on the efficacy of radiation therapy for head and neck cancer. N Engl J Med 1993;328:159–63.

45. Fakhry C, Gillison ML, D'Souza G. Tobacco use and oral HPV-16 infection. JAMA 2014;312:1465–67.

46. Winn DM, Blot WJ, Shy CM, et al. Snuff dipping and oral cancer among women in the Southern United States. N Engl J Med 1981;304:745–9.

47. Klein BEK, Klein R, Lee KE, Meuer SM. Socioeconomic and lifestyle factors and the 10-year incidence of age-related cataracts. Am J Ophthalmol 2003;136:506–12.

48. Age-Related Eye Disease Study Research Group. Risk factors associated with age-related macular degeneration. Ophthalmology 2000;107:2224–32.

49. Pauwels RA, Rabe KF. Burden and clinical features of chronic obstructive pulmonary disease. Lancet 2004;364:613–20.

50. Løkke A, Lange P, Scharling H, et al. Developing COPD: a 25-year follow-up study of the general population. Thorax 2006;61:935–9.

51. Lundback B, Lindberg A, Lindstrom M, et al. Not 15 but 50% of smokers develop COPD? Report from the Obstructive Lung Diseases in Northern Sweden Studies. Respir Med 2003;97:115–22.

52. Rodriguez J, Jiang R, Johnson WC, et al. The association of pipe and cigar use with cotinine levels, lung function, and airflow obstruction: a cross-sectional study. Ann Intern Med 2010;152:201–10.

53. Althuis MD, Sexton M, Prybylski D. Cigarette smoking and asthma symptom severity among adult asthmatics. J Asthma 1999;36:257–64.

54. Chadhuri R, Livingston E, McMahon AD, et al. Cigarette smoking impairs the therapeutic response to oral corticosteroids in chronic asthma. Am J Respir Crit Care Med 2003;168:1308–11.

55. Hogg JC. Pathophysiology of airflow limitation in chronic obstructive pulmonary disease. Lancet 2004;364:709–21.

56. Janus ED, Phillips NT, Carrell RW. Smoking, lung function, and alpha 1-antitrypsin deficiency. Lancet 1985;1:152–4.

57. Dahl M, Tybjaerg-Hansen A, Lange P, et al. Change in lung function and morbidity from chronic obstructive pulmonary disease in alpha1-antitrypsin MZ heterozygotes: a longitudinal study of the general population. Ann Intern Med 2002;136:270–9.

58. Hunninghake GM, Cho MH, Tesfaigzi Y, et al. MMP12, lung function, and COPD in high risk populations. N Engl J Med 2009;361:2599–608.

59. Chinn S, Jarvis D, Melotti R, et al. Smoking cessation, lung function, and weight gain: a follow-up study. Lancet 2005;365:1629–35.

60. Hersh CP, DeMeo DL, Al-Ansari E, et al. Predictors of survival in severe, early onset COPD. Chest 2004;126:1443–51.

61. Alberg AJ, Samet JM. Epidemiology of lung cancer. Chest 2003;123(1 Suppl):21S–49S.

62. Tammemagi CM, Neslund-Dudas C, Simoff M, Kvale P. Smoking and lung cancer survival: the role of comorbidity and treatment. Chest 2004;125:27–37.

63. Mannino DM, Aguayo SM, Petty TL, Redd SC. Low lung function and incident lung cancer in the United States: data from the First National Health and Nutrition Examination Survey follow-up. Arch Intern Med 2003;163:1475–80.

64. Yang P, Zhifu S, Krowka MJ, et al. Alpha1-antitrypsin deficiency carriers, tobacco smoke, chronic obstructive pulmonary disease, and lung cancer risk. Arch Intern Med 2008;168:1097–1103.

65. International Early Lung Cancer Action Program Investigators. Women's susceptibility to tobacco carcinogens and survival after diagnosis of lung cancer. JAMA 2006;296:180–4.

66. Harris JE, Thun MJ, Mondul AM, Calle EE. Cigarette tar yields in relation to mortality from lung cancer in the cancer prevention study II prospective cohort, 1982–8. BMJ 2004;328:72.

67. Godtfredsen NS, Prescott E, Osler M. Effect of smoking reduction on lung cancer risk. JAMA 2005;294:1505–49.

68. Kark JD, Lebiush M, Rannon L. Cigarette smoking as a risk factor for epidemic a(H1N1) influenza in young men. N Engl J Med 1982;307:1042–6.

69. Almirall J, Gonzalez CA, Balanzo X, Bolibar I. Proportion of community-acquired pneumonia cases attributable to tobacco smoking. Chest 1999;116:375–9.

70. Nuorti JP, Butler JC, Farley MM, et al. Cigarette smoking and invasive pneumococcal disease. N Engl J Med 2000;342:681–9.

71. Bates MN, Khalakdina A, Pai M, et al. Risk of tuberculosis from exposure to tobacco smoke: a systematic review and meta-analysis. Arch Intern Med 2007;167:335–42.

72. Greenland P, Knoll MD, Stamler J, et al. Major risk factors as antecedents of fatal and nonfatal coronary heart disease events. JAMA 2003;290:891–7.

73. Teo KK, Ounpuu S, Hawken S, et al. Tobacco use and risk of myocardial infarction in 52 countries in the INTERHEART study: a case-control study. Lancet 2006;368:647–58.

74. Zeiher AM, Schachinger V, Minners J. Long-term cigarette smoking impairs endothelium-dependent coronary arterial vasodilator function. Circulation 1995;92:1094–100.

75. Cullen P, Schulte H, Assman G. Smoking, lipoproteins and coronary disease risk. Eur Heart J 1998;19:1632–41.

76. Rea TD, Heckbert SR, Kaplan RC, et al. Smoking status and risk for recurrent coronary events after myocardial infarction. Ann Intern Med 2002;137:494–500.

77. Goldenberg I, Jonas M, Tenenbaum A, et al. Current smoking, smoking cessation, and the risk of sudden cardiac death in patients with coronary artery disease. Arch Intern Med 2003;163:2301–5.

78. Boffetta P, Straif K. Use of smokeless tobacco and risk of myocardial infarction and stroke: systematic review with meta-analysis. BMJ 2009;339:h3060.

79. Gupta R, Gurm H, Bartholomew JR. Smokeless tobacco and cardiovascular risk. Arch Intern Med 2004;164:1845–9.

80. Arefalk G, Hambraeus K, Lind L, et al. Discontinuation of smokeless tobacco and mortality risk after myocardial infarction. Circulation 2014;130(4):325–32.

81. Conen D, Everett BM, Kurth T, et al. Smoking, smoking status and risk for symptomatic peripheral artery disease in women. Ann Intern Med 2011;154:719–26.

82. Meijer WT, Grobbee DE, Hunink M, et al. Determinants of peripheral arterial disease in the elderly. Arch Intern Med 2000;160:2934–8.

83. Olin JW, Young JR, Graor RA, et al. The changing clinical spectrum of thromboangiitis obliterans (Buerger's disease). Circulation 1990;82(5 Suppl):IV3–IV8.

84. Lederle FA, Nelson DB, Joseph AM. Smokers' relative for aortic aneurysm compared with other smoking-related diseases: a systematic review. J Vasc Surg 2003;38:329–34.

85. Goldoni M, Bonini S, Urban ML, et al. Asbestos and smoking as risk factors for idiopathic retroperitoneal fibrosis: a case-control study. Ann Intern Med 2014; 161:181–8.

86. Brown LM, Hoover R, Silverman D, et al. Excess incidence of squamous cell esophageal cancer among US black men: role of social class and other risk factors. Am J Epidemiol 2001;153:114–22.

87. Wu AH, Wan P, Bernstein L. A multiethnic population-based study of smoking, alcohol and body size and risk of adenocarcinomas of the stomach and esophagus (United States). Cancer Causes Control 2001;12:721–32.

88. Coughlin SS, Calle EE, Patel AV, Thun MJ. Predictors of pancreatic cancer mortality among a large cohort of United States adults. Cancer Causes Control 2000;11:915–23.

89. Botteri E, Iodice S, Bagnardi V, et al. Smoking and colorectal cancer: a meta-analysis. JAMA 2008; 300:2765–78.

90. Chao A, Thun J, Jacobs EJ, et al. Cigarette smoking and colorectal cancer mortality in the cancer prevention study II. J Natl Cancer Inst 2000;92:1888–96.

91. Chao A, Thun MJ, Jacobs EJ, et al. Cigarette smoking, use of other tobacco products and stomach cancer mortality in US adults. Int J Cancer 2002;101:380–9.

92. Daling JR, Madeleine MM, Johnson LG, et al. Human papillomavirus, smoking, and sexual practices in the etiology of anal cancer. Cancer 2004;101:270–80.

93. Rosenstock S, Jorgensen T, Bonnevie O, Anderson L. Risk factors for peptic ulcer disease: a population based prospective cohort study comprising 2416 Danish adults. Gut 2003 52:186–93.

94. Kulig M, Nocon M, Vieth M, et al. Risk factors for gastroesophageal reflux disease: methodology and first epidemiological results of the proGERD study. J Clin Epidemiol 2004;57:580–9.

95. Mahid SS, Minor KS, Soto RE, et al. Smoking and inflammatory bowel disease: a meta-analysis. Mayo Clin Proc 2006;81:1462–71.

96. McGrath J, McDonald JW, Macdonald JK. Transdermal nicotine for induction of remission in ulcerative colitis. Cochrane Database Syst Rev 2004;4:CD004722.

97. Tolstrup JS, Kristiansen L, Becker U, Grønbæk M. Smoking and risk of acute and chronic pancreatitis among men and women: a population-based cohort study. Arch Intern Med 2009;169:603–9.

98. Yadav D, Hawes RH, Brand RE, et al. Alcohol consumption, cigarette smoking, and the risk of recurrent acute and chronic pancreatitis. Arch Intern Med 2009;169:1035–45.

99. Yokoyama H, Tomonaga O, Hirayama M, et al. Predictors of the progression of diabetic nephropathy and the beneficial effect of angiotensin-converting enzyme inhibitors in NIDDM patients. Diabetologia 1997;40:405–11.

100. Bleyer AJ, Shemanski LR, Burke GL, et al. Tobacco, hypertension, and vascular disease: risk factors for renal function in an older population. Kidney Int 2000;57:2072–9.

101. Baggio B, Budakovic A, Casara D, et al. Renal involvement in subjects with peripheral atherosclerosis. J Nephrol 2001;14:286–92.

102. Hunt JD, van der Hel OL, McMillian GP, et al. Renal cell carcinoma in relation to cigarette smoking: a meta-analysis of 24 studies. Int J Cancer 2005;114:101–8.

103. Bacon CG, Mittleman MA, Kawachi I, et al. Sexual function in men older than 50 years of age: results from the health professionals follow-up study. Ann Intern Med 2003;139:161–8.

104. McVary KT, Carrier S, Wessells H, et al. Smoking and erectile dysfunction: evidence based analysis. J Urol 2001;166:1624–32.

105. Freedman ND, Silverman DT, Hollenbeck AR, et al. Association between smoking and risk of bladder cancer among men and women. JAMA 2011;306:737–45.

106. Giovannucci E, Rimm EB, Ascherio A, et al. Smoking and risk of total and fatal prostate cancer in United States health professionals. Cancer Epidemiol Biomarkers Prev 1999;8:277–82.

107. Kenfield SA, Stampfer MJ, Chan JM, Giovannucci E. Smoking and prostate cancer survival and recurrence. JAMA 2011;305:2548–55.

108. Shields TS, Brinton LA, Burk RD, et al. A case-control study of risk factors for invasive cervical cancer among U.S. women exposed to oncogenic types of human papillomavirus. Cancer Epidemiol Biomarkers Prev 2004;13:1574–82.

109. Zhou B, Yang L, Sun Q, et al. Cigarette smoking and the risk of endometrial cancer: a meta-analysis. Am J Med 2008;121:501–8.

110. Xue F, Willet WC, Rosner BA, et al. Cigarette smoking and the incidence of breast cancer. Arch Intern Med 2011;171:125–33.

111. Willi C, Bodenmann P, Ghali WA, et al. Active smoking and the risk of type 2 diabetes: a systematic review and meta-analysis. JAMA 2007 298:2654–64.

112. Shinton R, Beevers G. Meta-analysis of relation between cigarette smoking and stroke. BMJ 1989;298:789–94.

113. Rothwell PM, Slattery J, Warlow CP. Clinical and angiographic predictors of stroke and death from carotid endarterectoy: systematic review. BMJ 1997;315:1571–7.

114. Van Duijin CM, Hofman A. Relation between nicotine intake and Alzheimer's disease. BMJ 1991;302:1491–4.

115. Ott A, Slooter AJ, Hofman A, et al. Smoking and risk of dementia and Alzheimer's disease in a population-based cohort study: the Rotterdam Study. Lancet 1998;351:1840–3.

116. Rusanen M, Kivipelto M, Quesenberry CP, et al. Heavy smoking in midlife and long-term risk of Alzheimer disease and vascular dementia. Arch Intern Med 2011;171:333–9.

117. Doll R, Peto R, Boreham J, Sutherland I. Smoking and dementia in male British doctors: prospective study. BMJ 2000;320:1097–102.

118. Ascherio A. Munger AL. Environmental risk factors for multiple sclerosis, part II: noninfectious factors. Ann Neurol 2007;61:504–13.

119. Healy BC, Ali EN, Guttman CR, et al. Smoking and disease progression in multiple sclerosis. Arch Neurol 2009;66:858–64.

120. Costenbader KH, Feskanich D, Mandl LA, Karlson EW. Smoking intensity, duration, and cessation, and the risk of rheumatoid arthritis in women. Am J Med 2006;119:503–11.

121. Manfredsdottir VF, Vikingsdottir T, Jonsson T, et al. The effects of tobacco smoking and rheumatoid factor seropositivity on disease activity and joint damage in early rheumatoid arthritis. Rheumatology (Oxford) 2006;45:734–40.

122. Schectman G, Byrd JC, Gruchow HW. The influence of smoking on vitamin C status in adults. Am J Public Health 1989;79:158–62.

123. Olmedo JM, Yiannias JA, Windgassen EB, Gornet MK. Scurvy: a disease almost forgotten. Int J Dermatol 2006;45:909–13.

124. Dube SR, Caraballo RS, Dhingra SS, et al. The relationship between smoking status and serious psychological distress: findings from the 2007 Behavioral Risk Factor Surveillance System. Int J Public Health 2009;54(Suppl 1):68–74.

125. John U, Meyer C, Rumpf HJ, Hapke U. Smoking, nicotine dependence and psychiatric comorbidity—a population-based study including smoking cessation after three years. Drug Alcohol Depend 2004;76:287–95.

126. Taylor G, McNeill A, Girling A, et al. Change in mental health after smoking cessation: systematic review and meta-analysis. BMJ 2014;348:g1151.

127. Augood C, Duckitt K, Templeton AA. Smoking and female infertility: a systematic review and meta-analysis. Hum Reprod 1998;13:1532–9.

128. DiFranza JR, Lew RA. Effect of maternal cigarette smoking on pregnancy complications and sudden infant death syndrome. J Fam Pract 1995;40:385–94.

129. Shah NR, Bracken MB. A systematic review and meta-analysis of prospective studies on the association between maternal cigarette smoking and preterm delivery. Am J Obstet Gynecol 2000;182:465–72.

130. Castles A, Adams EK, Melvin CL, et al. Effects of smoking during pregnancy. Five meta-analyses. Am J Prev Med 1999;16:208–15.

131. Hayatbakhsh MR, Sadasivam S, Mamun AA, et al. Maternal smoking during and after pregnancy and lung function in early adulthood: a prospective study. Thorax 2009;64:810–4.

132. McEvoy CT, Schilling D, Clay N, et al. Vitamin C supplementation for pregnant smoking women and pulmonary function in their newborn infants: a randomized clinical trial. JAMA 2014;311:2074–82.

133. United States Preventive Services Task Force. Counseling and Interventions to Prevent Tobacco Use and Tobacco-Caused Disease in Adults and Pregnant Women: U.S. Preventive Services Task Force Reaffirmation Recommendation Statement. Ann Intern Med 2009;150:551–5.

134. **Critchley JA, Capewell S. Mortality risk reduction associated with smoking cessation in patients with coronary heart disease: a systematic review. JAMA 2003;290:86–97.** *Data from 20 studies indicated that those who quit reduce their risk of mortality from coronary heart disease by 36%.*

135. Fiore MC, Jaén CR, Baker TB, et al. *Treating Tobacco Use and Dependence: 2008 Update. Clinical Practice Guideline.* Rockville, MD: U.S. Department of Health and Human Services. Public Health Service; May 2008.

136. Lindson-Hawley N, Aveyard P, Hughes JR. Reduction versus abrupt cessation in smokers who want to quit. Cochrane Database Syst Rev 2012;11:CD008033.

137. Thomas RE, McLellan J, Perera R. School-based programmes for preventing smoking. Cochrane Database Syst Rev 2013;4:CD001293.

138. Johnston V, Liberato S, Thomas D. Incentives for preventing smoking in children and adolescents. Cochrane Database Syst Rev 2012;10:CD008645.

139. Bala MM, Strzeszynski L, Topor-Madry R, Cahill K. Mass media interventions for smoking cessation in adults. Cochrane Database Syst Rev 2013;6:CD004704.

140. Thomson CC, Fisher LB, Winickoff JP, et al. Statewide tobacco excise taxes and adolescent smoking behaviors in the United States. J Public Health Manag Pract 2004;10:490–6.

141. Fichtenberg CM, Glantz SA. Effect of smoke-free workplaces on smoking behavior: systematic review. BMJ 2002;325:188–95.

142. **Volpp KG, Troxel AB, Pauly MV, et al. A randomized, controlled trial of financial incentives for smoking cessation. N Engl J Med 2009;360:699–709.** *Employees of a company who volunteered for a smoking-cessation study (n = 878) were randomly assigned to receive information about a smoking cessation program with or without financial incentives to complete the program ($100), to quit within 6 months ($250), and to remain abstinent for another 6 months ($400). Those assigned to financial incentives were more likely to enroll in the smoking cessation program (15% vs. 5%) and to quit within 6 months (21% vs. 12%; NNT = 11); they were also more likely to be abstinent at 9 or 12 months (15% vs. 5%; NNT = 10) and 15 or 18 months after enrollment (9% vs. 4%; NNT = 20).*

143. **Hartmann-Boyce J, Lancaster T, Stead LF. Print-based self-help interventions for smoking cessation. Cochrane Database Syst Rev 2014;(6):CD001118.** *Based on 11 trials comparing self-help materials to no intervention, the risk ratio of quitting was 1.19 (95% CI: 1.04–1.37); there was no evidence of benefit when the materials were used to supplement a face-to-face encounter or as an adjunct to nicotine replacement therapy.*

144. Stead LF, Bultrago D, Preciado N, et al. Physician advice for smoking cessation. Cochrane Database Syst Rev 2013;5:CD000165.

145. **Rice VH, Hartmann-Boyce J, Stead LF. Nursing interventions for smoking cessation. Cochrane Database Syst Rev 2013;8:CD001188.** *The pooled relative risk of quitting from 35 studies comparing a nursing intervention with control or usual care was 1.29 (95% CI: 1.20–1.39).*

146. **Stead LF, Hartmann-Boyce J, Perera R, Lancaster T. Telephone counselling for smoking cessation. Cochrane Database Syst Rev**

2013;8:CD002850. *In nine studies of smokers who contacted quit lines, those randomized to receive multiple call-back counseling sessions were more likely to have long-term smoking cessation; the relative risk was 1.37 (95% CI: 1.26–1.50).*

147. Rigotti NA, Clair C, Munafo MR, Stead LF. Interventions for smoking cessation in hospitalised patients. Cochrane Database Syst Rev 2012;5:CD001837.

148. **Stead F, Lancaster T. Group behavioral therapy programmes for smoking cessation. Cochrane Database Syst Rev 2005;2:CD001007.** *Group programs were found to be better than no intervention (pooled OR: 2.17; 95% CI: 1.37–3.45) and self-help (pooled OR: 2.04; 95% CI: 1.60–2.60).*

149. **Lancaster T, Stead F. Individual behavioral counselling for smoking cessation. Cochrane Database Syst Rev 2002;3:CD001292.** *The pooled odds ratio from 15 trials comparing individual counseling with minimal intervention was 1.62 (95% CI: 1.35–1.94). Four studies comparing different levels of intensity of counseling failed to show a significant effect.*

150. Civjak M, Stead F, Hartmann-Boyce J, et al. Internet-based interventions for smoking cessation. Cochrane Database Syst Rev 2013;7:CD007078.

151. Quinn VP, Hollis JF, Smith KS, et al. Effectiveness of the 5A's tobacco cessation treatments in nine HMOs. J Gen Intern Med 2009;24:149–54.

152. Stead LF, Lancaster T. Behavioural interventions as adjuncts to pharmacotherapy for smoking cessation. Cochrane Database of Syst Rev 2012;12:CD009670.

153. **Stead LF, Perera R, Bullen C, et al. Nicotine replacement therapy for smoking cessation. Cochrane Database Syst Rev 2012;11:CD000146.** *The pooled risk ratio from 150 trials comparing all forms of nicotine replacement therapy (NRT) with placebo or a non-NRT group was 1.6.*

154. **Schnoll RA, Patterson F, Wileyto EP, et al. Effectiveness of extended-duration transdermal nicotine therapy: a randomized trial. Ann Intern Med 2010;152:144–51.** *In this study 568 smokers were randomized to receive 8 or 24 weeks of a 21 mg nicotine patch; all received behavioral counseling. Those assigned to an active patch were more likely to be abstinent at week 24 (42% vs. 27%), but not at week 52 (14% in both arms).*

155. **Kenford SL, Fiore MC, Jorenby DE, et al. Predicting smoking cessation: who will quit with and without the nicotine patch. JAMA 1994;271:589–94.** *Among 210 smokers from two trials of nicotine patch for smoking cessation, smoking status during week 2 was the strongest predictor of 6-month outcomes.*

156. Lawson GM, Hurt RD, Dale LC, et al. Application of serum nicotine and plasma cotinine concentrations to assessment of nicotine replacement in light, moderate, and heavy smokers undergoing transdermal therapy. J Clin Pharmacol 1998;38:502–9.

157. Caponneto P, Campagna D, Cibella F, et al. Efficiency and safety of an electronic cigarette (ECLAT) as tobacco cigarettes substitute: a prospective 12-month randomized control design study. PLoS One 2013;8:e66317.

158. Bullen C, Howe C, Laugesen M, et al. Electronic cigarettes for smoking cessation: a randomized controlled trial. Lancet 2013;382:1629–37.

159. Grana RA, Popova L, Ling PM. A longitudinal analysis of electronic cigarette use and smoking cessation. JAMA Intern Med 2014;174:812–3.

160. Brown J, Beard E, Kotz D, et al. Real-world effectiveness of e-cigarettes when used to aid smoking cessation: a cross-sectional population study. Addiction 2014;109:1531–40.

161. Goniewicz ML, Knysak J, Gawron M, et al. Levels of selected carcinogens and toxicants in vapour from electronic cigarettes. Tob Control 2014;23(2):133–9.

162. **Gonzales D, Rennard SI, Nides M, et al. Varenicline, a α4β2 nicotinic acetylcholine receptor partial agonist, vs. sustained-release bupropion and placebo for smoking cessation: a randomized controlled trial. JAMA 2006;296:47–55.** *In this study, 1,025 healthy volunteer smokers were randomized to (1) varenicline 1 mg bid, (2) bupropion 150SR bid, or (3) placebo for 12 weeks; all received brief counseling. Continuous abstinence weeks 9–12 was achieved by 44% on varenicline, 30% on bupropion, and 18% on placebo; for weeks 9–52, the rates were 22%, 16%, and 8%, respectively.*

163. **Jorenby DE, Hays JT, Rigotti NA, et al. Efficacy of varenicline, a α4β2 nicotinic acetylcholine receptor partial agonist, vs. placebo or sustained-release bupropion for smoking cessation: a randomized controlled trial. JAMA 2006;296:56–63.** *In this study, 1,027 healthy volunteer smokers were randomized to (1) varenicline 1 mg bid,*

(2) bupropion 150SR bid, or (3) placebo for 12 weeks; all received weekly brief counseling. Continuous abstinence weeks 9–12 was achieved by 44% on varenicline, 30% on bupropion, and 18% on placebo; for weeks 9–52, the rates were 23%, 15%, and 10%, respectively.

164. **Cahill K, Stead LF, Lancaster T. Nicotine receptor partial agonists for smoking cessation. Cochrane Database Syst Rev 2012;4:CD006103.** *The pooled risk ratio of quitting smoking at 6 months or longer was 2.3 when compared to placebo, 1.5 when compared with bupropion, and 1.1 when compared to NRT (95% CI: 0.9–1.4). Based on two trials, the pooled RR for cytisine was 4.0 (95% CI: 2.0–7.9).*

165. **Tonstad S, Tonnesen P, Hajek P, et al. Effect of maintenance therapy with varenicline on smoking cessation: a randomized controlled trial. JAMA 2006;296:64–71.** *Of 1,927 smokers treated with varenicline for 12 weeks, 1,236 (64%) did not smoke during the last week, and 1,210 (63%) were randomized to continue varenicline or placebo for an additional 12 weeks. Continuous abstinence for weeks 13–24 was 71% with varenicline vs. 50% with placebo; for weeks 13–52, the rates were 44% vs. 37%.*

166. Hajek P, McRobbie H, Smith KM, et al. Increasing varenicline dose in smokers who do not respond to the standard dosage: a randomized clinical trial. JAMA Intern Med 2015;175:266–71.

167. Oncken C, Gonzales D, Nides M, et al. Efficacy and safety of the novel selective nicotinic aceylcholine receptor partial agonist, varenicline for smoking cessation. Arch Intern Med 2006;186:1571–7.

168. Gunnell D, Irvine D, Wise L, et al. Varenicline and suicidal behavior: a cohort study based on data from the General Practice Research Database. BMJ 2009;339:b3805.

169. Anthenelli RM, Morris C, Ramey TS, et al. Effects of varenicline on smoking cessation in adults with stably treated current or past major depression: a randomized trial. Ann Intern Med 2013;159:390–400.

170. West R, Zatonski W, Cedzynska M, et al. Placebo-controlled trial of cytisine for smoking cessation. N Engl J Med 2011;365:1193–200.

171. Walker N, Howe C, Glover M, et al. Cytisine versus nicotine for smoking cessation. N Engl J Med 2014:371:2353–62.

172. **Hughes JR, Stead F, Hartmann-Boyce J, et al. Antidepressants for smoking cessation. Cochrane Database Syst Rev 2014;1:CD000031.** *The pooled risk ratio of quitting smoking from 44 trials of buproprion monotherapy was 1.6 and from six trials of nortriptyline, 2.0.*

173. **Jorenby DE, Leischow SJ, Nides MA, et al. A controlled trial of sustained-release bupropion, a nicotine patch or both for smoking cessation. N Engl J Med 1999;340:685–91.** *Smokers (n = 893) were randomized to (1) bupropion SR, (2) nicotine patch, (3) bupropion + nicotine patch, or (4) placebo for 9 weeks. The 12-month abstinence rates were 30% (B), 16% (N), 36% (B+N), and 16% (P), respectively.*

174. Glassman AH, Stetner F, Walsh BT, et al. Heavy smokers, smoking cessation and clonidine. Results of a double-blind, randomized trial. JAMA 1988;259:2863–6.

175. Prochazka AV, Petty TL, Nett L, et al. Transdermal clonidine reduced some withdrawal symptoms but did not increase smoking cessation. Arch Intern Med 1992;152:2065–9.

176. **Gourlay SG, Stead LF, Benowitz NL. Clonidine for smoking cessation. Cochrane Database Syst Rev 2004;3:CD000058.pub2.** *The pooled odds ratio of quitting smoking from six trials was 1.9 (95% CI: 1.3–2.7), but the "quality of the trials was poor" and side effects were common.*

177. **Ebbert JO, Hatsukami DK, Corghan IT, et al. Combination varenicline and bupropion SR for tobacco-dependence treatment in cigarette smokers: a randomized trial. JAMA 2014;311:155–63.** *Smokers (n = 506) were randomized to varenicline alone or with bupropion and were treated for 12 weeks and followed for 52 weeks. Those on combination therapy were more likely to achieve prolonged abstinence at 12 weeks (53% vs. 43%) but not at 52 weeks (31% vs. 25%).*

178. **Hajek P, Smith KM, Dhanji AR, McRobbie H. Is a combination of varenicline and nicotine patch more effective than varenicline alone? A randomized controlled trial. BMC Medicine 2013;11:140.** *Smokers (n = 117) were randomized to varenicline with nicotine or placebo patch; abstinence rates at 12 weeks were higher with the combination, but not significantly so (36% vs. 29%). Side effects and withdrawal symptoms were also similar.*

179. **Koegelenberg CF, Noor F, Bateman ED, et al. Efficacy of varenicline combined with nicotine replacement therapy vs. varenicline alone for smoking cessation: a randomized clinical trial. JAMA 2014;312:155–61.** *Smokers (n = 456) were randomized to varenicline with nicotine or placebo patch for 12 weeks. Continuous abstinence was higher with the combination at 12 weeks (55% vs. 41%) and 24 weeks (49% vs. 33%). The most common side effects were nausea and insomnia; these*

tended to be higher with the combination, but the difference was not statistically significant.

180. He D, Melbø JI, Høstmark AT. Effect of acupuncture on smoking cessation or reduction: an 8-month and 5-year follow-up study. Prev Med 2001;33:364–72.

181. Bier ID, Wilson J, Studt P, Shakleton M. Auricular acupuncture, education and smoking cessation: a randomized, sham-controlled trial. Am J Public Health 2002;92:1642–7.

182. White AR, Rampes H, Liu JP, et al. Acupuncture and related interventions for smoking cessation. Cochrane Database Syst Rev 2014;1:CD000009.

183. Elkins GR, Rajab MH. Clinical hypnosis for smoking cessation: preliminary results of a three-session intervention. Int J Clin Exp Hypn 2004;52:73–81.

184. Barnes J, Dong CY, McRobbie H, et al. Hypnotherapy for smoking cessation. Cochrane Database Syst Rev 2010;10:CD001008.

185. Joseph AM, Willenbring ML, Nugent SM, Nelson DB. A randomized trial of concurrent versus delayed smoking intervention for patients in alcohol dependence treatment. J Stud Alcohol 2004;65:681–91.

8

Cocaine, Methamphetamine, and Other Stimulants

community reinforcement. Long-acting amphetamines have been shown to reduce other stimulant use but not complications.

Caffeine   265
Caffeine has mild stimulant effects and may lead to a mild dependence syndrome.

Background

The *stimulants* are class of drugs with sympathomimetic effects and include cocaine and amphetamines. *Cocaine* is an alkaloid derived from the leaves of the Coca plant, which is indigenous to South America. The leaves have been chewed by natives for centuries as a mild stimulant. In the mid-1800s, cocaine was extracted from the leaves by Europeans and subsequently used as an anesthetic and as an additive to beverages and patent medicines. The nonprescription use of cocaine was banned in the United States by the passage of the Harrison Narcotics Act in 1914.

Amphetamine-like compounds (technically, phenylethylamines) also have a long history dating back to the use of the alkaloid ephedrine derived from *Ephedra ma-huang* in China. Medicinal amphetamines were developed in the early 20th century and were originally used for the treatment of rhinitis and asthma. They were subsequently employed as a stimulant for soldiers in combat during World War II and later to treat obesity. Methamphetamine is easily synthesized from readily available precursors, such as ephedrine or pseudoephedrine.

There are a number of so-called designer drugs that are pharmacologically similar to the amphetamines, such as MDA, MDEA, and MDMA (ecstasy); these have stimulant properties but are used more for their hallucinogenic effect. These agents are covered in Chapter 9, on hallucinogens.

Cathinones are another class of stimulants that are used in a variety of forms. Khat (or "qat") is a plant that has been traditionally used on the Arabian Peninsula and in East Africa. The leaves of this plant (*Catha edulis*) contain an alkaloid—cathinone—that resembles amphetamines.[1] The leaves are typically chewed and have mild effects similar to those of other stimulants. A related drug, methacathinone, can be synthesized from ephedrine. This yellowish-white powder is injected, snorted, or ingested, with effects similar to those of methamphetamine. Methacathinone is sometimes referred to as "cat" or "ephedrone" and is one of the most commonly abused stimulants in Russia. More recently, synthetic cathinones have been marketed as "bath salts" or "plant food" to circumvent drug regulations.[2]

Areca nuts come from tropical palm trees (of the genus *Areca*) and are often chewed with betel leaf, lime (calcium oxide), and sometimes tobacco; they are also referred to as "betel nuts" and the combination is referred to as "betel quid." This mixture is most commonly used in South and Southeast Asia and appears to have mild stimulant effects.[3]

Caffeine, another mild stimulant, is the most commonly used psychoactive substance worldwide; this is briefly covered at the end of this chapter.

Stimulants have a number of therapeutic uses, including the treatment of attention-deficit hyperactivity disorder (ADHD), depression, and narcolepsy and to promote weight loss. Table 8.1 provides a list of some of the available prescription stimulants and medications with stimulant effects.

Epidemiology

According to the 2013 National Survey on Drug Use and Health (NSDUH),[4] approximately 37.6 million Americans reported lifetime use of cocaine (14.3% of those aged 12 or older); 4.2 million had used in the past year (1.6%), and 1.5 million had used in the past month (0.6%). Over 21 million Americans reported lifetime nonmedical use of other stimulants, including methamphetamine (8.3% of those aged 12 or older); 3.5 million had used in the past year (1.3%), and 1.4 million in the past month (0.5%).

TABLE 8.1 Selected Prescription and Over-the-Counter Stimulants

Generic Name	Trade Name(s)	Usual Daily Dose	Indication/Use
Amphetamine	Adderall	5–60 mg	ADHD
Dexmethylphenidate	Focalin	5–20 mg	ADHD
Dextroamphetamine	Dexedrine, Dextrostat	5–30 mg	ADHD, Narcolepsy
Lisdexamfetamine	Vyvanse	30–50 mg	ADHD
Methylphenidate	Methylin, Ritalin, Concerta, Metadate, Daytrana	10–60 mg	ADHD
Modafinil	Provigil, Nuvigil	100–200 mg	Narcolepsy
Benzphetamine	Didrex	25–300 mg	Obesity
Diethylpropion	Tenuate	75 mg	Obesity
Phendimetrazine	Adipost, Bontril, Melflat	70–210 mg	Obesity
Phentermine	Adipex-P, Ionamin	15–37.5 mg	Obesity
Theophylline	Theo-24, Uniphyl	100–600 mg	Chronic obstructive pulmonary disease
Caffeine	Cafergot, Norgesic Fiorecet/ Fiorinal*	40–600 mg	Headache, musculoskeletal pain
Ephedrine	Rynatuss*	10–40 mg	Decongestant

(*continued*)

TABLE 8.1 (Continued)

Generic Name	Trade Name(s)	Usual Daily Dose	Indication/Use
Phenylephrine	Dimetapp, Sudafed PE, Triaminic	15–60 mg	Decongestant
Pseudoephedrine	Dimetapp, Duratuss, Entex, Robitussin-CF*, Sudafed	30–240 mg	Decongestant

Not all trade names are listed.
*Combination medications.

According to the Drug Abuse Warning Network (DAWN),[5] in 2011, cocaine was associated with the highest number of illicit drug-related emergency department (ED) visits. Cocaine accounted for an estimated 162 ED visits per 100,000 population, while for methamphetamine, the number was 33 and for amphetamines, 23.

Drug Effects

Acute Effects

Cocaine is used in the hydrochloride (crystal), sulfated (powder), or alkaloid (crack) form; the latter has a lower melting point, which makes it conducive to smoking. The effects of cocaine peak after 60–90 minutes with oral use, and within a few minutes of snorting, intravenous use, or smoking, and the effects wear off after 15–30 minutes.

Methamphetamine is used in a powder or crystal form and can also be ingested, snorted, smoked, or injected; there are even reports of transrectal use.[6] The acute effects of methamphetamine are similar to those of cocaine but are longer lasting (generally 4–8 hours).

The stimulants exert their effect by increasing levels of catecholamines through stimulation of release or blockage of reuptake; direct stimulation of receptors may also play a role. Users of cocaine and methamphetamine experience a "high" or "rush" of intense euphoria accompanied by tachycardia and elevated blood pressure and followed by depression, which may lead to repeated use. Cocaine also has a local anesthetic effect when applied to the mucus membranes.

Oral amphetamines promote wakefulness, alertness, concentration, as well as psychomotor functioning and speed.[7] Amphetamines (and other stimulants) are sometimes used by athletes to improve physical performance, although there is limited evidence to support this and their use is prohibited or monitored by most athletic organizations.[8] Amphetamines also suppress appetite. Prolonged use is often followed by depression and fatigue.

Acute Toxicity and Overdose

High doses of stimulants produce generalized sympathomimetic effects. The DSM-5 criteria for stimulant intoxication require the presence of "clinically significant problematic behavioral or psychological changes" plus two (or more) of the following signs or symptoms occurring during or shortly after stimulant use: (1) tachycardia or bradycardia, (2) pupillary dilation, (3) elevated or lowered blood pressure, (4) perspiration or chills, (5) nausea or vomiting, (6) evidence of weight loss, (7) psychomotor agitation or retardation, (8) muscular weakness, respiratory depression, chest pain, or cardiac arrhythmias, and (9) confusion, seizures, dyskinesias, dystonias, or coma.[9] The ICD-10 code varies depending on whether cocaine (F14) or another stimulant (F15) was used, whether it was accompanied by a perceptual disturbance, and whether there is a comorbid use disorder and on the severity of the disorder.

The cardiovascular effects may lead to myocardial infarction, aortic dissection, or stroke (as discussed later in this chapter); hyperthermia and rhabdomyolysis can also occur. In one study of 146 cocaine-related deaths over a 10-year period in Australia, most of the fatalities were associated with injection use (86%), and in most cases, other substances were also involved (81%).[10] In a case-control study in Spain of 311 sudden cardiovascular deaths among individuals aged 15–49, 9% had used cocaine recently and, on multivariable analysis, recent cocaine use had the strongest association with deaths, with an adjusted odds ratio of 4.1.[11] Despite the association of cocaine use with fatalities, in a cohort of U.S. adults surveyed in 1991, baseline cocaine use was not associated with a significantly increased 15-year mortality (compared to those who did not use illicit drugs).[12]

There is no specific antidote for stimulant overdose—benzodiazepines are frequently used for agitation and phenothiazines for psychotic symptoms. Beta-blockers should generally be avoided because they may potentiate coronary artery vasoconstriction. One animal study suggests that activated charcoal may reduce methamphetamine toxicity after ingestion of the drug.[13]

Withdrawal

Regular users of stimulants seem to experience withdrawal symptoms upon cessation, but they do not have a clear-cut, easily observable syndrome as can be seen with opioid, sedative, or alcohol withdrawal. The DSM-5 criteria for stimulant withdrawal require the presence of two or more of the following symptoms in the setting of cessation or reduction of long-term stimulant use: (1) fatigue, (2) vivid, unpleasant dreams, (3) insomnia or hypersomnia, (4) increased appetite, and (5) psychomotor retardation or agitation.[9] The symptoms may also include depressed mood and generally dissipate over 1–2 weeks.[14]

Assessment

The DSM-5 diagnostic criteria for a substance use disorder with cocaine or other stimulants are the same as for other substances;

see Chapter 1 for further details.[9] The ICD-10 divides this category between cocaine (F14) and other stimulants (F15). The ICD-10 code for cocaine use disorder is F14.10 if is mild and F14.20 if moderate-severe; for other stimulants, it is F15.10 if mild and F15.20 if moderate-severe.

Physical Exam

Stimulant users may exhibit signs of use such as tachycardia, elevated blood pressure, or agitation. They may present with one of the medical complications discussed in the next section. Intranasal users may have nasoseptal erosions or perforation. Injection drug users may have the stigmata of needle use on their arms, legs, or other sites.

Laboratory Testing

While cocaine has a short half-life, its metabolites (specifically benzoylecgonine) can be detected in the urine for 2–3 days after last use and up to 8 days with heavy use. False-positive results are very uncommon, but coca tea consumption has been reported to cause a positive urine cocaine assay.[15] Amphetamines can likewise be detected in the urine for 23 days after last use. There are a number of drugs that can cause false-positive amphetamine screen, including ephedrine, pseudoephedrine, trazodone, bupropion, desipramine, amantadine, and ranitidine.[16] Urine drug testing is discussed further in Chapter 2.

Medical Complications

Most of the complications of stimulant use are related to their effect on the vascular system and damage to various organs that occurs as a result. Some of the medical complications are due to the use of needles, not the drug per se. The medical complications of injection drug use are covered in more detail in Chapter 14.

Cutaneous Complications

Cocaine is sometimes cut with levamisole, an anthelminthic drug. Use of levamisole-contaminated cocaine has been associated with cutaneous necrosis, purpura, and neutropenia.[17]

Eye, Ear, Nose, and Throat Complications

Intranasal use of cocaine has been associated with a variety of nasopharyngeal complications, including nasal septal erosions and perforation, oronasal fistulas,[18] perforation of the hard palate,[19] and saddle-nose deformity. The clinical presentation may mimic a vasculitis such as Wegner's granulomatosis.[20] There are also reports of severe dental disease among methamphetamine users ("meth mouth");[21] it is not clear if this is due to a drug effect or simply neglect.

Smoking "crack" cocaine has been associated with corneal ulcerations and infections;[22] similar complications have been reported with methamphetamine use.[23] There also may be an association between cocaine use and open-angle glaucoma.[24]

Pulmonary Complications

Smoking the alkaloid (crack) form of cocaine causes acute bronchoconstriction and may lead to wheezing and asthma attacks.[25] It has been found (on bronchoalveolar lavage) to be associated with alveolar hemorrhage and microvascular injury; however, the clinical significance of this finding is unclear.[26] There is a case report of bronchiolitis obliterans organizing pneumonia (BOOP) associated with free-base cocaine use.[27]

Pulmonary hypertension has been reported in association with intravenous cocaine use,[28] as well as inhaled methamphetamine use.[29] By contrast, cocaine smoking has not been found to have significant acute or chronic effects on diffusing capacity of the lung.[30]

Drug users who inject talc-containing crushed tablets are at risk for pulmonary granulomatosis, which may lead to pulmonary hypertension[31] and chronic obstructive lung disease.[32] This complication has been generally (but not exclusively) associated with intravenous methylphenidate (Ritalin) use.

Cardiovascular Complications

Myocardial Infarction

Cocaine users often experience chest pain with use, and cocaine-related chest pain is a frequent reason for ED visits. In one study, 17% of all patients presenting to four emergency departments with nontraumatic chest pain had used cocaine; among those 18–30 years old, 29% had used cocaine, and among those 31–40 years old, 48% had used it.[33] A minority of these patients will suffer a myocardial infarction; in one series, approximately 6% experienced this complication.[34]

Cocaine-induced myocardial infarction is thought to be due to vasoconstriction of coronary arteries (in turn, due to stimulation of alpha-adrenergic receptors) as well as increased myocardial oxygen demand (due to increased heart rate, arterial pressure, and ventricular contractility).[35] Cocaine-induced vasoconstriction is potentiated by beta-blockade in physiological experiments;[36] this is thought to be due to unopposed alpha-adrenergic stimulation. Therefore, it has been recommended that selective beta-blockers be avoided when treating patients with cocaine-associated chest pain or myocardial infarction.[37] A recent observational study has raised questions about the clinical significance of this observation. This study of 331 cocaine users with chest pain found that those who received beta-blockers did not have increased complications or mortality; in fact, those who were discharged on a beta-blocker had a lower subsequent cardiovascular mortality.[38] While, theoretically, beta-blockers with alpha-blocking activity—such as labetolol or carvedilol—may be safer, labetolol does not reverse cocaine-induced coronary vasoconstriction.[39] On the other hand, labetolol[40] and carvedilol[41] have been shown to attenuate the increased blood pressure and pulse associated with cocaine use.

Most of those who experience myocardial infarction are male cigarette smokers and many have preexisting coronary artery disease; however, myocardial infarction can occur in those with normal coronary arteries.[42] Furthermore, one cannot reliably predict which patients will experience myocardial infarction on the basis of clinical presentation or ECG findings.[34] Patients with cocaine-associated chest pain should be evaluated with serum troponin measurement; serum creatinine kinase is less reliable, since it can be elevated due to rhabdomyolysis. For those who have normal troponin levels, no new ischemic changes on ECG, and no evidence of cardiovascular complications, a 9- to 12-hour observation period is probably sufficient.[43]

Less is known about the cardiac effects of methamphetamine, but there have been reports of chest pain and myocardial infarction associated with its use as well.[44] There is also one study from the Middle East that reports that khat users presenting with an acute coronary syndrome experienced a higher morbidity and mortality rate than others.[45]

Cardiomyopathy

Cocaine users may be at increased risk for the development of cardiomyopathy.[46] Although some of these cases are due to myocardial damage from coronary artery disease and myocardial infarction, others occur in the absence of any evidence of ischemia and may be due to myocarditis[47] or the direct toxic effect of cocaine.[48] Similarly, there have been reports of cardiomyopathy with methamphetamine use,[49] and a case-control study of hospitalized patients age 45 or younger reported that methamphetamine use was associated with an increased risk of cardiomyopathy (adjusted odds ratio: 3.7).[50]

Arrhythmia

Cocaine use has also been associated with a variety of arrhythmias, often in the setting of cardiac ischemia or myocardial infarction, or in patients with cardiomyopathy, hypotension, or hypoxemia.[35] These may lead to syncope or sudden death.

Aortic Dissection

Cocaine use has been associated with acute aortic dissection. In one series, 37% of cases of acute aortic dissection were associated with cocaine use; many of these patients also had untreated hypertension.[51] In an analysis of the International Registry of Acute Aortic Dissection from 1996 to 2012, 1.8% had documented cocaine use. Those who used cocaine were younger and were more likely to smoke and to be male.[52]

Endocarditis

While all injection drug users are at risk for endocarditis, those who use cocaine appear to be at higher risk for this complication.[53] Endocarditis is discussed in more detail in Chapter 14.

Peripheral Vascular Disease

Cocaine use has been associated with limb ischemia; this can occur acutely after inadvertent injection into an artery[54] or even after intranasal use.[55] There may also be an association between cocaine use and thromboangiitis obliterans (Buerger disease).[56]

Gastrointestinal Complications

The vasoconstrictive effects of cocaine can affect the gastrointestinal tract and lead to ischemic colitis;[57] this has also been observed with methamphetamine[58] and prescription stimulants.[59]

Renal Complications

Cocaine use has been associated with declines in kidney function[60] and kidney failure,[61] especially among hypertensive patients. Cocaine-induced rhabdomyolysis may also be complicated by renal failure.[62] Renal infarction associated with cocaine use has also been reported.[63]

Neuromuscular Complications

Stroke

Cocaine use has been associated with ischemic and hemorrhagic stroke.[64] In a study of 371 amphetamine-related fatalities in Australia, 20% had evidence of cerebrovascular pathology.[65] An analysis of hospitalizations in Texas found that cocaine use was associated with an increased risk of hemorrhagic and ischemic stroke; while amphetamine use was also associated with an increased risk of hemorrhagic stroke, it was not associated with ischemic stroke.[66]

Subarachnoid Hemorrhage

Cocaine use has also been associated with subarachnoid hemorrhage. In an analysis of 1,134 patients admitted with aneurysmal subarachnoid hemorrhage, 13% had recent cocaine exposure by urine drug testing; these patients were younger and had a higher risk of aneurysm re-rupture and in-hospital mortality.[67]

Rhabdomyolysis

Cocaine and methamphetamine users are at risk for rhabdomyolysis, which can be complicated by renal failure or compartment syndrome and can occur with any route of use.[68] In one California series of nontraumatic rhabdomyolysis, 43% of the patients had positive drug tests for methamphetamines; those with methamphetamine-associated rhabdomyolysis tended to be younger and were more likely to be agitated on presentation.[69]

Hyperthermia/Heat Stroke

Epidemiological studies have noted an association between high ambient temperature (>88°F) and mortality associated with cocaine use.[70] This is probably at least partly due to an increased risk of hyperthermia among cocaine users; cocaine has been found to impair heat dissipation by inhibiting sweating and cutaneous vasodilation.[71] Athletes who use stimulants are also at risk for this complication, and there have been a number of highly publicized deaths of athletes who were using stimulants and developed hyperthermia.

Movement Disorders

In animal studies, methamphetamine damages dopaminergic neurons in the substantia nigra, which leads to motor impairment characteristic of Parkinsonism.[72] Two cohort studies have found that methamphetamine or amphetamine use was associated with an increased risk of Parkinsonism, whereas cocaine use was not.[73,74]

Seizures

Seizures have been associated with cocaine use, but a 2013 systematic review on the topic concluded "no rigorous scientific evidence supports a causal relationship between cocaine and seizures."[75]

Psychiatric Complications

Cocaine users may develop a variety of psychiatric symptoms, including anxiety, agitation, paranoia, and psychosis. Cocaine-induced psychosis and paranoia appear to be a relatively common experience for users.[76] This phenomenon seems to be partly dose related,[77] but individual predisposition probably also plays a role.[78] Amphetamine users can experience similar complications, but they tend to be longer in duration. Synthetic cathinones ("bath salts") may be associated with more severe psychiatric side effects,[79] but there are limited comparative data.

Cocaine use, particularly crack cocaine use, has been blamed for violent behavior. A study published in 2010 found that individuals who used crack cocaine were more likely than other cocaine users to have engaged in violent behavior, but the difference appeared to be entirely due to other sociodemographic differences.[80]

As with other substances, those with stimulant use disorder are at increased risk of a variety of psychiatric illnesses, including depression, bipolar disorder, anxiety disorders, personality disorders, and schizophrenia, though a cause-and-effect relationship has not been established.[81] Psychiatric co-occurring disorders are covered further in Chapter 15.

Pregnancy

There has been a great deal of concern about the effects of cocaine on the developing fetus and alarm about an epidemic of crack babies. However, studies have not supported an association between cocaine exposure in utero and serious developmental disorders. Many of the children born to these mothers do have poorer outcomes than others, but these are likely due to other factors, such as their environment and exposure to other substances, particularly alcohol and tobacco.[82] There are some data that suggest an association between cocaine use and placental abruption and premature rupture of membranes.[83] Less is known about the effects of methamphetamine on pregnancy. It does not appear to increase the risk of birth defects[84] but has been associated with fetal growth restriction.[85] Substance use disorders and pregnancy are covered further in Chapter 16.

Treatment

Most of the research done on the treatment of stimulant use disorders has been performed on individuals using cocaine There are fewer data on the treatment of methamphetamine and other stimulant use disorders, but given their similarity to cocaine, it is reasonable to postulate that treatment effects would be comparable.[86] The treatment modalities that have been utilized can be roughly divided into two types: (1) psychosocial treatment and (2) pharmacotherapy and other interventions. There are a variety of psychosocial interventions that appear to be effective for selective individuals. No medical agent has consistently been shown to be effective, but long-acting amphetamines, disulfiram, and topiramate may be beneficial. Combinations of psychosocial treatment and pharmacotherapy may prove to be the most effective approach.

Psychosocial Treatment

A variety of psychosocial modalities have been used in treating cocaine and other stimulant use disorders. Participation in self-help groups is associated with improved outcomes. Individual and group drug counseling also appear to be helpful. A number of other behavioral approaches have been found to be modestly effective.

Brief Interventions

The data on the effectiveness of brief interventions for cocaine and other stimulant use are mixed. One trial of a single-session motivational intervention for cocaine or heroin use reported effectiveness,[87] while other trials of drug users (including cocaine and amphetamines) have failed to show a benefit.[88,89] Brief interventions are discussed further in Chapter 2.

Self-Help Groups

As with other forms of addiction, self-help (or mutual-help) groups are a commonly used form of treatment; Narcotics Anonymous (www.na.org) and Cocaine Anonymous (www.ca.org) both sponsor meetings throughout North America. These groups use the 12-step approach developed by Alcoholics Anonymous, but it may vary depending on the makeup of their members. The data on the effectiveness of these groups are limited but suggest a benefit for some individuals. In one observational study of patients in a variety of treatment modalities, those who after treatment participated in self-help groups twice weekly or greater for more than 6 months had better outcomes in terms of drug use and illegal activity. This effect was sustained even when correcting for measures of motivation and demographic factors.[90] Another observational study similarly found that participation at least weekly in 12-step groups was associated with lower drug and alcohol use, even when motivational measures were taken into account; less than weekly participation was no better than no participation at all.[91] A recent study suggests that cocaine-dependent individuals who actively participate in the self-help process—in the form of speaking or performing duties at meetings, talking with a sponsor, reading 12-step literature, or working on a step—have better outcomes than those of people who simply attend meetings.[92] An important factor to keep in mind here is that these studies generally looked at individuals who had gone through another form of drug treatment before (or while) attending these groups.

Drug Counseling

Drug counseling is another commonly used therapeutic modality and can be offered in a group or individual setting. Simple screening and counseling of outpatients who use cocaine (and heroin) has been found to be modestly effective at reducing subsequent drug use.[93] A study of intensive group counseling (three 3-hour sessions/week for 12 weeks) found no better outcomes when compared with weekly individual counseling alone or with a weekly group session.[94] Individual drug counseling may offer some benefit over traditional group therapy. In one study of cocaine-dependent adults, this type of treatment (when combined with group drug counseling) was associated with (modestly) better outcomes than with cognitive therapy, supportive-expressive therapy, or group drug counseling alone.[95]

Behavioral Therapy

There are a variety of behavioral approaches that appear to provide modest benefits, though the data on their effectiveness are mixed.

Coping skills therapy was associated with reduced cocaine use in a short-term study,[96] but this effect appeared to dissipate after a year.[97] A subsequent study failed to find any benefit associated with coping skills therapy but did find that motivational enhancement therapy appeared to benefit individuals with lower initial motivation.[98] In another study (mentioned earlier), the addition of cognitive therapy to group drug counseling did not appear to offer any additional benefit and performed worse than individual drug counseling.[95] On the other hand, a study of amphetamine users reported that 2–4 sessions of cognitive behavioral therapy was effective at reducing amphetamine use.[99] Finally, in a study of the treatment of methamphetamine dependence, an approach that combines cognitive-behavioral therapy with family education, social support, and individual counseling (the "Matrix Model") was found to perform better than treatment as usual in the short term but not beyond the treatment phase.[100]

The application of incentives contingent on abstinence, or "contingency management," appears to be a useful approach, although the long-term effectiveness (i.e., beyond the period of incentives) has not been established. For example, in one 24-week trial, contingency management with vouchers (in combination with behavioral treatment and community reinforcement) was found to reduce cocaine use.[101] The use of community reinforcement with vouchers (compared to vouchers alone) appears to reduce cocaine use further, at least during the treatment phase.[102] In a study of individuals on methadone maintenance therapy, however, cognitive-behavioral therapy performed as well as contingency management, and the combination of the two was no better than either alone.[103] Nevertheless, a recent systematic review of community reinforcement concluded that this approach is effective, especially when combined with abstinence-contingent incentives (such as vouchers).[104]

Analytic Psychotherapy

For those who are addicted to stimulants, there is little evidence that analytic psychotherapeutic approaches are effective. In one study, once-weekly psychotherapy was not shown to be effective; this was true for once-weekly family therapy and group therapy as well.[105] Another study (mentioned earlier) found no benefit associated with the addition of supportive-expressive therapy to group drug counseling for cocaine-dependent individuals.[95] Furthermore, another study found that outcomes with interpersonal therapy were poorer than with cognitive-behavioral therapy.[106]

Residential Treatment

The most intensive form of treatment for cocaine dependence is residential treatment; this is generally in the form of a therapeutic community, but a variety of approaches are used. A large observational study of treatment outcomes reported that long-term residential treatment, when compared with short-term outpatient and outpatient drug-free programs, was associated with lower cocaine use for a subset of individuals with a high level of addiction severity, provided they stayed 90 days or longer in treatment.[107]

Pharmacotherapy (and Acupuncture)

There have been many studies of numerous agents in search of one that would help reduce cocaine use; unfortunately, there is little evidence that any of these interventions is effective. Recent studies suggest that disulfiram, topiramate, modafinil, and long-acting amphetamines may be effective, but more research needs to be done to confirm initial observations and to assess their long-term impact. The development of vaccines against cocaine or methamphetamine is another intriguing therapeutic option that is being explored.[108]

Antidepressants/Anxiolytics

Studies on the use of antidepressants for cocaine dependence have generally failed to show a benefit.[109] A 2011 Cochrane review concluded that the current data "do not support the efficacy of antidepressants in the treatment of cocaine abuse/dependence."[110]

Likewise, the anxiolytic buspirone was not found to be effective in a clinical trial.[111]

Dopamine Agonists

Some early trials suggested that dopamine agonists, such as amantadine and bromocriptine, were effective for treatment of cocaine withdrawal symptoms.[112] However, subsequent studies of their chronic administration did not find any reduction in cocaine use.[113,114] A 2011 Cochrane review of the use of dopamine agonists for cocaine dependence concluded that the current evidence "does not support the use of dopamine agonists for treating cocaine dependence."[115]

Dopamine Antagonists

Dopamine may be responsible for the reinforcing effects of cocaine. As a result, it has been postulated that dopamine antagonists, such as the antipsychotics olanzapine and risperidone, may reduce cocaine craving and use; unfortunately, clinical trials have shown no benefit.[116,117]

Disulfiram

Many cocaine-dependent individuals also have problems with alcohol. Studies of disulfiram treatment of individuals with concurrent alcohol and cocaine dependence have indicated that use of this medication was associated with reduced cocaine use.[118] It was subsequently reported that disulfiram reduced cocaine use in individuals (on methadone maintenance) who were *not* alcohol dependent.[119] A 12-week trial found significantly greater reduction in cocaine use with disulfiram, especially when combined with cognitive-behavioral therapy.[106] However, a 2010 Cochrane systematic review concluded that "there is low evidence, at the present, supporting the clinical use of disulfiram for the treatment of cocaine dependence."[120]

It has been hypothesized that disulfiram may reduce cocaine use through inhibition of dopamine β-hydroxylase (DβH). A study published in 2014 suggests that the drug may be more effective in individuals with genetically low DβH levels.[121]

Carbamazepine

One study of carbamazepine reported a reduction in cocaine use over a 12-week period.[122] However, other studies did not find any benefit, and a 2003 Cochrane review of five studies on the use of carbamazepine for cocaine dependence concluded that there is "no current evidence supporting the clinical use of carbamazepine in the treatment of cocaine dependence."[123]

Topiramate

The gamma amino butyric acid (GABA) system is thought to play a role in mediating the reinforcing effects of cocaine. Thus, it has been postulated that the GABAergic anticonvulsant topiramate may reduce cocaine craving. A 2004 pilot study of a cohort with mild cocaine dependence found that its use was associated with significant reduction in cocaine-positive urine drug tests but not other measures of cocaine use.[124] A 2013 clinical trial reported that topiramate was modestly efficacious at "increasing the weekly proportion of cocaine nonuse days."[125] On the other hand, a study of topiramate for methamphetamine addiction did not find increased abstinence,[126] and in another study of cocaine-dependent subjects, topiramate did not improve outcomes.[127] Moreover, topiramate was not effective in studies of topiramate for cocaine dependence during methadone maintenance[128] or for treatment of comorbid cocaine and alcohol dependence.[129]

Atomoxetine

Atomoxetine is a norepinephrine reuptake inhibitor, which is used to treat attention deficit disorder. In contrast to stimulants, it appears to have low abuse potential. Unfortunately, in one clinical trial, atomoxetine did not have any effect on cocaine use.[130]

Modafinil

Modafinil is a glutamate-enhancing agent that promotes wakefulness and is approved for treatment of narcolepsy. Since cocaine depletes extracellular glutamate, it has been postulated that this agent may help reduce craving and use. Moreover, modafinil appears to have low abuse potential. An 8-week pilot study reported that its use was associated with a reduction in cocaine use, without serious side effects.[131] However, its effectiveness and long-term safety need to be studied further.

Stimulants

Some have proposed the use of long-acting agonists for individuals dependent on stimulants, analogous to the use of methadone to treat opioid addicts. A pilot study of dexamethamphetamine reported favorable results in 30 cocaine-dependent adults over a period of 14 weeks;[132] a subsequent larger randomized controlled trial (using sustained-release D-amphetamine) supported this initial evaluation.[133] Sustained-release dexamphetamine has also been shown to reduce methamphetamine use.[134] It should be noted that these studies were for limited periods of time (12–14 weeks) and did not assess clinical or psychosocial outcomes. Cochrane systematic reviews of psychostimulants for cocaine dependence in 2010[135] and amphetamine abuse or dependence in 2013[136] did not find sufficient evidence to support their use. A 14-week trial of sustained-release methylphenidate, published in 2014, reported modest improvements in some secondary measures among methamphetamine-dependent subjects.[137]

Naltrexone

In one small 12-week trial, naltrexone was reported to be effective at reducing amphetamine use.[138] However, two other studies found no change in cocaine use among cocaine- and alcohol-dependent individuals who were treated with oral[139] or injectable extended-release naltrexone.[140]

Acupuncture

An initial study of 82 cocaine-dependent subjects on methadone maintenance reported a reduction in cocaine use among subjects who received auricular acupuncture.[141] However, a subsequent larger trial with 620 subjects found that it was no more effective than sham needle insertion or relaxation controls.[142] A 2005 meta-analysis of nine studies concluded that the evidence "does not support the use of acupuncture for the treatment of cocaine dependence."[143]

Table 8.2 provides a summary of studies on treatment for stimulant use disorders.

TABLE 8.2 Summary of Stimulant Use Disorder Treatment Studies

Intervention	Studies	Outcomes
Psychosocial		
Brief advice	RCT	Effective for reducing cocaine use in one RCT
Self-help groups	Observational	Participation is associated with better outcomes
Group counseling	RCTs	Effective, more intensive (3 times/week), no more effective than weekly
Individual counseling	RCTs	Effective, may offer some benefit when added to group counseling
Cognitive-behavioral therapy (CBT)	RCTs	Effective (in some studies)

(continued)

TABLE 8.2 (Continued)

Intervention	Studies	Outcomes
Psychosocial		
Contingency management	RCTs	Effective (while incentives are offered)
Analytic psychotherapy	RCTs	No benefit when added to group counseling; outcomes better with CBT
Residential treatment	Observational	>90 days participation associated with better outcomes
Pharmacotherapy		
Antidepressants	RCTs Meta-analysis	Not effective
Dopamine agonists	RCTs Meta-analysis	Not effective
Dopamine antagonists	RCTs Meta-analysis	Not effective
Disulfiram	RCTs Meta-analysis	Effective in some studies
Topiramate	RCTs	Modestly effective in some studies
Stimulants	RCTs Meta-analysis	Effective in some studies
Acupuncture	RCTs Meta-analysis	Not effective

Most studies were of cocaine users; see text for references and more details.
RCT: randomized controlled trial.

Caffeine

Background

Caffeine (1,3,7-trimethylxanthine) is a naturally occurring methylxanthine, similar to the drug theophylline. It blocks adenosine receptors, leading to release of dopamine. Caffeine is found in coffee, tea, and chocolate and as an additive in a variety of beverages. It is also an ingredient in a variety of over-the-counter and prescription medications, including headache preparations and drugs to promote wakefulness. A cup (8 ounces) of coffee can contain 50–200 mg of caffeine; tea, 15–80 mg; and soft drinks, 20–60 mg (12 ounces). "Energy drinks" typically contain 80–160 mg, but some may have 250–500 mg of caffeine.[144] Over-the-counter preparations may have as much as 300 mg of caffeine in each dose.

Drug Effects

Low to moderate doses of caffeine produce a number of positive subjective effects, including an increased sense of well-being, energy, and alertness. The toxic effects of caffeine include nausea, vomiting, tremulousness, anxiety, and agitation. Caffeine appears to promote cardiac arrhythmias, but probably not at the doses usually consumed.[145] Caffeine overdose generally only occurs with consumption of caffeine-containing medications or ingestion of caffeine powders and can be fatal in some cases.[146,147] While caffeine does increase blood pressure acutely, it does not appear to increase the risk of hypertension.[148] The DSM-5 includes criteria for "caffeine intoxication" (ICD-10 code: F15.929) under "caffeine-related disorders."[9]

Withdrawal

Many regular caffeine users experience mild withdrawal symptoms with cessation of use, including headaches, fatigue, and drowsiness,[149] as well as symptoms of depression and anxiety and diminished motor performance.[150] The DSM-5 includes criteria for caffeine withdrawal (ICD-10 code: F15.93). Some believe that caffeine use can lead to dependence; it appears that some users exhibit signs of dependence, including unsuccessful attempts to cut down and continued use despite harmful effects.[151] However, the DSM-5 does not recognize a caffeine use disorder.

Health Effects

Caffeinated beverages may have a number of beneficial health effects. Coffee can ameliorate the driving impairment associated with sleep deprivation.[152] Coffee and tea also appear to have a protective effect against development of type II diabetes,[153] although this is probably not due to caffeine.[154,155] Coffee consumption also appears to protect against cirrhosis of the liver, especially among heavy alcohol drinkers,[156] and is associated with a lower risk of liver disease progression among persons with hepatitis C.[157] Moreover, a recent study in Finland found that coffee drinkers had a lower risk of developing dementia.[158]

There have been mixed data on the association of coffee consumption and mortality. A 2008 cohort study of over 13,000 men and women found that the unadjusted risk of mortality increased with higher coffee consumption.[159] However, this appeared to be largely due to an association between heavier coffee consumption and smoking. When adjusting for smoking and other risk factors for cardiovascular disease and cancer, coffee consumption was not associated with an increased risk of mortality and, in fact, appeared to confer a modest benefit. This benefit is probably not due to caffeine, because it was also observed among those who drank decaffeinated coffee. A 2012 study of over 400,000 men and women found that coffee consumption was inversely associated with total and cause-specific mortality, even among those who drank more than 6 cups/day.[160] By contrast, a longitudinal study of over 43,000 participants found that heavy coffee consumption (>28 cups/week) was associated with increased mortality in men of all ages and women younger than 55 years.[161]

Notes

1. Mateen FJ, Cascino GD. Khat chewing: a smokeless gun? Mayo Clin Proc 2010;85:971–3.

2. Prosser JM, Nelson LS. The toxicology of bath salts: a review of synthetic cathinones. J Med Toxicol 2012;8:33–42.

3. Chu NS. Neurological aspects of areca and betel chewing. Addict Biol 2002;7:111–4.

4. Substance Abuse and Mental Health Services Administration. *Results from the 2013 National Survey on Drug Use and Health: National Findings*. NSDUH Series H-48, HHS Publication No. (SMA) 14-4863. Rockville, MD: Substance Abuse and Mental Health Services Administration; 2014.

5. Substance Abuse and Mental Health Services Administration, Drug Abuse Warning Network, 2011. *National Estimates of Drug-Related Emergency Department Visits*. HHS Publication No. (SMA) 13-4760, DAWN Series D-39. Rockville, MD: Substance Abuse and Mental Health Services Administration; 2013.

6. Cantrell FL, Breckenridge HM. Transrectal methamphetamine use: a novel route of exposure. Ann Intern Med 2006;145:78–9.

7. Silber BY, Croft RJ, Papafotiou K, Stough C. The acute effects of d-amphetamine and methamphetamine on attention and psychomotor performance. Psychopharmacology (Berl) 2006;187:154–69.

8. Avois L, Robinson N, Saudan C, et al. Central nervous system stimulants and sport practice. Br J Sports Med 2006;40(Suppl 1):i16–i20.

9. American Psychiatric Association. *Diagnostic and Statistical Manual of Mental Disorders*, Fifth Edition. Arlington, VA: American Psychiatric Publishing; 2013.

10. Darke S, Kaye S, Duflou J. Cocaine-related fatalities in New South Wales, Australia 1993-2002. Drug Alcohol Depend 2005;77:107–14.

11. Morentin B, Ballesteros J, Callado LF, Meana JJ. Recent cocaine use is a significant risk factor for sudden cardiovascular death in 15-49 year-old subjects: a forensic case-control study. Addiction 2014;109:2071–8.

12. Muhuri PK, Gfroerer BA. Mortality associated with illegal drug use among adults in the United States. Am J Drug Alcohol Abuse 2011;37:155–64.

13. McKinney PE, Tomaszewski C, Phillips S, et al. Methamphetamine toxicity prevented by activated charcoal in a mouse model. Ann Emerg Med 1994;24:220–3.

14. Gorelick DA, Baumann MH. The phamacology of cocaine, amphetamines and other stimulants. In Ries RK, Fiellin DA, Miller SC, Saitz R, eds. *The ASAM Principles of Addiction Medicine*, 5th ed. Philadelphia: Wolters Kluwer; 2014:151–79.

15. Mazor SS, Mycyk MB, Willis BK, et al. Coca tea consumption causes positive urine cocaine assay. Eur J Emerg Med 2006;13:340–1.

16. Tests for drugs of abuse. The Medical Letter 2002;44:71–3.

17. Bradford M, Rosenberg B, Moreno J. Bilateral necrosis of earlobes and cheeks: another complication of cocaine contaminated with levamisole. Ann Intern Med 2010;152:758–9.

18. Vilela RJ, Langford C, McCullagh L, Kass ES. Cocaine-induced oronasal fistulas with external nasal erosion but without palate involvement. Ear Nose Throat 2002;81:562–3.

19. Mattson-Gates G, Jabs AD, Hugo NE. Perforation of the hard palate associated with cocaine use. Ann Plast Surg 1991;26:466–8.

20. Friedman DR, Wolfsthal SD. Cocaine-induced pseudovasculitits. Mayo Clin Proc 2005;80:671–3.

21. Curtis EK. Meth mouth: a review of methamphetamine abuse and its oral manifestations. Gen Dent 2006;54:125–9.

22. Sachs R, Zagelbaum BM, Hersh PS. Corneal complications associated with the use of crack cocaine. Ophthalmalogy 1993;100:187–91.

23. Poulsen EJ, Mannis MJ, Chang SD. Keratitis in methamphetamine abusers. Cornea 1996;15:477–82.

24. French DD, Margo CE, Harman LE. Substance use disorder and the risk of open-angle glaucoma. J Glaucoma 2011;20:452–7.

25. Tashkin DP, Kleerup EC, Koyal SN, et al. Acute effects of inhaled and IV cocaine on airway dynamics. Chest 1996;110:904–10.

26. Baldwin GC, Choi R, Roth MD, et al. Evidence of chronic damage to the pulmonary microcirculation in habitual users of alkaloidal ("crack") cocaine. Chest 2002;121:1231–8.

27. Patel RC, Dutta D, Schonfeld SA. Free-base cocaine use associated with bronchiolitis obliterans organizing pneumonia. Ann Intern Med 1987;107:186–7.

28. Yakel DL, Eisenberg MJ. Pulmonary artery hypertension in chronic intravenous cocaine users. Am Heart J 1995;130:398–9.

29. Chin KM, Channick RN, Rubin LJ. Is methamphetamine use associated with idiopathic pulmonary arterial hypertension? Chest 2006;130:1657–63.

30. Kleerup EC, Koyal SN, Marques-Magallanes JA, et al. Chronic and acute effects of "crack" cocaine on diffusing capacity, membrane diffusion, and pulmonary capillary blood volume in the lung. Chest 2002;122:629–38.

31. Arnett EN, Battle WE, Russo JV, Roberts WC. Intravenous injection of talc-containing drugs intended for oral use. A cause of pulmonary granulomatosis and pulmonary hypertension. Am J Med 1976;60:711–8.

32. Sherman CB, Hudson LD, Pierson DJ. Severe precocious emphysema in intravenous methylphenidate (Ritalin) abusers. Chest 1987;92:1085–7.

33. **Hollander JE, Todd KH, Green G, et al. Chest pain associated with cocaine: an assessment of prevalence in suburban and urban emergency departments. Ann Emerg Med 1995;26:671–6.** *Among 359 patients with chest pain (8% had a myocardial infarction), 29% of those age 18–30 had a positive urine test for cocaine, 48% age 31–40, 18% age 41–50, 3% age 51–60, and 0% age 61 or older.*

34. Hollander JE, Hoffman RS, Gennis P, et al. Prospective multicenter evaluation of cocaine-associated chest pain. Acad Emerg Med 1994;1:330–9.

35. Lange RA, Hillis LD. Cardiovascular complications of cocaine use. N Engl J Med 2001;345:351–8.

36. Lange RA, Cigarroa RG, Flores ED, et al. Potentiation of cocaine-induced coronary vasoconstriction by beta-adrenergic blockade. Ann Intern Med 1990;112:897–903.

37. McCord J, Jneid H, Hollander JE, et al. Management of cocaine-associated chest pain and myocardial infarction: a scientific statement from the American Heart Association Acute Cardiac Care Committee of the Council on Clinical Cardiology. Circulation 2008;117:1897–907.

38. Rangel C, Shu RG, Lazar LD, et al. Beta-blockers for chest pain associated with recent cocaine use. Arch Intern Med 2010;170:874–9.

39. Boehrer JD, Moliterno DJ, Willard JE, et al. Influence of labetolol on cocaine-induced coronary vasoconstriction in humans. Am J Med 1993;94:608–10.

40. Sofuoglu M, Brown S, Babb DA, et al. Effects of labetolol treatment on the physiologic and subjective response to smoked cocaine. Pharmacol Biochem Behav 2000;65:255–9.

41. Sofuglu M, Brown S, Babb DA, et al. Carvedilol affects the physiologic and behavioral response to smoked cocaine in humans. Drug Alcohol Depend 2000;60:69–76.

42. **Minor RL, Scott BD, Brown DD, Winniford MD. Cocaine-induced myocardial infarction in patients with normal coronary arteries. Ann Intern Med 1991;115:797–806.** *Of 114 cases of cocaine-associated myocardial infarction, 92 had angiography or autopsy and 38% of these had normal coronary arteries.*

43. **Weber JE, Shofer FS, Larkin GL, et al. Validation of a brief observation period for patients with cocaine-associated chest pain. N Engl J Med 2003;348:510–7.** *Consecutive patients with cocaine-associated chest pain were evaluated; 42/344 (12%) were admitted. Those with normal troponin-I levels, no new ischemic ECG changes, and no cardiovascular complications during a 9- to 12-hour observational period (n = 302) were discharged. At 30-day follow-up, none had died of a cardiovascular event; 4 of 256 (1.6%) had had a nonfatal myocardial infarction—all 4 had continued to use cocaine.*

44. Turnipseed SD, Richards JR, Kirk JD, et al. Frequency of acute coronary syndrome in patients presenting to the emergency department with chest pain after methamphetamine use. J Emerg Med 2003;24:369–73.

45. Ali WM, Zubaid M, Al-Motarreb A, et al. Association of khat chewing with increased risk of stroke and death in patients presenting with acute coronary syndrome. Mayo Clin Proc 2010;85:974–80.

46. **Roldan CA, Aliabadi D, Crawford MH. Prevalence of heart disease in asymptomatic chronic cocaine users. Cardiology 2001;95:25–30.** *In comparison with 32 age-matched controls, 35 cocaine users were more likely to have a positive stress test (34% vs. 9%) and decreased LV function (14% vs. 0%, p = 0.055). They were also more likely to smoke (47% vs. 19%).*

47. Turnicky RP, Goodin J, Smialek JE, et al. Incidental myocarditis with intravenous drug use: the pathology, immunopathology, and potential implications for human immunodeficiency virus-associated myocarditis. Hum Pathol 1992;23:138–43.

48. Peng SK, French WJ, Pelikan PC. Direct cocaine cardiotoxicity demonstrated by endomyocardial biopsy. Arch Pathol Lab Med 1989;113:842–5.

49. Hong R, Matsuyama E, Nur K. Cardiomyopathy associated with the smoking of crystal methamphetamine. JAMA 1991;265:1152–4.

50. Yeo KK, Wijetunga M, Ito H, et al. The association of methamphetamine use and cardiomyopathy in young patients. Am J Med 2007;120:165–71.

51. Hsue PY, Salinas CL, Bolger AF, et al. Acute aortic dissection related to crack cocaine. Circulation 2002;105:1592–5.

52. Dean JH, Woznicki EM, O'Gara P, et al. Cocaine-related aortic dissection: lessons from the International Registry of Acute Aortic Dissection. Am J Med 2014;127:878–85.

53. Chambers HF, Morris DL, Täuber MG, Modin G. Cocaine use and the risk for endocarditis in intravenous drug users. Ann Intern Med 1987;106:833–6.

54. Silverman SH, Turner WW. Intraarterial drug abuse: new treatment options. J Vasc Surg 1991;14:111–6.

55. Mizrayan R, Hanks SE, Weaver FA. Cocaine-induced thrombosis of common iliac and popliteal arteries. Ann Vasc Surg 1998;12:476–81.

56. Marder VJ, Mellinghoff IK. Cocaine and Buerger disease: is there a pathogenic association? Arch Intern Med 2000;160:2057–60.

57. Linder JD, Monkemuller KE, Raijman I, et al. Cocaine-associated ischemic colitis. South Med J 2000;93:909–13.

58. Johnson TD, Berenson MM. Methamphetamine-induced ischemic colitis. J Clin Gastroenterol 1991;13:687–9.

59. Comay D, Ramsay J, Irvine EJ. Ischemic colitis after weight-loss medication. Can J Gastroenterol. 2003;17:719–21.

60. **Vupputuri S, Batuman V, Munter P, et al. The risk for mild kidney function decline associated with illicit drug use among hypertensive men. Am J Kidney Dis 2004;43:629–35.** *Among 647 hypertensive veterans followed for a median of 7 years, cocaine use was associated with mild kidney function decline (adjusted relative risk 3.0).*

61. **Norris KC, Thornhill-Joynes M, Robinson C, et al. Cocaine use, hypertension, and end-stage renal disease. Am J Kidney Dis 2001;38:523–8.** *Among 201 subjects at two urban dialysis units, cocaine*

use was associated with a diagnosis of hypertension-related renal failure (odds ratio of 9.4).

62. Singhal P, Horowitz B, Quinones MC, et al. Acute renal failure following cocaine abuse. Nephron 1989;52:76–8.

63. Sharff JA. Renal infarction associated with intravenous cocaine use. Ann Emerg Med 1984;13:1145–7.

64. Sordo L, Indave BI, Degenhardt L, et al. Cocaine use and risk of stroke: a systematic review. Drug Alcohol Depend 2014;142:1–13.

65. Kaye S, Darke S, Duflou J, McKetin R. Methamphetamine-related fatalities in Australia: demographics, circumstances, toxicology and major organ pathology. Addiction 2008;103:1353–60.

66. **Westover AN, McBride S, Haley RW. Stroke in young adults who abuse amphetamines or cocaine: a population-based study of hospitalized patients. Arch Gen Psych 2007;64:495–502.** *Among 812,247 hospitalizations in 2003, the adjusted odds ratio of hemorrhagic stroke was 5.0 for amphetamines and 2.3 for cocaine; for ischemic stroke, the respective odds ratios were 1.04 and 2.0.*

67. Chang TR, Kowalski RG, Caserta F, et al. Impact of acute cocaine use on aneurysmal subarachnoid hemorrhage. Stroke 2013;44:1825–9.

68. Horowitz BZ, Panacek EA, Jouriles NJ. Severe rhabdomyolysis with renal failure after intranasal cocaine use. J Emerg Med 1997;15:833–7.

69. Richards JR, Johnson EB, Stark RW, Derlet RW. Methamphetamine abuse and rhabdomyolysis in the ED: a 5-year study. Am J Emerg Med 1999;17:681–5.

70. Marzuk PM, Tardiff K, Leon AC, et al. Ambient temperature and mortality from unintentional cocaine overdose. JAMA 1998;279:1795–800.

71. Crandall CG, Vongpatanasin W, Victor RG. Mechanism of cocaine-induced hyperthermia in humans. Ann Intern Med 2002;136:785–91.

72. Granado N, Ares-Santos S, Moratalla R. Methamphetamine and Parkinson's disease. Parkinsons Dis 2013;2013:308052.

73. Callaghan RC, Cunningham JK, Sykes J, Kish SJ. Increased risk of Parkinson's disease in individuals hospitalized with conditions related to the use of methamphetamine or other amphetamine-type drugs. Drug Alcohol Depend 2012;120:35–40.

74. Curtin K, Fleckenstein AE, Robison RJ, et al. Methamphetamine/amphetamine abuse and risk of Parkinson's disease in Utah: a population-based assessment. Drug Alcohol Depend 2015;146:30–8.

75. Sordo L, Indave BI, Degenhardt L, et al. A systematic review of evidence on the association between cocaine use and seizures. Drug Alcohol Depend 2013;133:795–804.

76. Brady KT, Lydiard RB, Malcom R, Ballenger JC. Cocaine-induced psychosis. J Clin Psychiatry 1991;52:509–12.

77. Batki SL, Harris DS. Quantitative drug levels in stimulant psychosis: relationship to symptom severity, catecholamines and hyperkinesia. Am J Addict 2004;13:461–70.

78. Satel SL, Edell WS. Cocaine-induced paranoia and psychosis proneness. Am J Psychiatry 1991;148:1708–11.

79. **Spiller HA, Ryan ML, Weston RG, Jansen J. Clinical experience with and analytic confirmation of "bath salts" and "legal highs" (synthetic cathinones) in the United States. Clin Toxicol 2011;49:499–505.** *In this analysis of 236 cases reported to poison control centers, complications included agitation (82%), combative behavior (57%), hallucinations (40%), paranoia (36%), and confusion (35%).*

80. Vaughn MG, Fu Q, Perron BE, et al. Is crack cocaine use associated with greater violence than powdered cocaine use? Results from a national sample. Am J Drug Alcohol Abuse 2010;36:181–6.

81. Regier DA, Farmer ME, Rae DS, et al. Comorbidity of mental disorders with alcohol and other drug abuse. Results from the Epidemiologic Catchment Area study. JAMA 1990;264:2511–8.

82. Frank DA, Augustyn M, Knight WG, et al. Growth, development, and behavior in early childhood following prenatal cocaine exposure: a systematic review. JAMA 2001;285:1613–25.

83. Addis A, Moretti ME, Ahmed Syed F, et al. Fetal effects of cocaine: an updated meta-analysis. Reprod Toxicol 2001;15:341–69.

84. Little BB, Snell LM, Gilstrap LC. Methamphetamine abuse during pregnancy: outcome and fetal effects. Obstet Gynecol 1988;72:541–4.

85. Smith LM, LaGasse LL, Derauf C, et al. The infant development, environment, and lifestyle study: effects of prenatal methamphetamine exposure, polydrug exposure, and poverty on intrauterine growth. Pediatrics 2006;118:1149–56.

86. Cretzmeyer M, Sarrazin MV, Huber DL, et al. Treatment of methamphetamine abuse: research findings and clinical directions. J Subst Abuse Treat 2003;24:267–77.

87. Bernstein J, Bernstein E, Tassiopoulos K, et al. Brief motivational intervention at a clinic visit reduces cocaine and heroin use. Drug Alcohol Depend 2005;77:49–59.

88. Saitz R, Palfai TPA, Cheng DM, et al. Screening and brief intervention for drug use in primary care-The ASPIRE randomized clinical trial. JAMA 2014;312:502–13.

89. Roy-Byrne P, Bumgardner K, Krupski A, et al. Brief interventions for problem drug in safety-net primary care settings—a randomized clinical trial. JAMA 2014;312:492–501.

90. Etheridge RM, Craddock SG, Hubbard RL, Rounds-Bryant JL. The relationship of counseling and self-help participation to patient outcomes in DATOS. Drug Alcohol Depend 1999;57:99–112.

91. Fiorentine R. After drug treatment: are 12-step programs effective in maintaining abstinence? Am J Drug Alcohol Abuse 1999;25:93–116.

92. **Weiss RD, Griffin ML, Gallop RJ, et al. The effect of 12-step self-help group attendance and participation on drug use outcomes among cocaine-dependent patients. Drug Alcohol Depend 2005;77:177–84.** *This observational study included 336 cocaine-dependent adults from a randomized controlled trial of different treatment modalities. Active participation in 12-step activities was associated with reduced subsequent drug use, whereas attendance alone was not.*

93. **Bernstein J, Bernstein E, Tassiopoulos K, et al. Brief motivational intervention at a clinic visit reduces cocaine and heroin use. Drug Alcohol Depend 2005;77:49–59.** *Patients attending walk-in clinics were screened for heroin and cocaine use and were randomized to (1) brief intervention by a trained counselor consisting of a motivational interview, active referrals, and a handout with a list of treatment resources, followed by a phone call 10 days later, or (2) handout only. Of 23,669 screened, 1,232 (5%) were eligible, 1,175 enrolled, and 778 were used in the final analysis. At 6-month follow-up, those in the intervention group were more likely to be abstinent from cocaine alone (22% vs. 17%), heroin alone (40% vs. 31%), and both drugs (17% vs. 13%).*

94. **Gottheil E, Weinstein SP, Sterling RC, et al. A randomized controlled study of the effectiveness of intensive outpatient treatment for cocaine dependence. Psychiatr Serv 1998;49:782–7.**

Cocaine-dependent adults (447 of 862 offered treatment) were randomized to (1) weekly individual counseling, (2) individual counseling plus a weekly group session, and (3) intensive group treatment (three 3-hour sessions/ week). There was no difference after 12 weeks of treatment and at 9-month follow-up; the 24% who completed treatment did better, regardless of type.

95. **Crits-Christoph P, Siqueland L, Blaine J, et al. Psychosocial treatments for cocaine dependence**. Arch Gen Psychiatry **1999;56:493–502**. *Cocaine-dependent adults (487 of 2197 screened) were randomized to (1) individual drug counseling + group drug counseling (GDC), (2) cognitive therapy + GDC, (3) supportive-expressive therapy +GDC, or (4) GDC alone; 28% of the total completed the 6-month treatment. Over 12 months, the mean addiction severity index (ASI) scores and cocaine use in all four arms decreased, but more so in the first arm.*

96. Monti PM, Rohsenow DJ, Michalec E, et al. Brief coping skills treatment for cocaine abuse: substance use outcomes at three months. Addiction 1997;92:1717–28.

97. Rohsenow DJ, Monti PM, Martin RA, et al. Brief coping skills treatment for cocaine abuse: 12-month substance use outcomes. J Consult Clin Psychol 2000;68:515–20.

98. Rohsenow DJ, Monti PM, Martin RA, et al. Motivational enhancement and coping skills training for cocaine abusers: effects on substance use outcomes. Addiction 2004;99:862–74.

99. **Baker A, Lee NK, Claire M, et al. Brief behavioural interventions for regular amphetamine users: a step in the right direction**. Addiction **2005;100:367–78**. *Amphetamine users (n = 214) were randomized to (1) two sessions of cognitive-behavioral therapy (CBT), (2) four sessions of CBT, or (3) a self-help booklet. At 6-month follow-up, abstinence rates were 34%, 38%, and 18% respectively.*

100. **Rawson RA, Marinelli-Casey P, Anglin MD, et al. A multi-site comparison of psychoscocial approaches for the treatment of methamphetamine dependence**. Addiction **2004;99:708–17**. *Methamphetamine-dependent adults (n = 978) were randomized to (1) Matrix Model (MM) or (2) treatment as usual—a variety of community treatment programs. Overall, those assigned to MM were more likely to complete their program (41% vs. 34%), had longer periods of abstinence, and were more likely to have methamphetamine-negative urine tests over 16 weeks. The 86% who completed 6-month follow-up (in both groups) reported reduced use and 69% had negative urine tests, but there was no significant difference between the groups.*

101. **Higgins ST, Budney AJ, Bickel WK, et al. Incentives improve outcome in outpatient behavioral treatment of cocaine dependence. Arch Gen Psychiatry 1994;51:568–76.** *Cocaine-dependent adults (n = 40) were randomized to behavioral treatment and community reinforcement with or without voucher incentives over 12 weeks. Both received the same treatment for the second 12 weeks. The voucher group had higher 12-week retention (90% vs. 65%) and 24-week retention (75% vs. 40%); they were also more likely to be cocaine-abstinent during both 12-week periods (but this declined in both groups).*

102. **Higgins ST, Sigmon SC, Wong CJ, et al. Community reinforcement therapy for cocaine-dependent outpatients. Arch Gen Psychiatry 2003;60:1043–52.** *Cocaine-dependent adults (n = 100) were randomized to (1) community reinforcement + vouchers (CR) or (2) vouchers alone. All received 24 weeks of treatment followed by 6 months aftercare and were assessed at 12, 15, and 24 months. Those assigned to CR had better treatment retention (84% vs. 51%) and were more likely to have cocaine-negative urine tests at 12 weeks (78% vs. 51%) but not subsequently. CR subjects had more paid employment days during treatment and at 9- to 12-month follow-up, but not at 15- to 24-month follow-up. Legal, medical, psychiatric, and family problems were about the same.*

103. **Rawson RA, Huber A, McCann M, et al. A comparison of contingency management and cognitive-behavioral approaches during methadone maintenance treatment for cocaine dependence. Arch Gen Psychiatry 2002;59:817–24.** *Cocaine-dependent adults on methadone maintenance (n = 120) were randomized to (1) cognitive-behavioral therapy (CBT), (2) contingency management, that is, vouchers for cocaine-negative urine tests (CM), (3) CBT + CM, or (4) usual care. During 16 weeks of treatment, the two CM arms had the highest rate of cocaine-negative urine tests (54% vs. 40% with CBT and 23% with usual care). At 52-week follow-up, the CBT-only group had the highest rate (60%), followed by CM only (53%), CBT + CM (40%), and usual care (27%).*

104. Roozen HG, Boulogne JJ, Tulder MW, et al. A systematic review of the effectiveness of the community reinforcement approach in alcohol, cocaine and opioid addiction. Drug Alcohol Depend 2004;74:1–13.

105. **Kang SY, Kleinman PH, Woody GE, et al. Outcomes for cocaine abusers after once-a-week psychosocial therapy. Am J Psychiatry 1991;148:630–5.** *Cocaine abusers (n = 168) were randomized weekly: (1) individual supportive-expressive psychotherapy, (2) family therapy, or (3) group therapy. Of the 122 who had 6-month and 1-year*

follow-up, 23 (19%) reported ≥3 months of abstinence, but there was no difference between the three arms.

106. **Carroll KM, Fenton LR, Ball SA, et al. Efficacy of disulfiram and cognitive behavior therapy in cocaine-dependent outpatients. Arch Gen Psychiatry 2004;61:264–72.** *Cocaine-dependent outpatients (n = 121) were randomized in a 2×2 factorial trial to (1) disulfiram or placebo, and (2) cognitive-behavioral therapy (CBT) or interpersonal psychotherapy (IPT) for 12 weeks. About half had alcohol dependence/abuse. There was greater reduction in cocaine use among those assigned to disulfiram versus placebo and those assigned CBT versus IPT.*

107. Simpson DD, Joe GW, Fletcher BW at al. A national evaluation of treatment outcomes for cocaine dependence. Arch Gen Psychiatry 1999;56:507–14.

108. Haney M, Kosten TR. Therapeutic vaccines for substance dependence. Expert Rev Vaccines 2004;3:11–8.

109. Oliveto AH, Feingold A, Schottenfeld R, et al. Desipramine in opioid-dependent cocaine abusers maintained on buprenorphine vs. methadone. Arch Gen Psychiatry 1999;56:812–20.

110. Pani PP, Trogu E, Vecchi S, Amato L. Antidepressants for cocaine dependence and problematic cocaine use. Cochrane Data Syst Rev 2011;12:CD002950.

111. Winhusen TM, Kropp F, Lindblad R, et al. Multisite, randomized, double-blind, placebo-controlled pilot clinical trial to evaluate the efficacy of buspirone as a relapse-prevention treatment for cocaine dependence. J Clin Psychiatry 2014;75:757–64.

112. Tennant FS Jr, Sagherian AA. Double-blind comparison of amantadine and bromocriptine for ambulatory withdrawal from cocaine dependence. Arch Intern Med 1987;147:109–12.

113. Handelsman L, Limpitlaw L, Williams D, et al. Amantadine does not reduce cocaine use or craving in cocaine-dependent methadone maintenance patients. Drug Alcohol Depend 1995;39:173–80.

114. Handelsman L, Rosenblum A, Palij M, et al. Bromocriptine for cocaine dependence. A controlled clinical trial. Am J Addict 1997;6:54–64.

115. Amato L, Minozzi M, Pani PP, et al. Dopamine agonists for cocaine dependence. Cochrane Data Syst Rev 2011;12:CD003352.

116. Kampman KM, Pettinati H, Lynch KG, et al. A pilot trial of olanzapine for the treatment of cocaine dependence. Drug Alcohol Depend 2003;70:265–73.

117. Grabowski J, Rhoades H, Stotts A, et al. Agonist-like and antagonist-like treatment for cocaine dependence with methadone for heroin dependence: two double-blind randomized clinical trials. Neuropsychopharmacology 2004;29:969–81. *Cocaine- and heroin-dependent adults were recruited for two parallel trials—all received methadone maintenance and cognitive-behavioral therapy. Trial I: 94 were randomized to placebo or one of two doses of sustained release D-amphetamine (15–30 mg vs. 30–60 mg); 34 completed the 6-month trial. Those on the higher D-amphetamine dose had fewer cocaine (and opiate) positive toxicology screens. Trial II: 96 were randomized to placebo or one of two doses of risperidone (2 or 4 mg); after 6 months, there was no difference in cocaine (or opiate) positive drug screens.*

118. Carroll KM, Nich C, Ball SA, et al. Treatment of cocaine and alcohol dependence with psychotherapy and disulfiram. Addiction 1998;93:713–28.

119. Petrakis IL, Carroll KM, Nich C, et al. Disulfiram treatment for cocaine dependence in methadone-maintained opioid addicts. Addiction 2000;95:219–28. *Cocaine-dependent adults on methadone (n = 67) were randomized to disulfiram or placebo with their methadone; 78% completed 12 weeks of treatment. Both arms reported decreased cocaine and alcohol use. Those on disulfiram had a greater reduction in cocaine (but not alcohol) use. The absolute difference was modest (~5 vs. 7 days of use in the previous 30 days at the end of treatment).*

120. Pani PP, Trogu E, Vacca R, et al. Disulfiram for the treatment of cocaine dependence. Cochrane Database Syst Rev 2010;1:CD007024.

121. Schottenfeld RS, Chawarski MC, Cubells JF, et al. Randomized clinical trial of disulfiram for cocaine dependence or abuse during buprenorphine treatment. Drug Alcohol Depend 2014;136:36–42. *Buprenorphine-treated adults with cocaine use (n = 177) disorder were randomized to disulfiram or placebo and followed for 12 weeks; 155 were genotyped and 71 had genetically low DβH. Disulfiram was associated with significantly lower frequency of self-reported cocaine use, but not cocaine-negative urine samples. In the subsample with genetic testing, those with genetically low DβH had significant declines in self-reported cocaine use, while others did not; again, there was no significant difference in cocaine-negative urine samples.*

122. Halikas JA, Crosby RD, Pearson VL, Graves NM. A randomized double-blind study of carbamazepine in the treatment of cocaine abuse. Clin Pharmacol Ther 1997;62:89–105.

123. Lima Reisser A, Lima MS, Soares BGO, Farrell M. Carbamazepine for cocaine dependence. Cochrane Data Syst Rev 2002;2:CD002023.

124. Kampman KM, Pettinati H, Lynch KG, et al. A pilot trial of topiramate for the treatment of cocaine dependence. Drug Alcohol Depend 2004;75:233–40.

125. **Johnson BA, Alt-Daoud N, Wang XQ, et al. Topiramate for the treatment of cocaine addiction: a randomized clinical trial. JAMA Psychiatry 2013;70:1338–46.** *Cocaine-dependent adults (n = 142) were randomized to topiramate titrated from 50 mg to 300 mg/day or placebo and followed for 12 weeks. The primary outcome was proportion of cocaine nonuse days during weeks 6–12, which was significantly lower with topiramate (13% vs. 5% if missing data were not imputed to the baseline value, 9% vs. 4% if they were). Those assigned to topiramate were also more likely to achieve cocaine-free weeks on drug testing (17% vs. 6%).*

126. **Elkashef A, Kahn R, Yu E, et al. Topiramate for the treatment of methamphetamine addiction: a multicenter placebo-controlled trial. Addiction 2012;107:1297–306.** *Methamphetamine-dependent adults (n = 140) were randomized to placebo or topiramate, titrated from 25 to 200 mg/day. The primary outcome was abstinence from methamphetamine during weeks 6–12, which was not significantly different. Topiramate was associated with improvements in two secondary outcomes: reduced weekly median urine methamphetamine levels and observer-rated severity of dependence scores.*

127. Nultjen M, Blanken P, van den Brink W, Hendriks V. Treatment of crack-cocaine dependence with topiramate: a randomized controlled feasibility trial in The Netherlands. Drug Alcohol Depend 2014;138:177–84.

128. **Umbricht A, DeFullo A, Winstanley EL, et al. Topiramate for cocaine dependence during methadone maintenance treatment: a randomized controlled trial. Drug Alcohol Depend 2014;140:92–100.** *This trial used a factorial design to assign 171 cocaine-dependent subjects on methadone maintenance to one of four arms: topiramate vs. placebo and monetary voucher incentives that were either contingent or noncontingent on drug abstinence. Neither intervention had a significant effect.*

129. Kampman KM, Pettinati HM, Lynch KG, et al. A double-blind, placebo-controlled trial of topiramate for the treatment of comorbid cocaine and alcohol dependence. Drug Alcohol Depend 2013;133:94–9.

130. Walsh SL, Middleton LS, Wong CJ, et al. Atomoxetine does not alter cocaine use in cocaine dependent individuals: A double-blind randomized trial. Drug Alcohol Depend 2013;130:150–7.

131. **Dackis CA, Kampman KM, Lynch KG, et al. A double-blind placebo-controlled trial of modafinil for cocaine dependence. Neuropsychopharmacology 2005;30:205–11.** *Cocaine-dependent adults (n = 62) were randomized to 400 mg/day of modafinil or placebo; 64% completed the 8-week study. Those on modafinil had more cocaine-negative urine tests (mean 42% vs. 24%) but did not report less use or craving.*

132. Shearer J, Wodak A, van Beek I, et al. Pilot randomized double-blind placebo-controlled study of dexamethamphetamine for cocaine dependence. Addiction 2003;98:1137–41.

133. Grabowski J, Rhoades H, Schmitz J, et al. Dextroamphetamine for cocaine-dependence treatment: a randomized clinical trial. J Clin Psychopharmacol 2001;21:522–6.

134. **Long M, Wickes W, Smout M, et al. Randomized controlled trial of dexamphetamine maintenance for the treatment of methamphetamine dependence. Addiction 2010;105:146–54.** *In this 12-week trial with 49 methamphetamine-dependent subjects, those who received directly observed daily doses of 110 mg of dexamphetamine had better treatment retention (average 86 days vs. 49 days with placebo) and reduction in methamphetamine use. There were no serious adverse events.*

135. Castells X, Casas M, Perez-Mana C, et al. Efficacy of psychostimulant drugs for cocaine dependence. Cochrane Database Syst Rev 2010;2:CD007380.

136. Perez-Mana C, Castells X, Torrens M, et al. Efficacy of psychostimulant drugs for amphetamine abuse or dependence. Cochrane Database Syst Rev 2013;9:CD009695.

137. Ling W, Chang L, Hillhouse M, et al. Sustained-release methylphenidate in a randomized trail of treatment of methamphetamine use disorder. Addiction 2014;109:1489–500.

138. Jayaram-Lindstrom N, Hammarberg A, Beck O, Franck J. Naltrexone for the treatment of amphetamine dependence: a randomized placebo-controlled trial. Am J Psychiatry 2008;165:1442–8.

139. Schmitz JM, Lindsay JA, Green CE, et al. High-dose naltrexone therapy for cocaine-alcohol dependence. Am J Addict 2009;18:356–62.

140. Pettinati HM, Kampmann KM, Lynch KG, et al. A pilot trial of injectable, extended release naltrexone for the treatment of co-occurring cocaine and alcohol dependence. Am J Addict 2014;23:591–7.

141. Avants SK, Margolin A, Holford TR, Kosten TR. A randomized controlled trial of auricular acupuncture for cocaine dependence. Arch Intern Med 2000;160:2305–12.

142. Margolin A, Kleger HD, Avants SK, et al. Acupuncture for the treatment of cocaine addiction. A randomized controlled trial. JAMA 2002;287:55–63.

143. Mills EJ, Wu P, Gagnier J, Ebbert JO. Efficacy of acupuncture for cocaine dependence: a systematic review and meta-analysis. Harm Reduct J 2005;17:4

144. Reissig CJ, Strain EC, Griffiths RR. Caffeinated energy drinks—a growing problem. Drug Alcohol Depend 2009;99:1–10.

145. Myers MG. Caffeine and cardiac arrhythmias. Ann Intern Med 1991;114:147–50.

146. Holmgren P, Nordén-Pettersson, Ahlner J. Caffeine fatalities—four case reports. Forensic Sci Internat 2004;139:71–3.

147. Jabbar SB, Hanly MG. Fatal caffeine overdose: a case report and review of literature. Am J Forensic Med Pathol 2013;34:321–4.

148. Winkelmayer WC, Stampfer MJ, Willett WC, Curhan GC. Habitual caffeine intake and the risk of hypertension in women. JAMA 2005:294:2330–5.

149. Hughes JR, Higgins ST, Bickel WK, et al. Caffeine self-administration, withdrawal, and adverse effects among coffee drinkers. Arch Gen Psychiatry 1991;48:611–7.

150. Silverman K, Evans SM, Strain EC, Griffiths RR. Withdrawal syndrome after the double-blind cessation of caffeine consumption. N Engl J Med 1992;327:1109–14.

151. Strain EC, Mumford GK, Silverman K, Griffiths RR. Caffeine dependence syndrome. Evidence from case histories and experimental evaluations. JAMA 1994;272:1043–8.

152. Philip P, Tailard J, Moore N, et al. The effects of coffee and napping on nighttime highway driving: a randomized trial. Ann Intern Med 2006;144:785–91.

153. van Dam RM, Hu FB. Coffee consumption and risk of type 2 diabetes: a systematic review. JAMA 2005;294:97–104.

154. Pereira MA, Parker ED, Folsom AR. Coffee consumption and risk of type 2 diabetes mellitus: an 11-year prospective study of 28 812 postmenopausal women. Arch Intern Med 2006;166:1311–6.

155. Huxley R, Lee CMY, Barzi F, et al. Coffee, decaffeinated coffee, and tea consumption in relation to incident type 2 diabetes mellitus: a systematic review with meta-analysis. Arch Intern Med 2009;169:2053–63.

156. Klatsky AL, Morton C, Udaltsova N, Friedman GD. Coffee, cirrhosis, and transaminase enzymes. Arch Intern Med 2006;166:1190–5.

157. Freedman ND, Everhart JE, Lindsay KL, et al. Coffee intake is associated with lower rates of liver disease progression in chronic hepatitis C. Hepatology 2009;50:1360–9.

158. Eskelinen MH, Ngandu T, Tuomilehto J, et al. Midlife coffee and tea drinking and the risk of late-life dementia: a population-based CAIDE study. J Alzheimers Dis 2009;16:85–91.

159. Lopez-Garcia E, van Dam RM, Li TY, et al. The relationship of coffee consumption with mortality. Ann Intern Med 2008;148:904–14.

160. Freedman ND, Park Y, Abnet CC, et al. Association of coffee drinking with total and cause-specific mortality. N Engl J Med 2012;366:1891–904.

161. Liu J, Sui X, Lavie CJ, et al. Association of coffee consumption with all-cause and cardiovascular disease mortality. Mayo Clin Proc 2013;88:1066–74.

9

Hallucinogens and Dissociatives

Background

Hallucinogens are a broad spectrum of substances that alter an individual's perception of reality, sometimes referred to as "psychedelics." There are a number of synthetic and naturally occurring agents that are used for their hallucinogenic effect. Phencyclidine (PCP) and related agents, such as ketamine, are technically dissociative anesthetics but share many characteristics with hallucinogens and will also be covered in this chapter. Nitrous oxide is an anesthetic with dissociative properties and is discussed in Chapter 11, on inhalants. The hallucinogens include methylenedioxymethamphetamine (MDMA, or ecstasy) and lysergic acid diethylamide (LSD); Table 9.1 lists some hallucinogenic and dissociative agents. Marijuana and its active ingredient, tetrahydrocannibinol (THC), as well as other cannabinoids, also have hallucinogenic effects but are covered separately in Chapter 10.

We will begin by reviewing the epidemiology of hallucinogen use in the United States and then provide a brief overview on the effects and complications of use. This will be followed by more detailed information on the different classes of hallucinogens. We will finish with a brief discussion on treatment options.

Epidemiology

According to the 2013 National Survey on Drug Use and Health, almost 40 million Americans have used hallucinogens (this category includes PCP) at some point in their lives; this is 15.1% of the population aged 12 or older.[1] An estimated 4.4 million used hallucinogens in the past year (1.7%), and 1.3 million had used one in the past month (0.5%). Lifetime use was highest for LSD (9.4%), followed by psilocybin (8.7%), MDMA (6.8%), PCP (2.5%), and peyote (2.2%). Although lifetime use of LSD was highest, MDMA was the most commonly used hallucinogen in 2013; 1.0% of Americans age 12 and older were estimated to have used MDMA in the past year, 0.4% had used LSD, and less than 0.1%, PCP. Hallucinogen use was highest in the 18–25 age group; 6.7% had used a hallucinogen in the past year. This percentage declined to 3% for those aged 26–29 and below 1% for those over 40.

TABLE 9.1 Selected Agents with Hallucinogenic and Dissociative Effects

Technical Names	Plant or Animal Sources (If Any)*	Street/Popular Names
Piperidines		
Phencyclidine (PCP)		Angel dust
Ketamine		Special K, Ket
Tiletamine		
Phenylethylamines		
3,4-Methylenedioxymethamphetamine (MDMA)		Ecstasy, Adam, STP, Molly
3,4-methylenedioxyamphetamine (MDA)		Eve
4-bromo-2,5-dimethoxyamphetamine (DOB)		Bromo, Nexus
4-methylthioamphetamine (4-MTA)		Flatliners
Paramethoxyamphetamine (PMA)		Death
Mescaline	Peyote (*Lophophora williamsii*)	Buttons, Cactus, Mesc
	San Pedro (*Trichocereus pachanoi*)	Cimora
Macromerine	Doña ana (*Coryphantha macromeris*)	Doñana, false peyote
Myristicin	Nutmeg (*Myristica fragrans*)	

(continued)

TABLE 9.1 (Continued)

Technical Names	Plant or Animal Sources (If Any)*	Street/Popular Names
Ergot alkaloids		
D-Lysergic acid diethylamide (LSD)		Acid
Lysergic acid amide (LSA, Ergine)	Morning glory (*Ipomoea violacea*, *Rivea corymbosa*)	Ololiuqui, Tlitliltzin
	Hawaiian baby woodrose (*Argyreia nervosa*)	
Tryptamines		
Psilocybin/psilocyn	*Psilocybe cubensis and other spp.*	Magic mushrooms
Dimethyltryptamine (DMT)	*Anadenanthera peregrina, Virola spp.*	Ayahuasca, Caapi, Yage
5-HO-DMT (Bufotenine)	*Colorado river toad (Bufo alvarius)*	Bufo
5-MeO-DIPT		Foxy, Foxy methoxy
Ibogaine	*Tabernanthe iboga*	Iboga

Piperazines		
Benzylpiperazine (BZP)		Legal E, Legal X, Rapture
Trifluoromethylphenylpiperazine (TFMPP)		Legal E, Legal X, Rapture
Anticholinergics		
Belladonna alkaloids	Jimsonweed (*Datura stramonium*) Angel's trumpet (*Datura suaveolens*) Mandrake (*Mandragora officinarum*) Henbane (*Hyoscyamus niger*) Deadly nightshade (*Atropa belladonna*)	
Terpenoids		
Tetrahydrocannibinol (THC)	Marijuana (*Cannabis sativa*)	Grass, Pot, Reefer, Blunt
Thujone	Wormwood (*Artemisia absinthium*)	Absinthe
Salvinorin-A	Diviner's Sage (*Salvia divinorum*)	Salvia, Yerba de la pastora

(*continued*)

TABLE 9.1 (Continued)

Technical Names	Plant or Animal Sources (If Any)*	Street/Popular Names
	Terpenoids	
Asarone	Calamus (*Acorus calamus*)	Sweet flag
Humulene	Hops (*Humulus lupulus*)	
Coleon	Coleus (*Coleus blumei and pumila*)	
	Others	
Muscimol	Fly agaric (*Amanita muscaria*)	Toadstool
Dextromethorphan (DXM)		Robo, Rojo, DM

*Not all sources are listed.

Drug Effects

Acute Effects

Hallucinogens, in general, alter sensory perception and change the qualities of thought or emotion. Users sometimes describe a slowing or speeding of their perception of time. An individual's experience can vary quite widely depending on the substance used, the person's mindset, and environmental factors. The experience may be intensely pleasurable or extremely frightening ("a bad trip"). Some may have a sense of profound insight or spirituality with use.[2]

Acute Toxicity and Overdose

Overall, serious complications or death from hallucinogen use are rare, especially when compared with alcohol, opioid, or stimulants. In a cohort of U.S. adults surveyed in 1991, those who reported lifetime hallucinogen use did not have significantly higher 15-year mortality than that of non-drug users.[3] Nevertheless, these substances can be dangerous. The perceptual and cognitive changes can result in impaired judgment and risky or violent behavior. Users may be delirious or psychotic for days after use of some substances.[4] The best treatment for most of these individuals is providing a calm and supportive environment; benzodiazepines or other sedatives may be helpful for some.

The DSM-5 provides separate diagnostic criteria for phencyclidine and other hallucinogen intoxication.[5] The ICD-10 does not differentiate between phencyclidine and other hallucinogens, and the code for intoxication depends on whether there is a comorbid hallucinogen use disorder and the severity of the disorder; the code is F16.929 if there is none, F16.129 if mild, and F16.229 if moderate-severe.

Withdrawal

Although cessation of hallucinogen use is generally not associated with a physical withdrawal syndrome, some regular users of MDMA report tolerance to the drug's effect and after cessation experience fatigue and low mood.[6] These are similar to the symptoms that some stimulant users report with cessation. The DSM-5 does not recognize a hallucinogen withdrawal syndrome.

Some hallucinogen users may transiently re-experience perceptual disturbances that were associated with previous hallucinogen use (flashbacks). This uncommon phenomenon, technically known as "hallucinogen persisting perception disorder" (HPPD), is most associated with LSD use and may occur months to years after last use. Little is known about the etiology, risk factors, or effective treatment of this disorder.[7] The DSM-5 provides diagnostic criteria for HPPD,[5] and the ICD-10 code is F16.983.

Assessment

Hallucinogen use should be suspected in individuals, especially adolescents or young adults, who present with acute psychosis, confusion, or obtundation. The specific medical complications discussed in the following sections may also be a clue to use.

Phencyclidine can be detected in urine drug testing and many commercially available assays test for its presence; ketamine and dextramethorphan may cause a false-positive test result. MDMA and LSD can also be detected in the urine, but are not generally included in the commonly used commercial urine drug tests.

The DSM-5 divides this class between phencyclidine and other hallucinogens; the diagnostic criteria for "phencyclidine use disorder" and "other hallucinogen use disorder" are the same as for other substances; see Chapter 1 for details.[5] The ICD-10 code for either disorder is the same: F16.10 for mild disorder, and F16.20 for moderate-severe.

Acute Effects and Complications of Specific Classes of Hallucinogens

Piperidines

Phencyclidine (PCP, or "angel dust") is an antagonist of the N-methyl-D-aspartate (NMDA) receptor and was initially developed in the 1920s and used as an anesthetic; however, its use declined after it was found to often cause psychosis and dysphoria and it is no longer used therapeutically. PCP is sold in the form of powder, pills, or rocks that can be smoked. It can be ingested, snorted, smoked, or injected. The powder is often added to marijuana, and cigarettes are sometimes dipped into formaldehyde with dissolved PCP. Two related agents, ketamine and tiletamine, are used as veterinary anesthetics and also used illicitly. Dextromethorphan (DXM), which is used as a cough suppressant, also has effects similar to those of PCP.[8] Users must consume large quantities of cough syrup (at least 4 oz) to achieve the desired effect; some use a powdered form of the drug. Many pills sold as "ecstasy" have been found to contain DXM.[9]

Acute Effects

PCP and related compounds typically cause dissociative symptoms: feelings of depersonalization, derealization, and analgesia. Users may manifest slurred speech and ataxia. Some users may quietly stare for extended periods, while others may become psychotic, paranoid, and even violent. The half-life of PCP is fairly long; in one study of oral and intravenous administration, the mean half-life was 17 hours, with a range of 7 to 46 hours.[10] There are some reports of ketamine users experiencing withdrawal symptoms with cessation of regular use. Symptoms include drug craving, anxiety, tremor, sweats, and fatigue.[11]

Toxicity and Overdose

PCP overdose can lead to seizures, stupor, catatonia, and even coma; cardiac or respiratory arrest may occur.[12] Ingestion of large amounts of dextromethorphan can cause stupor, ataxia, dystonia, psychosis, and coma.[13] Dextromethorphan ingestion has also been associated with serotonin syndrome among individuals who are taking selective serotonin reuptake inhibitors (SSRIs).[14] Naloxone may help reverse the toxicity of dextromethorphan.[13]

Medical Complications

PCP has been associated with rhabdomyolysis; in a case series published in 1981, 25 of 1,000 patients with PCP intoxication developed this complication, and in 10 it was complicated by acute renal failure.[15] PCP has also been associated with hyperthermia.[16] Severe liver damage has also been reported as a complication of PCP-associated malignant hyperthermia.[17] PCP use has also been associated with intracranial hemorrhage[18] and stroke; in one case series, 11 of 116 cases of stroke were associated with drug use and 2 of these were associated with PCP.[19]

Phenylethylamines

Methylenedioxymethamphetamine (MDMA, or ecstasy) and similar designer drugs are related to amphetamines and have many similar effects but are used primarily for their hallucinogenic effect. They are sometimes referred to as "enactogens" or "empathogens" because of their reported ability to induce feelings of empathy. MDMA is generally taken in a pill form; the MDMA content of these pills varies substantially and many pills contain other substances, including caffeine, ephedrine, methamphetamine, or ketamine.[20] Furthermore, there are a number of related phenylethylamines that have been identified and synthesized that have similar effects; some are sold illicitly as ecstasy.

Mescaline is the active hallucinogenic alkaloid that is found in peyote, a small cactus that grows in southwestern United States and northern Mexico; growths on the cactus, called "buttons," are removed and dried, then chewed and ingested. Native Americans have used these for religious ceremonies and as treatment for a variety of ailments. Mescaline can be extracted from peyote or synthesized and used in variety of forms; it can also be found in other cacti. Peyote is a schedule I substance, but members of the Native American Church are permitted to use it legally. Mescaline can also be found in lower concentrations in a South American cactus called San Pedro (*Tricherocerus pachanoi*). In Peru the skin is used to produce a drink called *cimora*.

Nutmeg (*Myristica fragrans*) is popular spice that can be hallucinogenic if consumed in large quantities. Myristicin is the primary hallucinogenic substance in the seeds and is metabolized to 3-methoxy-4,5-methylene-dioxyamphetamine (MMDA)—a phenylethylamine. Whole nuts or powder may be ingested or dissolved in water or alcohol before consumption; the psychogenic effect can be obtained with 1–3 whole nutmegs or 5–30 grams of the powder.[21]

Acute Effects

MDMA and related phenylethylamines are said to bring on feelings of energy, euphoria, openness, and heightened sensation. While users may experience changes in perception of time, hallucinations rarely (if ever) occur. Users may also experience restlessness, loss of appetite, and difficulty concentrating. The drug effect peaks about 2 hours after use and wears off in about 6 hours.[22] Combining MDMA with alcohol seems to prolong the euphoric effects of MDMA while negating the subjective sedative effect of alcohol alone.[23] Regular users seem to develop a tolerance to the drug and need to take higher doses or take it more frequently to achieve the desired effect.[24] Some regular users of MDMA experience fatigue and low mood after cessation;[6] these are similar to the symptoms that some stimulant users report with cessation. As noted earlier, DSM-5 does not recognize a hallucinogen withdrawal syndrome.[5]

Acute Toxicity and Overdose

The growing use of MDMA (ecstasy) has been accompanied by increasing reports of fatalities associated with its use; however, these numbers are still small in comparison to the fatalities associated with alcohol or other drugs.[25] Large doses of MDMA (and other phenylethylamines) can produce amphetamine-like effects, including hypertension, hyperthermia, rhabdomyolysis, and cardiac arrhythmias; some users may develop liver or renal failure. The combination of MDMA with MAO inhibitors appears to be particularly dangerous.[26] Some of the fatalities associated with MDMA use are due to hyponatremia complicated by cerebral edema. This is due to a combination of excessive fluid intake and inappropriate antidi-uretic hormone (ADH) secretion.[27] There are, however, reports of survival after ingestion of a large number of pills (40–50), without long-term sequelae.[28]

Medical Complications

Ecstasy is responsible for most of the reports of complications asso-ciated with hallucinogen use, in part because ecstasy is the most commonly used of these substances. Most of these complications are probably from the stimulant effect of this drug; however, given the varied content of pills sold, some of these complications may be due to substances other than MDMA. Furthermore, one must always keep in mind that case reports do not necessarily establish cause and effect, especially when the substance is commonly used.

Cardiovascular Complications

MDMA acutely increases heart rate, blood pressure, and myocar-dial oxygen consumption.[29] There have been case reports of myo-cardial infarction associated with ecstasy use, presumably due to these sympathomimetic effects.[30] MDMA users may be at risk for heart valve abnormalities: physiological studies have found that MDMA activates 5-HT_{2B} serotonin receptors,[31] and other 5-HT_{2B} agonists—pergolide, cabergoline, and the now-banned fenfluramine—have been associated with heart valve abnormali-ties, though this association has not been established with MDMA.

Gastrointestinal Complications

There are reports of severe hepatotoxicity associated with ecstasy use. In one series in Spain, of 62 patients admitted with acute liver failure, 5 (8%) cases were attributed to ecstasy use.[32]

Renal and Electrolyte Complications

There have been a number of reports of serious hyponatremia, some complicated by cerebral edema[33] and even death,[34] associated with ecstasy use. These incidents have generally occurred in the setting of "rave" dance parties. Ironically, advice given to these party goers to ingest large quantities of fluids to avoid dehydration may be partly to blame; inappropriate secretion of ADH also appears to contribute to this condition.[27] There is also one report of severe (and fatal) hyperkalemia associated with ecstasy use in the absence of renal failure.[35]

Neuromuscular Complications

HYPERTHERMIA

Like other stimulants, ecstasy use can be complicated by hyperthermia, which may in turn lead to rhabdomyolysis and renal failure.[36]

STROKE

Ecstasy use has been implicated in cerebral infarction[37] and hemorrhage. Many of the hemorrhages occur in individuals with underlying vascular malformations.[38]

MOVEMENT DISORDERS

There have been reports of Parkinsonism among ecstasy users,[39] and methamphetamine (which is related to MDMA) has also been associated with Parkinsonism. However, given the numbers of individuals who have used ecstasy, the association may be entirely coincidental.[40]

COGNITIVE IMPAIRMENT

There is some concern about the long-term effects of MDMA use on cognitive function. A number of studies suggest that ecstasy users have poorer short- and long-term memory, as well as impaired attention and processing speed on tests of cognitive function.[41] However, there are a number of possible confounding factors that may contribute to the observed differences, one being the use of other drugs. For example, one study found that ecstasy users tended to perform poorer on tests of memory; however, this difference disappeared when cannabis (marijuana) and amphetamine use was taken into account.[42] On the other hand, a study that recruited individuals with minimal exposure to other drugs reported a tendency toward poorer performance on tests of cognitive function (most were not statistically significant); a post hoc analysis of heavy users (60–450 lifetime doses) found significant impairment on a number of measures compared with that of nonusers or moderate users.[43]

Another possible confounding factor is that ecstasy users (or heavier users) may have lower baseline cognitive function—that is, those with poorer cognitive function may be more likely to use ecstasy, rather than ecstasy use itself causing poorer cognitive function. A recent study of memory performance among MDMA users found that those who stopped using MDMA had no improvement in memory, and those who continued had no deterioration in memory.[44]

PSYCHIATRIC COMPLICATIONS

As MDMA use has grown, so have concerns about its long-term psychiatric effects. There have been reports of chronic psychiatric symptoms associated with ecstasy use, including depression, anxiety, delusions, somatization, and even psychosis.[45] MDMA acutely promotes the release of serotonin (5-HT), and it also appears to stimulate dopamine receptors. However, in the long term, MDMA causes depletion of serotonin, and this may lead to chronic psychiatric complications. One study of 150 MDMA users presenting for addiction treatment reported that 53% had one or more psychiatric problems, including depression, psychotic disorders, panic disorders, and others.[46] This was a select group of users (those requesting drug treatment), and most had used other substances as well. As with the studies on the effect of MDMA on cognitive function, it is difficult to establish causality with these types of retrospective descriptive analyses.

Ergot Alkaloids

Background

Lysergic acid diethylamide (LSD), developed in the 1940s, is a colorless, odorless powder that it often sold in impregnated blotter-paper but may be distributed in tablet, capsule, powder, or crystal forms.

There are even accounts of using it in the form of eye drops. A closely related ergot alkaloid is produced by a fungus that infects rye and is the cause of ergotism, or "St. Anthony's fire." There are a number of other naturally occurring botanicals that contain lysergamides, including the seeds of the Hawaiian baby woodrose and a few species of morning glory. The seeds can be crushed or eaten whole; they are sometimes soaked in water and then the extract is drunk. The Aztecs used Mexican morning glory seeds ("ololiuqui") in their religious ceremonies. Commercially available seeds are often coated with an emetic toxin to discourage ingestion.

Acute Effects

When LSD is taken orally, the effects peak around 4 to 6 hours after use and generally wear off by 8 hours after use.[47] In one study of intravenous administration of LSD, the drug level peaked at 30 minutes and the half-life of the drug was calculated to be about 3 hours.[48]

Medical Complications

The main concern with LSD is with the possibility that it may have psychiatric effects that persist long after use has subsided. Unfortunately, there are few good data on long-term psychiatric complications. A 1999 review of this topic that used the results of nine studies of mostly LSD users concluded that the "general impression to emerge from these studies is that such [neuropsychological] effects, if present, are modest" and that "the dire predictions . . . appear unjustified."[49]

Tryptamines

There are number of naturally occurring hallucinogenic tryptamines (these are sometimes referred to as "indoles" or "indolealkylamines"). Psilocybin (4-phosphoryloxy-N,N-dimethyltryptamine) and psilocyn (4-hydroxy- N,N-dimethyltryptamine) are hallucinogenic tryptamines found in a variety of *Psilocybe* mushrooms that can be found in the southern and western United States, as well as other regions of the world. The dried mushrooms are typically ingested.

N,N-dimethyltryptamine (DMT) is found in a number of natural sources, including the bark of the Amazonian *Virola* species, referred to locally as "Yakee" or "Parica." It can also be found in other botanical sources worldwide. DMT can be inhaled, smoked, or injected; tribes in South America have traditionally used the ground bark of the *Virola* trees as a snuff. DMT is orally active only when combined with an MAO inhibitor; a brewed tea called "ayahuasca" is consumed in South America that combines DMT with a natural MAO inhibitor.

Bufotenine (5-hydroxydimethyltryptamine, or 5-OH-DMT) is found in the secretions and skin of "Bufo toads," including the Colorado River toad (*Bufo alvarius*), and has produced the strange (and perhaps apocryphal) practice of "toad-licking;" some individuals smoke the dried secretions, which are milked from the toad's secretory glands. A synthetic tryptamine, 5-methoxy-N, N-diisopropyltryptamine (5-MeO-DIPT), is reportedly sold under the name "Foxy" (or "Foxy methoxy") and can be purchased on the Internet.[50]

Ibogaine is derived from a West African shrub (*Tabernanthe iboga*); an extract of the root has been used by indigenous people in that region. Ibogaine is somewhat unique among hallucinogens because of its long duration of effect (18–24 hours). Some have claimed that it is an effective treatment for drug addiction.[51]

Anticholinergics

Background

There are a number of plants that contain the anticholinergics atropine and scopolamine that have been used for their hallucinogenic effect throughout the world. However, their toxicity has limited their use. These plants include jimsonweed (*Datura stramonium*), Angel's trumpet (*Datura suaveolens*), mandrake (*Mandragora officinarum*), henbane (*Hyoscyamus niger*), and deadly nightshade (*Atropa bella-donna*). Typically, the leaves are ingested or smoked.

Acute Effects

The belladonna alkaloids, in addition to their hallucinogenic effect, have significant anticholinergic effects that make them quite toxic. These include dilated pupils, blurred vision, nausea, tachycardia, ataxia, and delirium.

Terpenoids

There are a number of psychoactive terpene-like or terpenoid substances that are found in a variety of plants. The best known (and most used) of these is tetrahydrocannibinol (THC), which is found in marijuana and hashish.

Artemesia absinthum is a shrub in the wormwood family that has been used to flavor the liqueur absinthe. The psychoactive active ingredient, thujone, has hallucinogenic properties. Thujone is not soluble in water but can be dissolved in alcohol and has a distinctive menthol odor. Absinthe contains small amounts of thujone, but probably not enough to have significant effects.[52]

Salvinorin A is a hallucinogenic diterpene that is found in the leaves of *Salvia divinorum*, a plant in the mint family. Natives in Mexico have traditionally used it by chewing the leaves or ingesting the juice of the leaves. The dried leaves can be smoked, and it is also sold in the form of an extract. Studies have shown that salvinorin A is a potent kappa-opioid receptor agonist,[53] and the subjective effect has been described as intense but short-lived (generally less than 15 minutes).[54] This substance has not been scheduled by the Drug Enforcement Administration (DEA) but is being monitored as a possible emerging drug of abuse.

Hops (*Humulus lupulus*), which are used a flavoring agent in the production of beer, contain the terpenoid humulene and can have mild marijuana-like effects when smoked or ingested.

Other Hallucinogens

Fly agaric (*Amantia muscaria*) and panther cap (*Amantia panthera*) are mushrooms that also have hallucinogenic properties. There are a number of substances in the mushroom that are thought to produce this effect, including ibotenic acid, muscazone, and muscimol, which is a GABA agonist. These mushrooms are typically dried and ingested. Misidentification is risky and potentially lethal, since there are other poisonous *Amantia* varieties that often grow in close proximity.[55]

Treatment

There are few data on treatment for hallucinogen use. Counseling users on the (realistic) health risks associated with these substances would be prudent; research with other substances indicates that brief advice may be effective. As with other substances, treatment outcomes will likely be influenced by an individual's desire to stop and by other motivating factors. In one published study of outpatient group therapy for 37 PCP users, only 4 (11%) achieved a year of abstinence; 16 (48%) dropped out of treatment and 10 (30%) transferred to residential treatment or a recovery home.[56]

For MDMA users, it is thought that regular use depletes serotonin, therefore SSRIs may function as a kind of replacement therapy.[57] Moreover, studies have also found that SSRIs (including fluoxetine[58] and duloxetine[59]) inhibit the effects of MDMA. However, at this time, it is not known whether SSRIs are clinically useful for reducing MDMA use or toxicity.

Notes

1. Substance Abuse and Mental Health Services Administration. *Results from the 2013 National Survey on Drug Use and Health: National Findings.* NSDUH Series H-48, HHS Publication No. (SMA) 14-4863. Rockville, MD: Substance Abuse and Mental Health Services Administration; 2014.

2. Griffiths RR, Richards WA, McCann U, Jesse R. Psilocybin can occasion mystical-type experiences having substantial and sustained personal meaning and spiritual significance. Psychopharmacology (Berl) 2006;187:268–83.

3. Muhuri PK, Gfroerer JC. Mortality associated with illegal drug use among adults in the United States. Am J Drug Alcohol Abuse 2011;37:155–64.

4. Brvar M, Mozina M, Bunc M. Prolonged psychosis after *Amanita muscaria* ingestion. Wien Klin Wochenschr 2006;118:294–7.

5. American Psychiatric Association. *Diagnostic and Statistical Manual of Mental Disorders*, Fifth Edition. Arlington, VA: American Psychiatric Publishing; 2013.

6. Jansen KLR. Ecstasy (MDMA) dependence. Drug Alcohol Depend 1999;53:121–4.

7. Halpern JH, Opoe HG. Hallucinogen persisting perception disorder: what do we know after 50 years? Drug Alcohol Depend 2003;69:109–19.

8. Morris H, Wallach J. From PCP to MXE: a comprehensive review of the non-medical use of dissociative drugs. Drug Test Anal 2014;6:614–32.

9. Baggot M, Heifets B, Jones RT, et al. Chemical analysis of ecstasy pills. JAMA 2000;284:2190.

10. Cook CE, Brine DR, Jeffcoat AR, et al. Phencyclidine disposition after intravenous and oral doses. Clin Pharmacol Ther 1982;31:625–34.

11. Crithchlow DG. A case of ketamine dependence with discontinuation symptoms. Addiction 2006;101:1212–3.

12. McCarron MM, Schulze BW, Thompson GA, et al. Acute phencyclidine intoxication: incidence of clinical findings in 1,000 cases. Ann Emerg Med 1981;10:237–42.

13. Chyka PA, Erdman AR, Manoguerra AS, et al. Dextromethorphan poisoning: an evidence-based consensus guideline for out-of-hospital management. Clin Toxicol 2007;45:662–77.

14. Schwartz AR, Pizon AF, Brooks DE. Dextromethorphan-induced serotonin syndrome. Clin Toxicol 2008;46:771–3.

15. Akmal M, Valdin JR, McCarron MM, Massry SG. Rhabdomyolysis with and without acute renal failure in patients with phencyclidine intoxication. Am J Nephrol 1981;1:91–6.

16. Jan KM, Dorsey S, Bornstein A. Hot hog: hyperthermia from phencyclidine. N Engl J Med 1978;299:722.

17. Armen R, Kanel G, Reynolds T. Phencyclidine-induced malignant hyperthermia causing submassive liver necrosis. Am J Med 1984;77:167–72.

18. Bessen HA. Intracranial hemorrhage associated with phencyclidine abuse. JAMA 1982;248:585–6.

19. Sloan MA, Kittner SJ, Rigamonti D, Price TR. Occurrence of stroke associated with use/abuse of drugs. Neurology 1991;41:1358–64.

20. Cole JC, Bailey M, Sumnall HR, et al. The content of ecstasy tablets: implications for the study of their long-term effects. Addiction 2002;97:1531–6.

21. Stein U, Greyer H, Hentschel H. Nutmeg (myristicin) poisoning—report on a fatal case and a series of cases recorded by a poison information centre. Forensic Sci Int 2001;118:87–90.

22. Cami J, Farre M, Mas M, et al. Human pharmacology of 3,4-methylenedioxymethamphetamine ("ecstasy"): psychomotor performance and subjective effects. J Clin Psychopharmacol 2000;20:455–66.

23. Hernandez-Lopez C, Farre M, Roset PN, et al. 3,4-Methylenedioxymethamphetamine (ecstasy) and alcohol interactions in humans: psychomotor performance, subjective effects, and pharmacokinetics. J Pharmacol Exp Ther 2002;300:236–44.

24. Parrott AC. Chronic tolerance to recreational MDMA (3,4-methylenedioxymethamphetamine) or ecstasy. J Psychopharmacol 2005;19:71–83.

25. McKenna C. Ecstasy is in low league table of major causes of death. BMJ 2002;325:296.

26. Vuori E, Henry JA, Ojanperä I, et al. Death following ingestion of MDMA (ecstasy) and moclobemide. Addiction 2002;98:365–8.

27. Hartung TK, Schofield E, Short AI, et al. Hyponatremic states following 3,4-methylenedioxymethamphetamine (MDMA, 'ecstasy') ingestion. Q J Med 2002;95:431–7.

28. Regenthal R, Krüger M, Rudolph K, et al. Survival after massive "ecstasy" (MDMA) ingestion. Intensive Care Med 1999;25:640–1.

29. Lester SJ, Baggott M, Welm S, et al. Cardiovascular effects of 3,4-methylenedioxymethamphetamine. A double-blind placebo-controlled trial. Ann Intern Med 2000;133:969–73.

30. Qasim A, Townsend J, Davies MK. Ecstasy-induced acute myocardial infarction. Heart 2001;85:e10.

31. Setola V, Hufeisen SJ, Grande-Allen KJ, et al. 3,4-methylenedioxymethamphetamine (MDMA, "ecstasy") induces fenfluramine-like proliferative actions on human cardiac valvular interstitial cells in vitro. Mol Pharmacol 2003;63:1223–9.

32. Andreu V, Mas A, Bruguera M, et al. Ecstasy: a common cause of severe hepatoxicity. J Hepatol 1998;29:394–7.

33. Traub SJ, Hoffman RS, Nelson LS. The "ecstasy" hangover: hyponatremia due to 3,4-methylenedioxymethamphetamine. J Urban Health 2002;79:549–55.

34. Parr MJ, Low HM, Botterill P. Hyponatremia and death after "ecstasy" ingestion. Med J Aust 1997;166:136–7.

35. Raviña P, Quiroga JM, Raviña T. Hyperkalemia in fatal MDMA ('ecstasy') toxicity. Int J Cardiol 2004;93:307–8.

36. Dar KJ, McBrien ME. MDMA-induced hyperthermia: report of a fatality and review of current therapy. Intensive Care Med 1996;22:995–6.

37. Manchanda S, Connolly MJ. Cerebral infarction in association with ecstasy abuse. Postgrad Med J 1993;69:874–5.

38. McEvoy AW, Kitchen ND, Thomas DG. Intracerebral haemorrhage and drug abuse in young adults. Br J Neurosurg 2000;14:449–54.

39. Mintzer S, Hickenbottom S, Gilman S. Parkinsonism after taking ecstasy. N Engl J Med 1999;340:1443.

40. Kish SJ. What is the evidence that ecstasy (MDMA) can cause Parkinson's disease? Mov Disorders 2003;18:1219–23.

41. Verbaten MN. Specific memory deficits in ecstasy users? The results of a meta-analysis. Human Psychopharmacol 2003;18:281–90.

42. Simon NG, Mattick RP. The impact of regular ecstasy use on memory function. Addiction 2002;97:1523–9.

43. Halpern JH, Pope HG, Shewood AR, et al. Residual neuropsychological effects of illicit 3,4-methylenedioxymethamphetamine (MDMA) in individuals with minimal exposure to other drugs. Drug Alcohol Depend 2004;75:135–47.

44. Gouzoulis-Mayfrank E, Fischermann T, Rezk M, et al. Memory performance in polyvalent MDMA (ecstasy) users who continue or discontinue use. Drug Alcohol Depend 2005;78:317–23.

45. Montoya AG, Sorrentino R, Lukas SE, Price BH. Long-term neuropsychiatric consequences of "ecstasy" (MDMA): a review. Harvard Rev Psychiatry 2002;10:212–20.

46. Schifano F, DiFuria L, Forza G, et al. MDMA ('ecstasy') consumption in the context of polydrug abuse: a report on 150 patients. Drug Alcohol Depend 1998;52:85–90.

47. Linton HB, Langs RJ. Subjective reactions to lysergic acid diethylamide (LSD-25). Arch Gen Psychiatry 1962;6:352–68.

48. Aghajanian GK, Bing OH. Persistence of lysergic acid diethylamide in the plasma of human subjects. Clin Pharmacol Ther 1964;5:611–4.

49. Halpern JH, Pope HG. Do hallucinogens cause residual neuropsychological toxicity? Drug Alcohol Depend 1999;53:247–56.

50. Meatherall R, Sharma P. Foxy, a designer tryptamine hallucinogen. J Anal Toxicol 2003;27:313–7.

51. Vastag B. Addiction research. Ibogaine therapy: a 'vast, uncontrolled experiment'. Science 2005;308:345–6.

52. Lanchenmeier DW, Emmert J, Kuballa T, Sartor G. Thujone—cause of absinthism? Forensic Sci Int 2006;158:1–8.

53. Chavkin C, Sud S, Jin W, et al. Salvinorin A, an active component of the hallucinogenic sage salvia divinorum is a highly efficacious kappa-opioid receptor agonist: structural and functional considerations. J Pharmacol Exp Ther 2004;308:1197–203.

54. Débora González, Jordi Riba, José Carlos Bouso, et al. Pattern of use and subjective effects of *Salvia divinorum* among recreational users. Drug Alcohol Depend 2006;85:157–62.

55. Halpern JH. Hallucinogens and dissociative agents naturally growing in the United States. Pharmacol Ther 2004;102:131–8.

56. Gorelick DA, Wilkins JN, Wong C. Outpatient treatment of PCP abusers. Am J Drug Alcohol Abuse 1989;15:367–74.

57. Lingford-Hughes A, Nutt D. Neurobiology of addiction and implications for treatment. Br J Psychiatry 2003;182:97–100.

58. Tancer M, Johanson CE. The effects of fluoxetine on the subjective and physiological effects of 3,4-methylenedioxymethamphetamine (MDMA) in humans. Psychopharmacology (Berl) 2007;189:565–73.

59. Hysek CM, Simmler LD, Nicola VG, et al. Duloxetine inhibits effects of MDMA ("ecstasy") in vitro and in humans in a randomized placebo-controlled laboratory study. PLoS One 2012;7:e36476.

10

Marijuana and Other Cannabinoids

Background

Marijuana (cannabis) comes from plants in the genus *Cannabis* that are found worldwide. Humans have used the leaves for thousands of years. The leaves are typically smoked but can be ingested. A concentrated preparation of the resin, known as hashish, is also used. The main psychoactive ingredient of marijuana and hashish is tetrahydrocannabinol (THC); the isomer delta-9-tetrahydrocannabinol is considered to be the most active form of this substance. Another main constituent of marijuana is cannabidiol (CBD); this does not seem to have any psychoactive effects[1] but may have some therapeutic uses.

THC is part of a broad class of agents known as terpenoids. There are a number of other terpenoids that are found in plants and are used for their psychoactive effects. These plants include wormwood (used in absinthe), salvia, calamus, coleus, and hops; they are covered further in Chapter 9, on hallucinogens.

Recently, a number of synthetic cannabinoids have been developed and have been marketed as herbal blends or incense to circumvent drug laws. The compounds are sprayed onto plant matter and are sold in packets under a variety of brand names, including Spice and K2. Unlike THC, which is a partial cannabinoid receptor agonist, many of the synthetic cannabinoids are full agonists and are more potent as a result.[2]

Epidemiology

According to the 2013 National Survey on Drug Use and Health,[3] marijuana is the most commonly used illicit drug in the United States; 115 million people have ever used marijuana (or hashish) (43.7% of those aged 12 or older), 33 million reported use in the past year (12.6%), and 19.8 million Americans (7.5%) reported past-month use. Rates have steadily increased since 2007, when 5.8% reported using marijuana in the past month. An estimated 8.1 million Americans (3.1% of those age 12 or older) use marijuana on a daily or almost daily basis; this has increased steadily since 2005, when 5.1 million reported regular use. An estimated 2.4 million Americans aged 12 or older used marijuana for the first time in 2013; 1.4 million were under age 18. Marijuana is the most commonly used illicit drug; among current illicit drug users, 81% use marijuana and 65% use only marijuana.

There are fewer data on the emerging use of synthetic cannabinoids. In a 2014 analysis of urine drug tests performed on U.S. military personnel, 1.4% were found to have synthetic cannabinoids.[4] In a survey of 18- to 25-year-old marijuana and alcohol users, 9% reported using synthetic cannabinoids in the past month. Use was associated with male gender, not being in school, smoking, binge alcohol use, daily and weekly marijuana use, and use of other illicit drugs.[5]

Drug Effects

Cannabinoids appear to exert their effects through the stimulation of endogenous cannabinoid receptors. These receptors are thought to have an analgesic effect and to inhibit nociceptive responses in the central nervous system.[6]

Acute Effects

Users may feel a sense of relaxation and euphoria, while others may experience anxiety, nausea, and dizziness. Cannabinoids may also produce hallucinogenic effects such as depersonalization, visual distortions, and perceptual changes. Users typically report an increased sense of hunger; a prescription form of THC (dronabinol) is used as an appetite stimulant and antiemetic.

Acute Toxicity and Overdose

The DSM-5 criteria for "cannabis intoxication" requires "clinically significant behavioral or psychological changes" and the presence of two (or more) of the following signs or symptoms after recent use: (1) conjunctival injection, (2) increased appetite, (3) dry mouth, and (4) tachycardia.[7] The ICD-10 code depends on whether there is perceptual disturbance and comorbid use disorder, as well as the severity of the disorder.

Serious toxicity after marijuana use is uncommon. Nevertheless, users can experience significant side effects, including drowsiness, ataxia, nausea and vomiting, as well cardiovascular complications including tachycardia and other arrhythmias, hypotension, and even syncope. The risk of toxicity appears to be higher with edible marijuana products because of the variable content and potency and the fact that the full effects may not be felt until a few hours after ingestion. This is particularly a concern for children, and there are reports of coma in young children after eating cookies or other edibles containing marijuana.[8]

The recently developed synthetic cannabinoids appear to be more potent than THC. Common side effects included dry mouth, difficulty thinking, memory disturbance, lightheadedness, and headache. They have also been associated with more severe toxicity, including agitation, hallucinations, psychosis, seizures, nausea, and vomiting.[9]

Withdrawal

Abstinence from regular marijuana use does not cause an observable physical withdrawal syndrome. Nevertheless, the DSM-5 recognizes "cannabis withdrawal" and the diagnostic criteria require the presence of three (or more) of the following signs or symptoms after cessation or reduction of heavy and prolonged use: (1) irritability, anger, or aggression; (2) nervousness or anxiety; (3) sleep difficulty; (4) decreased appetite or weight loss; (5) restlessness; (6) depressed mood; and (7) at least one of the following symptoms causing significant discomfort: abdominal pain, shakiness/tremors, sweating, fever, chills, or headache.[7] The ICD-10 code for cannabis withdrawal is F12.288. These symptoms generally begin during the first day or two of abstinence and peak during the first week; most symptoms resolve after 2 weeks, but some may linger for a month or longer.[10] Marijuana withdrawal symptoms are ameliorated by oral administration of THC,[11] indicating that this is the psychoactive component responsible for withdrawal symptoms. Less is known about withdrawal from synthetic cannabinoids, but early reports suggest that it may be more severe than withdrawal from marijuana.[12]

Assessment

A metabolite of THC can be detected in urine for 1–7 days after use; for heavy users, it may be detected up to a month after last use. A number of other drugs may cause false-positive results, including efavirenz, ibuprofen, and naproxen.[13] Dronabinol, which is a synthetic form of THC, will also trigger a positive result on drug testing. Hemp seed oil, which is found in some foods, may cause a false-positive screen, but this is unlikely at the levels usually consumed.[14] The synthetic cannabinoids are not detected in standard urine drug tests for THC metabolites, but their metabolites can be detected with specific testing.[15]

The DSM-5 criteria for "cannabis use disorder" are the same as those for other substances; see Chapter 1 for details on these criteria.[7] The ICD-10 code for a mild disorder is F12.10 and for moderate-severe, F12.20.

Medical Complications

While serious medical complications with marijuana use are uncommon, there are increasing reports of serious complications associated with synthetic cannabinoid use. In a cohort of U.S. adults surveyed in 1991, baseline marijuana use was not associated with an increased 15-year mortality (compared to those who did not report any illicit drug use).[16]

Head and Neck Complications

Marijuana smoke may, like tobacco, contain a number of carcinogens. In one case-control study, marijuana use was associated with an increased risk of head and neck cancers.[17] A prospective cohort study reported that marijuana users were at increased risk for periodontal disease, even when controlling for tobacco smoking and irregular use of dental services.[18]

Pulmonary Complications

Studies suggest that smoking marijuana is associated with an increased frequency of respiratory symptoms such as wheezing, cough, and sputum production, similar to that seen in tobacco smokers. However, it has not been shown that marijuana smoking leads to an irreversible decline in lung function in the way that tobacco smoking does.[19] In a study of a cohort of young adults over 20 years, occasional and low cumulative marijuana use was not associated with adverse effects on pulmonary function, but the data suggested an adverse effect with heavier levels of marijuana smoking.[20] While there is no clear evidence that marijuana smokers are at increased risk for lung cancer, some studies have found an association between marijuana smoking and premalignant lung changes.[21]

Cardiovascular Complications

Marijuana use acutely stimulates sympathetic activity with increased heart rate and blood pressure; at higher doses, parasympathetic effects may predominate, resulting in bradycardia and orthostatic hypotension.[22] Chronic users develop tolerance to these effects. These effects do not generally lead to serious complications for young, healthy users, but there are reports of acute, sometimes fatal, cardiovascular events in association with marijuana use,[23] and it may be a (rare) trigger for myocardial infarction for individuals with other risk factors.[24]

Gastrointestinal Complications

Marijuana, specifically THC, has a number of effects on the gastrointestinal system that are mediated by cannabinoid receptors in the gut and have generated interest in its therapeutic use.[25] Cannabinoids have been shown to be effective antiemetics,[26] but some chronic users may paradoxically develop hyperemesis; individuals with this syndrome often report improvement with bathing or showering in hot water.[27,28] Cannabinoids may be beneficial for irritable bowel syndrome, Crohn's disease, and secretory diarrhea by reducing gastrointestinal motility.

Genitourinary Complications

In case-control studies, marijuana use has been associated with testicular cancer, particularly nonseminomatous testicular cancer.[29,30,31]

Renal Complications

Although marijuana does not appear to have renal toxicity, there are reports of acute kidney injury among individuals using synthetic cannabinoids and presenting with nausea and flank pain.[32]

Metabolic Effects

Marijuana may have beneficial metabolic effects. Despite the appetite-stimulating effects of marijuana, use is associated with lower levels of obesity[33] and diabetes.[34] In an analysis of data from the National Health and Nutrition Survey from 2005–2010, marijuana use was associated with lower levels of fasting insulin, less insulin resistance, and smaller waist circumference.[35]

Neuromuscular Complications

Heavy marijuana use (generally defined as daily use or more) impairs neurocognitive function,[36] and these effects may persist for a day or longer after last use.[37] However, regular users seem to develop some tolerance and have less impairment with use than occasional users.[38] Whether marijuana leads to residual or irreversible cognitive deficits is controversial. Some studies have found cognitive deficits among heavy users after 28 days of abstinence,[39] particularly among those with early onset of use (before age 17).[40] It is possible that this may be due to innate differences in heavy users—that is, that those with poorer cognitive function are more likely to become heavy users.[41] However, a longitudinal study published in 2012 found that adolescent-onset persistent marijuana use was associated with neuropsychological decline and that cessation of use did not fully restore function; these effects were not seen among adult-onset users.[42]

Acute marijuana use impairs driving skills and increases the risk of collisions.[43] A 2012 meta-analysis concluded that "driving while under the influence of cannabis was associated with an almost doubling of risk of being involved in a motor vehicle collision that resulted in serious death or injury."[44]

Psychiatric Complications

A number of studies have found an association between marijuana use and psychiatric illness, including depression,[45] anxiety,[46] and psychosis.[47,48] There are a few possible explanations for these observations: (1) those at higher risk for psychiatric illness are more likely to use marijuana (use is a consequence, not a cause), (2) marijuana exacerbates or unmasks mental illness among those with preexisting illness or a predisposition, or (3) marijuana use causes mental illness. A 2011 systematic review concluded that the available evidence supports "the hypothesis that cannabis use plays a causal role in the development of psychosis in some patients."[49]

Other Drug Use

There is debate about whether marijuana use leads to the use of other "hard" drugs; this is a prominent argument against the legalization of marijuana. An association between marijuana use and subsequent use of hard drugs has been demonstrated.[50] The argument for a cause-and-effect relationship is strengthened by the association of hard drug use with marijuana use among twins who are discordant for marijuana use (i.e., one uses, the other does not); this finding suggests that shared environmental and genetic factors do not account for the connection.[51] However, it is difficult (if not impossible) to establish a causal relationship with these types of observational studies. Furthermore, it is possible that the so-called gateway effect may be entirely explained by a "common-factor model"—a model in which individuals have a random propensity to use drugs (both marijuana and hard drugs) and one does not necessarily lead to the other.[52,53]

Another concern with marijuana use is that it may worsen outcomes of treatment of other drug dependence. In one study, marijuana use was associated with lower likelihood of abstinence from heavy alcohol or other drug use.[54] However, in a study of youths receiving treatment for opioid dependence with buprenorphine, marijuana use was not associated with poorer opioid treatment outcomes.[55]

Treatment

Overall, there has been comparatively little research done on the treatment of persons who abuse or are dependent on marijuana. Most of the available research is on psychosocial approaches. There are no medications that have been shown to be effective.

Brief Interventions

To date, studies on brief interventions for marijuana use have been disappointing. One randomized controlled trial of two brief counseling sessions in primary care found no effect on subsequent unhealthy drug use; 63% reported that marijuana was their main drug.[56] Another trial of brief intervention followed by a telephone booster for primary care patients found no change in subsequent drug use; 76% reported marijuana use.[57] In a third randomized controlled trial of drug-using patients seen in emergency departments, of whom marijuana was the primary substance for 44%, a brief intervention followed by telephone boosters did not have a significant effect on subsequent use.[58]

Self-Help Groups

As with other substances, there are self-help groups for individuals who want help with marijuana use. These groups are typically modeled on Alcoholics Anonymous and use the 12-step approach. Marijuana Anonymous (www.marijuana-anonymous.org) is one such group and holds meetings in many states, as well as in Australia and some European countries, and online. We were unable to find any data on its effectiveness, but these groups appear to help some individuals who have problems with other substances.

Psychosocial Treatment

There have been a number of studies on psychosocial treatments for individuals who want treatment for their marijuana use. These studies have generally reported short-term reduction in use with a variety of strategies that have been used previously for alcoholism and other substance use problems. These approaches include motivational enhancement, cognitive-behavioral therapy, and contingency management (voucher-based incentives). However, these studies were performed on volunteers who wanted treatment and excluded individuals who had alcohol or other drug problems. Furthermore, most of these studies are limited by the use of a best-case scenario; those who did not complete follow-up were not counted as treatment failures.

A randomized controlled trial of treatment for marijuana users "who wanted help quitting" (this study excluded those who were marijuana dependent) compared cognitive-behavioral sessions with a therapist-led social support group. Individuals in both groups who completed the follow-up (79% of original cohort) reported significantly reduced marijuana use over 12 months; however, the treatment effect seemed to dissipate over time, and neither treatment modality was superior to the other.[59] A subsequent trial reported that a brief two-session individual motivational enhancement intervention performed as well as a 14-session group cognitive-behavioral treatment; abstinence rates with either treatment were better than those with no treatment.[60] Another trial comparing a brief (one-session) cognitive-behavioral intervention with a six-session treatment reported improved outcomes among those who completed follow-up (74% of the original cohort); outcomes with the six-session treatment were marginally better than the one-session treatment by some measures.[61] Similarly, a study found that five sessions of motivational enhancement and cognitive-behavioral therapy performed as well as 12 sessions; the addition of family education and therapy did not improve outcomes further.[62]

In contrast to earlier studies that indicated that brief interventions were as effective as longer treatment, a 2004 study suggested that a longer and more intensive course of treatment may be more effective. This multicenter randomized, controlled trial compared two sessions of motivational enhancement with a nine-session treatment that included motivational enhancement, cognitive-behavioral therapy, and case management. Among those who completed follow-up (only 59% of the original cohort), the nine-session intervention performed better (at least in the short term).[63]

The addition of abstinence-contingent rewards (sometimes referred to as "contingency management") also appears to improve abstinence rates. A small randomized, controlled trial reported higher short-term abstinence rates among individuals given vouchers for cannabinoid-negative urine samples than rates of others who received motivational enhancement or cognitive-behavioral treatment.[64] Another study reported higher abstinence rates with the combination of motivational enhancement and incentives for marijuana-free urines.[65] However, another trial found that cognitive behavioral therapy and contingency management did not improve outcomes for cannabis-dependent youths referred by the criminal justice system.[66]

An emerging approach is the use of Web-based programs to treat substance use disorders; a study of one such program targeted to individuals who wanted to stop or reduce their marijuana use reported some short-term benefits in terms of use and dependence symptoms.[67]

Pharmacotherapy

There are comparatively few data on pharmacotherapy for marijuana dependence, and most studies to date have failed to show any benefit. Medications that have been studied in controlled trials and have not been effective include divalproex sodium,[68] nefazodone and bupropion,[69] buspirone,[70] quetiapine,[71] and venlafaxine.[72]

Rimonabant, a cannabinoid receptor antagonist had been developed and shown to block the effects of smoked marijuana.[73] It has been studied as a weight loss medication, but a trial investigating its use to prevent cardiovascular events was terminated early due to an increased risk of psychiatric side effects and, possibly, suicide.[74] The use of cannabinoid antagonists in the treatment of marijuana abuse or dependence has not been established, and it is very unlikely that this medication will ever be approved for this use.

Dronabinol is a synthetic form of THC, which is FDA approved for treatment of anorexia associated with weight loss in patients with AIDS, and nausea and vomiting associated with cancer chemotherapy. In a 12-week placebo controlled trial, those who received dronabinol had less withdrawal symptoms and were more likely to remain in treatment, but there was no significant difference in the proportion of participants who achieved 2 weeks of marijuana abstinence at the end of the maintenance phase.[75]

Notes

1. Martin-Santos R, Crippa JA, Batalla A, et al. Acute effects of a single, oral dose of d9-tetrahydrocannabinol (THC) and cannabidiol (CBD) administration in health volunteers. Curr Pharm Des 2012;18:4966–79.

2. Castaneto MS, Gorelick DA, Desrosiers NA, et al. Synthetic cannabinoids: epidemiology, pharmacodynamics, and clinical implications. Drug Alcohol Depend 2014;144:12–41.

3. Substance Abuse and Mental Health Services Administration. *Results from the 2013 National Survey on Drug Use and Health: National Findings.* NSDUH Series H-48, HHS Publication No. (SMA) 14-4863. Rockville, MD: Substance Abuse and Mental Health Services Administration; 2014.

4. Wohlfarth A, Scheldweller KB, Castaneto M, et al. Urinary prevalence, metabolite detection rates, temporal patterns and evaluation of suitable LC-MS/MS targets to document synthetic cannabinoid intake in US military specimens. Clin Chem Lab Med 2015;53:423–34.

5. Caviness CM, Tzilos G, Anderson BJ, Stein MD. Synthetic cannabinoids: use and predictors in a community sample of young adults. Subst Abus 2014 [Epub ahead of print].

6. Welch SP, Malcom R. The pharmacology of marijuana. In Ries RK, Fiellin DA, Miller SC, Saitz R, eds. *The ASAM Principles of Addiction Medicine*, 5th ed. Philadelphia: Wolters Kluwer; 2014:217–34.

7. American Psychiatric Association. *Diagnostic and Statistical Manual of Mental Disorders*, Fifth Edition. Arlington, VA: American Psychiatric Publishing; 2013.

8. Boros CA, Parsons DW, Zoanetti GD, et al. Cannabis cookies: a cause of coma. J Paediatr Child Health 1996;32:194–5.

9. Hermanns-Clausen M, Kneisel S, Szabo B, Auwarter V. Acute toxicity due to the confirmed consumption of synthetic cannabinoids: clinical and laboratory findings. Addiction 2013;108:534–44.

10. Budney AJ, Hughes JR, Moore BA, Vandrey R. Review of the validity and significance of cannabis withdrawal syndrome. Am J Psychiatry 2004;161:1967–77.

11. Budney AJ, Vandrey RG, Hughes JR, et al. Oral delta-9-tetrahydrocannabinol suppresses cannabis withdrawal symptoms. Drug Alcohol Depend 2007;86:22–9.

12. Nacca N, Vatti D, Sullivan R, et al. The synthetic cannabinoid withdrawal syndrome. J Addict Med 2013;7:296–8.

13. Tests for drugs of abuse. The Medical Letter. 2002;44:71–3.

14. Leson G, Pless P, Grotenhermen F, et al. Evaluating the impact of hemp food consumption on workplace drug tests. J Anal Toxicol 2001;25:691–8.

15. Hutler M, Broecker S, Kneisel S, Auwarter V. Identification of the major urinary metabolites in man of seven synthetic cannabinoids of the aminoalkylindole type present as adulterants in 'herbal mixtures' using LC-MS/MS techniques. J Mass Spectrom 2012;47:54–65.

16. Muhuri PK, Gfroerer JC. Mortality associated with illegal drug use among adults in the United States. Am J Drug Alcohol Abuse 2011;37:155–64.

17. Zheng ZF, Morgenstern H, Spitz MR, et al. Marijuana use and increased risk of squamous cell carcinoma of the head and neck. Cancer Epidemiol Biomarkers Prev 1999;8:1071–8.

18. Thompson WM, Poulton R, Broadbent JM, et al. Cannabis smoking and periodontal disease among young adults. JAMA 2008;299:525–31.

19. Tetrault JM, Crothers K, Moore BA, et al. Effects of marijuana smoking on pulmonary function and respiratory complications: a systematic review. Arch Intern Med 2007;167:221–8.

20. Pletcher MJ, Vittinghoff E, Kalhan R, et al. Association between marijuana exposure and pulmonary function over 20 years. JAMA 2012;307:173–81.

21. Mehra R, Moore BA, Crothers K, et al. The association between marijuana smoking and lung cancer: a systematic review. Arch Intern Med 2006;166:1359–67.

22. Jones RT. Cardiovascular system effects of marijuana. J Clin Pharmacol 2002;42:58S–63S.

23. Bachs L, Mørland H. Acute cardiovascular fatalities following cannabis use. Forensic Sci Int 2001;124:200–3.

24. Mittleman MA, Lewis RA, Maclure M, et al. Triggering myocardial infarction by marijuana. Circulation 2001;103:2805–9.

25. DiCarlo G, Izzo AA. Cannabinoids for gastrointestinal diseases: potential therapeutic applications. Expert Opin Investig Drugs 2003;12:39–49.

26. Tramèr MR, Carroll D, Campbell FA, et al. Cannabinoids for control of chemotherapy induced nausea and vomiting: quantitative systematic review. BMJ 2001;323:1–8.

27. Allen JH, de Moore GM, Heddle R, Twartz JC. Cannabinoid hyperemesis: cyclical hyperemesis in association with chronic cannabis abuse. Gut 2004;53:1566–70.

28. Simonetto DA, Oxentenko AS, Herman ML, Szostek JH. Cannabinoid hyperemesis: a case series of 98 patients. Mayo Clin Proc 2012;87:1114–9.

29. Daling JR, Doody DR, Sun X, et al. Association of marijuana use and the incidence of testicular germ cell tumors. Cancer 2009;115:1215–23.

30. Trabert B, Sigurdson AJ, Sweeney AM, et al. Marijuana use and testicular germ cell tumors. Cancer 2011;117:848–53.

31. Lacson JC, Carroll JD, Tuazon E, et al. Population-based case-control study of recreational drug use and testis cancer risk confirms an association between marijuana use and nonseminoma risk. Cancer 2012;118:5374–83.

32. Buser GL, Gerona RR, Horowitz BZ, et al. Acute kidney injury associated with smoking synthetic cannabinoid. Clin Toxicol 2014;52:664–73.

33. Le Strat Y, Le Foll B. Obesity and cannabis use: results from 2 representative national surveys. Am J Epidemiol 2011;174:929–33.

34. Rajavashisth TB, Shaheen M, Norris KC, et al. Decreased prevalence of diabetes in marijuana users: cross-sectional data from the National Health and Nutrition Examination Survey (NHANES) III. BMJ Open 2012;2:e000494.

35. Penner EA, Buettner H, Mittleman MA. The impact of marijuana use on glucose, insulin, and insulin resistance among US adults. Am J Med 2013;126:583–9.

36. Block RI, Ghoneim MM. Effects of chronic marijuana use on human cognition. Psychopharmacology 1993;110:219–28.

37. Pope HG Jr, Yurgelun-Todd D. The residual cognitive effects of heavy marijuana use in college students. JAMA 1996;275:521–7.

38. Ramaekers JG, Kauert G, Theunissen EL, et al. Neurocognitive performance during acute THC intoxication in heavy and occasional cannabis users. J Psychopharmacol 2009;23:266–77.

39. Bolla KI, Brown K, Eldreth BA, et al. Dose-related neurocognitive effects of marijuana use. Neurology 2002;59:1337–43.

40. Pope HG, Gruber AJ, Hudson JI, et al. Early-onset cannabis use and cognitive deficits: what is the nature of the association? Drug Alcohol Depend 2003;69:303–10.

41. Pope HG Jr. Cannabis, cognition, and residual confounding. JAMA 2002;287:1172–4.

42. **Meier MH, Caspi A, Ambler A, et al. Persistent cannabis users show neuropsychological decline from childhood to midlife. Proc Natl Acad Sci U S A 2012;109:E2657–64.** *Participants were members of the Dunedin study in New Zealand, a prospective cohort of 1,037 followed from birth to age 38. Researchers compared neuropsychological testing at age 13 and 38 and found that persistent marijuana use was associated*

with a decline in IQ testing and the Wechsler Adult Intelligence Scale–IV. Impairment was greater among those with more persistent use, but there was not a significant decline among those who did not develop cannabis dependence before the age of 18.

43. Hartman RL, Huestis MA. Cannabis effects on driving skills. Clin Chem 2013;59:478–92.

44. Ashbridge M, Hayden JA, Cartwright JL. Acute cannabis consumption and motor vehicle collision risk: systematic review of observational studies. BMJ 2012;344:e536.

45. Bovasso GB. Cannabis abuse as a risk factor for depressive symptoms. Am J Psychiatry 2001;158:2033–7.

46. Patton GC, Coffey C, Carlin JB, et al. Cannabis use and mental health in young people: cohort study. BMJ 2002;325:1195–8.

47. Zammit S, Allebeck P, Andreasson S, et al. Self-reported cannabis use as a risk factor for schizophrenia in Swedish conscripts of 1969: historical cohort study. BMJ 2002;325:1199–203.

48. Arseneault L, Cannon M, Poulton R, et al. Cannabis use in adolescence and risk for adult psychosis: longitudinal prospective study. BMJ 2002;325:1212–3.

49. Large M, Sharma S, Compton MT, et al. Cannabis use and earlier onset of psychosis. Arch Gen Psychiatry 2011;68:555–61.

50. Degenhardt L, Hall W, Lynskey M. The relationship between cannabis use and other substance use in the general population. Drug Alcohol Depend 2001;64:319–27.

51. Lynskey MT, Heath AC, Bucholz KK, et al. Escalation of drug use in early-onset cannabis users vs. co-twin controls. JAMA 2003;289:427–33.

52. Morral AR, McCaffrey DF, Paddock SM. Reassessing the marijuana gateway effect. Addiction 2002;97:1493–504.

53. Degenhardt L, Dierker L, Chiu WT, et al. Evaluating the drug use "gateway" theory using cross-national data: consistency and associations of the order of initiation of drug use among participants in the WHO World Mental Health Surveys. Drug Alcohol Depend 2010;108:84–97.

54. Mojarrad M, Samet JH, Cheng DM, et al. Marijuana use and achievement of abstinence from alcohol and other drugs among people with substance dependence: a prospective cohort study. Drug Alcohol Depend 2014;142:91–7.

55. Hill KP, Bennett HE, Griffin ML, et al. Association of cannabis use with opioid outcomes among opioid-dependent youth. Drug Alcohol Depend 2013;132:342–5.

56. Saitz R, Palfai TP, Cheng DM, et al. Screening and brief intervention for drug use in primary care: the ASPIRE randomized clinical trial. JAMA 2014;312:502–13.

57. Roy-Byrne P, Bumgardner K, Krupski A, et al. Brief intervention for problem drug use in safety-net primary care settings: a randomized clinical trial. JAMA 2014;312:492–501.

58. Bogenschutz MP, Donovan DM, Mandler RN, et al. Brief intervention for patients with problematic drug use presenting in emergency departments: a randomized clinical trial. JAMA Intern Med 2014;174:1736–45.

59. **Stephens RS, Roffman RA, Simpson EE. Treating adult marijuana dependence: a test of the relapse prevention model. J Consult Clin Psychol 1994;62:92–9.** *In this study, 212 adults who wanted help quitting marijuana were randomized to (1) a cognitive-behavioral group or (2) a therapist-led support group. Both were 10 sessions over 12 weeks followed by booster sessions 3 and 6 months later. There were no significant differences in attendance, completion, or abstinence rates. Of the 167 (79%) who completed all the assessments, 63% reported abstinence during the last 2 weeks of treatment; this fell to 49% at 3-month follow-up and 20% at 12 months.*

60. **Stepehens RS, Roffman RA, Curtin L. Comparison of extended versus brief treatments for marijuana use. J Consult Clin Psychol 2000;68:898–908.** *In this study, 291 treatment-seeking marijuana users were randomized to (1) 14 cognitive-behavioral group treatments over 18 weeks, (2) two 90-minute individual motivational interviewing sessions 1 month apart, or (3) delayed treatment (control). Of the 85% who completed 4-month follow-up, there was no difference between the active treatments, but both had higher abstinence rates than the control arm. There was no comparison between active and delayed treatment after 4 months, when the delayed arm could enter treatment. At 7-, 13-, and 16-month follow-up, the abstinence rates in the active treatment arms were about 34%, 27%, and 28%, respectively.*

61. **Copeland J, Swift W, Roffman R, Stephens R. A randomized controlled trial of brief cognitive-behavioral interventions for cannabis use disorder. J Subst Abuse Treat 2001;21:55–64.** *In this study, 229 treatment-seeking marijuana users were randomized to (1) six weekly individual sessions incorporating motivational interview with*

cognitive-behavioral therapy, (2) one 90-minute version of the same with a self-help booklet, or (3) 24-week delayed treatment (control). Of the 74% with complete follow-up, those in active treatment were more likely to report continuous abstinence, but there was no difference between the two active treatments. Those in active treatment also had lower "dependence severity scores," and these were significantly lower with six-session treatment than with one session.

62. **Dennis M, Godley SH, Diamond G, et al. The Cannabis Youth Treatment (CYT) Study: main findings from two randomized trials. J Subst Abuse Treat 2004;27:197–213.** *In this study, 600 adolescent marijuana users were assigned to one of five treatments at four sites: (1) five sessions of motivational enhancement/cognitive-behavioral therapy, (2) 12 sessions of the same, (3) #2 plus family education and therapy, (4) community reinforcement, or (5) multidimensional family therapy. Self-reported marijuana use declined significantly in all groups in the 12 months after assignment (~24% reported no past month drug use); no group was significantly better than any other, and there was no control group.*

63. **Marijuana Treatment Research Group. Brief treatments for cannabis dependence: findings from a randomized multisite trial. J Consult Clin Psychol 2004;72:455–66.** *In this study, 450 marijuana-dependent adults were randomized to (1) two sessions of motivational enhancement, 5 weeks apart; (2) nine sessions over 3 months, including motivational enhancement, case management, and cognitive-behavioral therapy; or (3) delayed treatment (control). The outcomes included only those who completed 4 months (59%) and 9 months (55%) of follow-up, respectively. At 4-month follow-up, subjects in both active arms did better than the control arm. The nine-session group had higher 90-day abstinence rates than those of the two-session group (23% vs. 9%), but this difference was no longer significant at 9 months (16% vs. 10%).*

64. **Budney AJ, Higgins ST, Radonovich KJ, Novy PL. Adding voucher-based incentives to coping skills and motivational enhancement improves outcomes during treatment for marijuana dependence. J Consult Clin Psychol 2000;68:1051–61.** *In this study, 60 marijuana-dependent adults were randomized to (1) four individual motivational enhancement sessions, (2) 14 weekly individual cognitive-behavioral sessions, or (3) cognitive-behavioral sessions (same as #2) plus financial vouchers for cannabinoid-negative urine drug tests. After 14 weeks, subjects in the third arm had higher rates of abstinence—40% achieved at least 7 weeks of abstinence compared with 5% in the first two arms.*

65. Carroll KM, Easton CJ, Nich C, et al. The use of contingency management and motivational/skills-building therapy to treat young adults with marijuana dependence. J Consult Clin Psychol 2006;74:955–66.

66. Carroll KM, Nich C, Lapaglia DM, et al. Combining cognitive behavioral therapy and contingency management to enhance their effects in treating cannabis dependence: less can be more, more or less. Addiction 2012;107:1650–9.

67. Rooke S, Copeland J, Norberg M, et al. Effectiveness of a self-guided Web-based cannabis treatment program: randomized controlled trial. J Med Internet Res 2013;15:e26.

68. Levin FR, McDowell D, Evans SM, et al. Pharmacotherapy for marijuana dependence: a double-blind placebo controlled pilot study of divalproex sodium. Am J Addict 2004;13:21–32.

69. Carpenter KM, McDowell D, Brooks DJ, et al. A preliminary trial: double-blind comparison of nefazodone, bupropion-SR, and placebo in the treatment of cannabis dependence. Am J Addict 2009;18:53–64.

70. McRae-Clark AL, Carter RE, Killeen TK, et al. A placebo-controlled trial of buspirone for the treatment of marijuana dependence. Drug Alcohol Depend 2009;105:132–8.

71. Cooper ZD, Foltin RW, Hart CL, et al. A human laboratory study investigating the effects of quetiapine on marijuana withdrawal and relapse in daily marijuana smokers. Addict Biol 2013;18:993–1002.

72. Levin FR, Mariani J, Brooks DJ, et al. A randomized double-blind, placebo-controlled trial of venlafaxine-extended release for co-occurring cannabis dependence and depressive disorders. Addiction 2013;108:1084–94.

73. Huestis MA, Boyd SJ, Heishman SJ, et al. Single and multiple doses of rimonabant antagonize acute effects of smoked cannabis in male cannabis users. Psychopharmacology 2007;194:505–15.

74. Topol EJ, Bousser MG, Fox KA, et al. Rimonabant for prevention of cardiovascular events (CRESCENDO): a randomised, multicentre, placebo-controlled trial. Lancet. 2010;376:517–23.

75. **Levin FR, Mariani JJ, Brooks DJ, et al. Dronabinol for the treatment of cannabis dependence: a randomized, double-blind, placebo controlled trial. Drug Alcohol Depend 2011;116:142–50.** *In this study, 156 cannabis-dependent adults were randomized to receive 20 mg*

of dronabinol twice daily or placebo. Doses were maintained for 8 weeks, then tapered over 2 weeks. At the end of the maintenance phase, treatment retention was higher among those on dronabinol (77% vs. 61% on placebo), but there was no significant difference in the proportion of participants who achieved 2 weeks of abstinence (18% with dronabinol vs. 16% with placebo).

11

Inhalants

Volatile Organic Compounds, Nitrites, and Anesthetics

Background

Inhalants are a pharmacologically heterogeneous group of substances that have been traditionally grouped together because of their predominant route of use. There is no technical definition for this group of agents, which is sometimes referred to as "volatile substances," but it generally includes three classes of chemicals: volatile organic compounds, volatile anesthetics, and nitrites. Table 11.1 lists some of these chemicals and their sources.

The volatile organic compounds are a diverse group of chemicals that can be found in fuels (gasoline, butane and propane), solvents (nail polish remover, paint thinner, correction fluid), cleaning agents, adhesives, aerosols (spray paint, hair spray), and refrigerants. Table 11.2 lists some of the organic compounds found in each of these substances. These organic compounds can be roughly divided into aromatic hydrocarbons, alkanes, chlorinated hydrocarbons, ketones, and fluorocarbons.

Abused volatile anesthetics include nitrous oxide (also known as "laughing gas"), which is also used a propellant in whipped cream. Other volatile anesthetics can be abused, including ether, halothane, enflurane, and propofol.

The nitrites include amyl, butyl, cyclohexyl, and isobutyl nitrite. These chemicals are volatile liquids with a yellowish color and fruity odor. Amyl nitrite was originally developed as a treatment for angina and was produced in glass capsules that were popped open to release the liquid and thus referred to as "poppers." Amyl, butyl, and isobutyl nitrite are sold (legally) in small bottles that are sometimes referred to as "poppers" as well. These agents can be purchased on the Internet or at stores (typically adult bookstores or head shops) and are sometimes labeled "room deodorizers" or "video head cleaners." Cyclohexyl nitrite is found in room deodorizers. Nitrites are often used in bars and nightclubs and for this

TABLE 11.1 Chemical Agents Found in Abused Inhalants

Substance	Source	Other Names
	Volatile Organic Compounds*	
Aromatic hydrocarbons		
Toluene	Airplane glue, rubber cement, nail polish and nail polish remover, paint thinner, gasoline	
Benzene		
Xylene		
Naphthalene	Mothballs	
Paradichlorobenzene	Toilet cake, room deodorizers	PDB, p-DCB
Alkanes		
Butane	Fuel for lighters, portable stoves, barbecues, and recreational vehicles	
Propane		
Isopropane	Spray paint, hair spray, deodorants, room fresheners, gasoline	
Hexane		
Chlorinated hydrocarbons		
Monochloroethane	Dry cleaning agents, video head cleaner, computer duster spray, spot removers, degreasers, correction fluid, gasoline	Ethyl chloride
Trichloroethane, Trichloroethene,		Methyl chloroform
Tetrachloroethylene,		Trichloroethylene
Dichloromethane		Perchloroethylene (PCE)
		Methylene chloride

(continued)

TABLE 11.1 (Continued)

Substance	Source	Other Names
Volatile Organic Compounds* (Continued)		
Ketones Acetone Methyl ethyl ketone Methyl butyl ketone	Nail polish remover, rubber cement, varnish, lacquers, paint remover	2-butanone 2-hexanone
Fluorocarbons	Asthma inhalers, air fresheners, hair spray, spray paint, fire extinguishers, refrigerants, electronic cleaning products (dusters)	Chlorofluorocarbons CFCs, Freon
Anesthetics		
Nitrous oxide Ether Halothane Enflurane Propofol	Whipping cream canisters	Whippets

Nitrites		
Amyl nitrite		Poppers, snappers
Butyl nitrite		Poppers, rush, bolt, video head cleaner
Isobutyl nitrite		Poppers
Cyclohexyl nitrite	Room deodorizers	

*Organic compounds are found in multiple sources. Many of the sources listed may contain more than one of the compounds listed; see Table 5.2 for the chemicals that can be found in specific sources.

TABLE 11.2 Organic Compounds Found in Abused Inhalants*

Source	Compounds
Fuels	
Gasoline	Aromatic hydrocarbons (benzene, xylene), alkanes (butane, hexane, octane, paraffins), alkenes, chlorinated hydrocarbons
Bottled fuel gas	Butane, isobutane, propane, isopropane
Lighter fluid	Butane, isopropane
Solvents	
Paint thinner	Toluene, xylene, methylene chloride, methanol
Nail polish remover	Acetone, toluene
Correction fluid	Trichloroethane, trichloroethylene
Cleaning agents	
Dry cleaning	Tetrachloroethylene, trichloroethylene
Spot removers	Tetrachloroethylene, trichloroethylene
Degreasers	Dichloromethane, trichloroethylene
Paint remover	Dichloromethane, toluene
Computer duster spray	Tetrafluoroethane, difluoroethane
Adhesives	
Airplane glue	Toluene, hexane, acetone
Rubber cement	Toluene, hexane, acetone, methyl ethyl ketone

(continued)

TABLE 11.2 (Continued)

Aerosols	
Spray paint	Methylene chloride, toluene, butane, propane, fluorocarbons
Hair spray	Butane, propane, fluorocarbons
Deodorants	Butane, propane, fluorocarbons
Room fresheners	Butane, propane, fluorocarbons
Others	
Varnish	Xylene, methyl ethyl ketone
Lacquers	Toluene, methyl ethyl ketone
Fingernail polish	Toluene
Mothballs	Naphthalene, paradichlorobenzene (p-DCB, PDB)
Room deodorizers	Paradichlorobenzene, cyclohexyl nitrite

*Note: Ingredients vary by manufacturer and brand.

reason are referred to as a "club drug," along with ecstasy, ketamine, gamma-hydroxybutyrate (GHB), and others.

Epidemiology

According to the 2013 National Survey on Drug Use and Health (NSDUH),[1] over 21 million Americans age 12 and over (8.0%) have used inhalants at some time in their lives; 1.5 million had used in the past year (0.6%) and 0.5 million had used in the past month (0.2%). An estimated 132,000 Americans abused or were dependent on inhalants. Among the inhalants, lifetime use of nitrous oxide was highest (12.4 million Americans; 4.7% of those age 12 or older), followed by amyl nitrite (7.4 million; 2.8%), glue, shoe polish, or toluene (2.8 million; 1.1%), and gasoline or lighter fluid (2.7 million; 1.0%).

According to the NSDUH, recent (past month) inhalant use declines with age; it was 0.6% among those aged 12–15, 0.3–0.4% among those 16–25, 0.2% among those aged 26–34, and 0.1% among those aged 35 or older. It appears that many adolescent inhalant users switch to other substances as they grow older.[2,3] Moreover, the risk of drug use and binge or frequent drinking among college students has been found to be strongly associated with early inhalant use, more so than early marijuana use.[4]

An analysis of data from the 2000 and 2001 NHDSA (now called the NSDUH) found that adolescent inhalant abuse or dependence was associated with participation in mental health treatment, delinquency, history of incarceration, history of foster care placement, and use of alcohol and other drugs, but not with gender, race/ethnicity, or family income.[5] An analysis of poison control center data indicated that inhalant cases declined 33% from 1993 to 2008; 74% of cases were boys, prevalence was highest for children aged 12–17 and peaked in 14-year-olds. Propellants, gasoline, and paint were the most commonly reported substances.[6]

The epidemiology of nitrite use appears to be different than that of other inhalants. Some studies have found comparatively high rates of nitrite use among cohorts of homosexual men[7] and an association between nitrite use and high-risk sexual behavior.[8]

The drug effects and complications of each of the three classes of inhalants will be covered separately. It should be noted that most of the information on complications is in the form of case reports or case series, which is not strong evidence for causation and suggests that serious medical complications are not common. There will be a brief discussion of treatment issues at the end of the chapter.

Assessment

The DSM-5 recognizes volatile hydrocarbons as inhalants, but does not include nitrites and anesthetics in this category.[9] The DSM-5 criteria for "inhalant use disorder" are the same as for other substances; see Chapter 1 for details. The ICD-10 code for a mild disorder is F18.10 and for moderate-severe, F18.20. DSM-5 also includes "unspecified inhalant-related disorder" (ICD-10: F18.99) but does not include withdrawal for this class. Other assessment issues specific to each class will be covered in their respective sections.

Volatile Organic Compounds: Fuels, Solvents, Adhesives, Cleaning Agents, and Aerosols

Drug Effects

The exact mechanism of the neuropsychological effects of volatile organic compounds is not well understood. These substances are typically "sniffed" from their original containers or "huffed" from a cloth that is soaked in the chemical; some users may place the substance in a plastic bag and inhale the fumes ("bagging").

Acute Effects

The acute effects of these substances are often likened to those of alcohol. Users typically experience a sense of euphoria followed by central nervous system (CNS) depression. They may also have visual or auditory hallucinations. Users may become hyperactive or agitated and do impulsive, even dangerous acts that lead to injuries.

Acute Toxicity and Overdose

The DSM-5 criteria for inhalant intoxication requires the presence of "clinically significant problematic behavioral or psychological changes" plus two (or more) of the following signs of symptoms occurring after inhalant use: (1) dizziness, (2) nystagmus, (3) incoordination, (4) slurred speech, (5) unsteady gait, (6) lethargy, (7) depressed reflexes, (8) psychomotor retardation, (9) tremor, (10) generalized muscle weakness, (11) blurred vision or diplopia, (12) stupor or coma, and (13) euphoria.[9] The ICD-10 code includes whether there is a comorbid inhalant use disorder and the severity of the disorder—F18.929 if there is no comorbid disorder, F18.129 if a mild disorder, and F18.229 if moderate-severe.

Deaths due to inhalant use are relatively uncommon; in a cohort from a national survey in 1991, those who reported lifetime inhalant use at baseline did not have an increased risk of mortality over 15 years of follow-up.[10] However, it is clear that fatalities do occur. A 1970 article reported on a series of 110 sudden deaths in the 1960s among adolescents and young adults who had inhaled organic compounds (toluene, benzene, gasoline, trichloroethane, and fluorocarbons); this phenomenon was dubbed "sudden sniffing death" and was postulated to be due to cardiac arrhythmia.[11] A later series in Virginia reported 39 deaths associated with inhalant use from 1987 to 1996; the majority were male (95%) and age 22 or younger (70%). Thirty-six (92%) of these fatalities were from inhaling organic compounds: butane (13), propane (5), fluorocarbons (10), trichloroethane (4), dichloromethane (1), toluene (2), and gasoline (1).[12] Another series from Texas reported 144 deaths related to inhalant use from 1988 to 1998; the mean age was 25.6, most were males (92%), and many were in occupations that employed these compounds. As in Virginia, most of these fatalities were associated with abuse of organic compounds: fluorocarbons (35%), chlorinated hydrocarbons (25%), toluene (17%), alkanes (3%), and gasoline (2%).[13] In a 20-year retrospective analysis of 18,880 autopsies in South Australia, 39 deaths were due to inhalants, with 11 of these being suicides; most were men, and the mean age of the accidental victims was 21 (range 13–45).[14]

The exact mechanism of death in these fatalities is often unclear; autopsies, when performed, generally show no anatomical abnormalities to explain the deaths. Many of these deaths appear to be due to fatal arrhythmias, others may be due to respiratory arrest[15] or aspiration.[16] Some cases are due to inadvertent asphyxiation, such as when a user places a plastic bag with the substance over their head and then loses consciousness.

Treatment of the intoxicated individual is generally supportive; there are no specific antidotes to these chemicals. Gastric lavage may be helpful in cases of ingestion.

Withdrawal

It appears that regular users of organic compounds develop tolerance to their effects over time. Some may experience unpleasant symptoms with abstinence. In one study, toluene and butane gas users reported insomnia, irritability, nausea, sweating, and tremulousness.[17] Another study that included all inhalant users found that hypersomnia, fatigue, and nausea were the most common symptoms.[18] As noted earlier, the DSM-5 does not recognize an inhalant withdrawal syndrome.[9]

Assessment

Organic compound abuse should be considered in anyone who presents with signs of intoxication, particularly among adolescents or individuals who work with these substances. Regular users may have a characteristic perioral rash. Other clues may include paint or solvent stains on clothing, a "chemical" odor on breath, and stained fingernails.

Solvents can be detected by gas chromatography in the serum, but this test is not widely available for clinical use. Organic compounds are not detected in routine urine drug tests although some of their metabolites can be detected in the urine, including phenol (metabolite of benzene), 2,5-dichlorophenol (paradichlorobenzene), hippuric acid (toluene), methylhippuric acid (xylene), and trichloroacetic acid (trichloroethylene).[19]

Medical Complications

It seems that serious, lasting complications from inhalant use are uncommon. Most of the information we have on medical complications is in the form of case reports or small case series. The most serious complication appears to be encephalopathy.

Cutaneous Complications

As mentioned earlier, an inhalant user may have perioral dermatitis from exposure to these substances. This is typically described as red spots or sores around the mouth and nose. Volatile inhalant users are also at risk for burns from accidental fires[20] and hypothermic injuries from aerosols or propellants,[21] including digital and oro-facial frostbite.[22] There is also a report of an "ichthyosis-like" dermatitis on the extremities associated with inhaling the fumes of mothballs containing paradichlorobenzene.[23]

Pulmonary Complications

Exposure to volatile organic compounds has been associated with (modestly) diminished lung function among asthmatics.[24] Furthermore, a number of studies on occupational exposure to solvents suggest that they are associated with respiratory complaints including wheezing[25] and asthma-related symptoms.[26] There is also a report of acute eosinophilic pneumonia after intentional inhalation of trichloroethane (in the commercial product Scotchguard).[27]

Cardiovascular Complications

Inhalation of organic compounds may lead to ventricular arrhythmias and sudden death. In some of these cases, death occurred in the setting of inhalant use followed by physical exertion, suggesting that endogenous catecholamines may play a role. Ventricular fibrillation has been observed after abuse of lighter fluid (butane),[28] air freshener (butane and isobutane),[29] and glue sniffing.[30] There is also a report of ventricular tachycardia in a child after accidental exposure to non-fluorocarbon propellants (isobutane, butane, and propane) in a deodorant.[31] There are case reports of cardiomyopathy associated with inhalation of volatile compounds.[32,33]

Gastrointestinal Complications

One case series of adults hospitalized with "problems related to paint sniffing" reported that 6 of the 25 individuals presented with gastrointestinal complaints, including abdominal pain, nausea, and vomiting.[34] There are also reports of hepatotoxicity associated with occupational exposure to chlorinated hydrocarbons[35] and hydrochlorofluorocarbons.[36]

Renal and Electrolyte Complications

Toluene exposure (typically among paint or glue sniffers) has been associated with Fanconi's syndrome and distal renal tubular acidosis, resulting in hypokalemia, hypocalcemia, hypophosphatemia, and hyperchloremic metabolic acidosis.[37,38] These individuals can present with profound generalized weakness.[39]

There are also reports of acute renal failure associated with toluene use;[40,41,42] however, one study of workers found no evidence of renal toxicity at a moderate level of exposure to toluene.[43]

Hematological Complications

Occupational exposure to benzene (especially at high levels) has been associated with aplastic anemia,[44] and there is a case report of aplastic anemia associated with glue sniffing.[45] Benzene exposure has also been linked with a number of hematological malignancies, including leukemia, lymphoma, and myelodysplastic syndrome.[46]

Neuromuscular Complications

The most serious long-term complications of exposure to organic compounds are the neurological sequelae. Acutely, users may exhibit a variety of neurological and cognitive deficits, including ataxia, tremor, chorea, myoclonus, nystagmus, delirium, and encephalopathy.[47,48] Many of these problems resolve with elimination of the substance from the body; however, some regular users may develop irreversible residual deficits. These include cognitive deficits (apathy, attention and memory impairment), peripheral neuropathy,[49] and cerebellar ataxia. Among individuals who sniff gasoline, some of these complications appear to be due to the toxicity of lead in the gasoline.[50] However, users of other organic compounds can have acute and chronic deficits. A case series in 1981 described 19 children aged 8–14 who were hospitalized with encephalopathy; presentations included coma, ataxia, convulsions, behavior disturbance, and diplopia—one developed persistent cerebellar ataxia.[51] Some of these chronic neurological deficits appear to correlate with white matter changes on MRI.[52] Encephalopathy generally resolves with cessation of use, but some individuals may have persistent impairment, particularly those who developed severe deficits after inhaling leaded gasoline.[53]

Psychiatric Complications

Inhalant encephalopathy may be mistaken for a primary psychiatric disorder such as depression.[54] Although this does not establish causality, inhalant users have a high prevalence of co-occurring psychiatric disorders. In an analysis of the 2001–2002 National Epidemiologic Survey on Alcohol and Related Conditions (NESARC), 70% met criteria for at least one lifetime mood (48%), anxiety (36%), or personality (45%) disorder.[55]

Volatile Anesthetics: Nitrous Oxide and Others

Drug Effects

Acute Effects

The acute effects of volatile anesthetics include euphoria, dizziness, drowsiness, ataxia, and blurred vision. Some users may experience visual illusions or hallucinations. Higher levels of exposure lead to loss of consciousness and respiratory depression.

Acute Toxicity and Overdose

The main hazard of volatile anesthetic abuse is hypoxia and asphyxiation due to inhalation of high concentrations of the anesthetic.

There have been a number of reports of fatalities due to use of these substances,[56] some among workers who handle nitrous oxide (such as food-serving establishments)[57] or other volatile anesthetics (hospital employees).[58] While use of nitrous oxide alone does not generally produce deep anesthesia, other volatile anesthetics can cause profound respiratory depression and death; the therapeutic window between anesthesia and death is fairly narrow. Nevertheless, the reports of deaths associated with volatile anesthetic abuse tend to be smaller in number than those associated with volatile organic compounds.[9,10]

Withdrawal

It appears that regular users of volatile anesthetics develop tolerance to their effects. There does not appear to be a well-defined withdrawal syndrome, but some users do experience drug craving. As noted earlier, one study that included inhalant users—and did not differentiate between drug classes—reported that hypersomnia, fatigue, and nausea were the most common symptoms with cessation.[15]

Assessment

Use of volatile anesthetics should be considered in individuals who present with an acute change in level of consciousness, especially those with occupational access to these agents (food preparation and healthcare workers). There are no specific physical findings or laboratory tests for detection of illicit use.

Medical Complications

Pulmonary Complications

Volatile anesthetics do not appear to have any pulmonary toxicity, but they may cause hypoxia due to inhalation of the anesthetic with insufficient quantities of oxygen.

Cardiovascular Complications

Nitrous oxide and other anesthetics can depress myocardial function[59] and there has been a case report of cardiovascular collapse associated with its therapeutic use.[60] There also have been reports of acute myocardial infarction associated with general anesthesia (enflurane and isoflurane).[61] It is possible that illicit users have also had these complications and that some of the fatalities associated with anesthetic use are due to these cardiovascular complications.

Gastrointestinal Complications

Case reports exist of hepatotoxicity (fatal in one case) associated with nonmedical halothane use among hospital personnel.[62]

Hematological Complications

Nitrous oxide irreversibly oxidizes the cobalt ion in cyanocobalamin (vitamin B12), thus inactivating cobalamin-dependent enzymes, leading to symptoms typical of vitamin B12 deficiency, including megaloblastic anemia.[63]

Neuromuscular Complications

When nitrous oxide causes clinical vitamin B12 deficiency, users may present with peripheral neuropathy, ataxia, and even cognitive changes.[64,65] There have been a number reports of seizures associated with (therapeutic) use of enflurane.[66]

Nitrites

Drug Effects

Nitrites are potent vasodilators and smooth muscle relaxers.

Acute Effects

Users describe a "rush" with a feeling of warmth, and giddiness. This is often accompanied by removal of inhibitions and heightened sensation and pleasure, especially when used during sexual intercourse. Some users may experience headaches and visual disturbances.

Acute Toxicity and Overdose

Nitrites may cause hypotension and even syncope. However, the most serious complication appears to be methemoglobinemia,[67] which can be fatal in some cases.[68] Methemoglobinemia presents with cyanosis, and the diagnosis can be established by the use of co-oximetry with arterial blood analysis. It can be reversed with intravenous methylene blue.[69]

Withdrawal

It is clear that, like nitrates, frequent exposure to nitrites leads to tolerance to its effects within a few days. There does not appear to be a withdrawal syndrome associated with cessation of use.

Assessment

Nonmedical nitrite use should be considered in individuals who present with complications such as hypotension or syncope and especially among those with unexplained methemoglobinemia. There are no specific physical findings or laboratory tests for nitrite use.

Medical Complications

Lasting medical complications from nitrites appear to be uncommon.

Ocular Complications

There are reports of retinal toxicity associated with nitrite use, which can result in transient (a few weeks) or permanent visual loss.[70]

Cutaneous Complications

There are reports of acrocyanosis associated with butyl nitrite use; this can present with painless, gray-bluish discoloration of the nose, ears, and distal extremities.[71]

Pulmonary Complications

Nitrite users can develop cyanosis due to methemoglobinemia (discussed earlier). There is one case report of severe tracheobronchitis associated with nitrite use.[72]

Cardiovascular Complications

As mentioned earlier, the vasodilatory effects of nitrites may lead to hypotension and even syncope. This effect may be potentiated by concurrent use of phosphodiesterase (PDE) inhibitors, such as sildenafil (Viagra).[73]

Hematological Complications

As noted earlier, nitrites can cause methemoglobinemia. The use of nitrites has also been associated with acute hemolytic anemia,[74] especially among individuals who have G6PD deficiency.[75]

Infectious Complications

A number of epidemiological studies have found that nitrite use among homosexual and bisexual men is associated with high-risk sexual behavior and sexually transmitted diseases, including HIV.[76] In fact, this association was noted before the discovery of the HIV virus, leading some to postulate (incorrectly) that AIDS was caused by amyl nitrite.[77]

Treatment

There are very few data on the treatment of inhalant use disorders. A 2010 Cochrane systematic review found no studies that fulfilled their inclusion criteria and could not reach any conclusions.[78] Brief counseling has been shown to be effective for alcohol (and other substance) misuse and may be effective for periodic inhalant users as well. It would be prudent to advise users of the health hazards of these substances and recommend that they stop using. However, the available data suggest poor response to conventional treatment. For example, one case series of 10 adults admitted for treatment of chronic solvent abuse reported that one half did not complete inpatient rehabilitation and all had relapsed by 6 months.[79] Another study reported on 14 adolescent chronic solvent abusers who were offered outpatient treatment (individual or family therapy); 11 kept appointments, and there was "no change" in 6 and "improvement" in 5 of these.[80] The poor outcomes observed may be partly due to selection of severe cases; the high prevalence of antisocial personality disorder among regular users may also be a factor.[81]

There are no data on treatment of nitrite users. However, given the association between nitrite use and unsafe sexual practices, users should be carefully evaluated for HIV infection and other sexually transmitted diseases and counseled on safe sexual practices.

Notes

1. Substance Abuse and Mental Health Services Administration. *Results from the 2013 National Survey on Drug Use and Health: National Findings.* NSDUH Series H-48, HHS Publication No. (SMA) 14-4863. Rockville, MD: Substance Abuse and Mental Health Services Administration; 2014.

2. Dinwiddie SH, Reich T, Cloninger CR. Solvent use as a precursor to intravenous drug abuse. Compr Psychiatry 1991;32:133–40.

3. Schultz CG, Chilcoat HD, Anthony JC. The association between sniffing inhalants and injecting drugs. Compr Psychiatry 1994;35:99–105.

4. Bennett ME, Walters ST, Miller JH, Woodall WG. Relationship of early inhalant use to substance use in college students. J Subst Abuse 2000;12:227–40.

5. Wu LT, Pilowsky DJ, Schlenger WE. Inhalant abuse and dependence among adolescents in the United States. J Am Acad Child Adolesc Psychiatry 2004;43:1206–14.

6. Marsolek MR, White NC, Litovitz TL. Inhalant abuse: monitoring trends by using poison control data, 1993–2008. Pediatrics 2010;125:906–13.

7. Woody GE, VanEtten-Lee ML, McKirnan D, et al. Substance use among men who have sex with men: comparison with a national household survey. J Acquir Immune Defic Syndr 2001;27:86–90.

8. Ostrow DG, Beltran ED, Joseph JG, et al. Recreational drugs and sexual behavior in the Chicago MACS/CCS cohort of homosexually active men. J Subst Abuse 1993;5:311–25.

9. American Psychiatric Association. *Diagnostic and Statistical Manual of Mental Disorders*, Fifth Edition. Arlington, VA: American Psychiatric Publishing; 2013.

10. Muhuri PK, Gfroerer JC. Mortality associated with illegal drug use among adults in the United States. Am J Drug Alcohol Abuse 2011;37:155–64.

11. Bass M. Sudden sniffing death. JAMA 1970;212:2075–9.

12. Bowen SE, Daniel J, Balster RL. Deaths associated with inhalant abuse in Virginia from 1987 to 1996. Drug Alcohol Depend 1999;53:239–45.

13. Maxwell JC. Deaths related to the inhalation of volatile substances in Texas: 1988–1998. Am J Drug Alcohol Abuse 2001;27:689–97.

14. Wick R, Gilbert JD, Felgate P, Byard RW. Inhalant deaths in South Australia: a 20-year retrospective autopsy study. Am J Forensic Pathol 2007;28:319–22.

15. Cronk SL, Barkley DEH, Farrell MF. Respiratory arrest after solvent abuse. BMJ 1985;290:897–8.

16. Shepherd RT. Mechanism of sudden death associated with volatile substance abuse. Hum Toxicol 1989;8:287–91.

17. Evans AC, Raistrick D. Phenomenology of intoxication with toluene-based adhesives and butane gas. Br J Psychiatry 1987;150:769–73.

18. Perron BE, Glass JE, Ahmedani BK, et al. The prevalence and clinical significance of inhalant withdrawal symptoms among a national sample. Subst Abuse Rehab 2011;2:69–76.

19. Broussard LA. The role of the laboratory in detecting inhalant abuse. Clin Lab Sci 2000;13:205–9.

20. Janežič TF. Burns following petrol sniffing. Burns 1997;23:78–80.

21. Kurbat RS, Pollack CV. Facial injury and airway threat from inhalant abuse: a case report. J Emerg Med 1998;16:167–9.

22. Koehelr MM, Henninger CA. Orofacial and digital frostbite caused by inhalant abuse. Cutis 2014;93:256–60.

23. Feuillet L, Mallet S, Spadari M. Twin girls with neurocutaneous symptoms caused by mothball intoxication. N Engl J Med 2006;335:423–4.

24. Harving H, Dahl R, Molhave L. Lung function and bronchial reactivity in asthmatics during exposure to volatile organic compounds. Am Rev Respir Dis 1991;143:751–4.

25. Hoppin JA, Umbach DM, London SJ, et al. Diesel exhaust, solvents, and other occupational exposures as risk factors for wheeze among farmers. Am J Respir Crit Care Med 2004;169:1308–13.

26. Cakmak A, Ekici A, Ekici M, et al. Respiratory findings in gun factory workers exposed to solvents. Respir Med 2004;98:52–6.

27. Kelly KJ, Ruffing R. Acute eosinophilic pneumonia following intentional inhalation of Scotchguard. Ann Allergy 1993;71:358–61.

28. Gunn J, Wilson J, Mackintosh AF. Butane sniffing causing ventricular fibrillation. Lancet 1989;333:617.

29. LoVecchio F, Fulton SE. Ventricular fibrillation following inhalation of Glade Air Freshener. Eur J Emerg Med 2001;8:153–5.

30. Cunninghan SR, Dalzell GW, McGirr P, Khan MM. Myocardial infarction and primary ventricular fibrillation after glue sniffing. BMJ 1987;294:739–40.

31. Wason S, Gibler WB, Hassan M. Ventricular tachycardia associated with non-freon aerosol propellants. JAMA 1986;256:78–80.

32. Vural M, Ogel K. Dilated cardiomyopathy associated with toluene abuse. Cardiology 2006;105:158–61.

33. Samson R, Kado H, Chapman D. Huffing-induced cardiomyopathy: a case report. Cardiovasc Toxicol 2012;12:90–2.

34. Streicher HZ, Gabow PA, Moss AH, et al. Syndromes of toluene sniffing in adults. Ann Intern Med 1981;94:758–62.

35. Hodgson MJ, Heyl AE, VanThiel DH. Liver disease associated with exposure to 1,1,1-trichloroethane. Arch Intern Med 1989;149:1793–8.

36. Hoet P, Graf ML, Bourdi M, et al. Epidemic of liver disease caused by hydrochlorofluorocarbons used as ozone-sparing substitutes of chlorofluorocarbons. Lancet 1997;350:556–9.

37. Taher SM, Anderson RJ, McCartney R, et al. Renal tubular acidosis associated with toluene "sniffing." N Engl J Med 1974;290:765–8.

38. Moss AH, Gabow PA, Kaehny WD, et al. Fanconi's syndrome and distal renal tubular acidosis after glue sniffing. Ann Intern Med 1980;92:69–70.

39. Camara-Lemarroy CR, Gonzalez-Moreno EI, Rodriguez-Gutierrez R, Gonzalez-Gonzalez JG. Clinical presentation and management in acute toluene intoxication: a case series. Inhal Toxicol 2012;24:434–8.

40. Will AM, McLaren EH. Reversible renal damage due to glue sniffing. BMJ 1981;283:525–6.

41. Taverner D, Harrison DJ, Bell GM. Acute renal failure due to interstitial nephritis induced by "glue-sniffing" with subsequent recovery. Scott Med J 1988;33:246–7.

42. Gupta RK, van der Meulen J, Johny KV. Oliguric renal failure due to glue-sniffing. Scand J Urol Nephrol 1991;25:247–50.

43. Nielsen HK, Krusell L, Baelum J, et al. Renal effects of acute exposure to toluene. A controlled clinical trial. Acta Med Scand 1985;218:317–21.

44. Smith MT. Overview of benzene-induced aplastic anemia. Eur J Haematol 1996;60:107–10.

45. Powars D. Aplastic anemia secondary to glue sniffing. N Engl J Med 1965;273:700–2.

46. Travis LB, Li CY, Zhang ZN, et al. Hematopoietic malignancies and related disorders among benzene exposed workers in China. Leuk Lymphoma 1994;14:91–102.

47. King MD. Neurologic sequelae of toluene abuse. Hum Toxicol 1982;1:281–7.

48. Cairney S, Maruff P, Burns C, Currie B. The neurobehavioral consequences of petrol (gasoline) sniffing. Neurosci Behav Rev 2002;26:81–9.

49. Burns TM, Shneker BF, Juel VC. Gasoline sniffing multifocal neuropathy. Pediatr Neurol 2001;25:419–21.

50. Cairney S, Maruff P, Burns CB, et al. Neurological and cognitive impairment associated with leaded gasoline encephalopathy. Drug Alcohol Depend 2004;73:183–8.

51. King MD, Day RE, Oliver JS, et al. Solvent encephalopathy. BMJ 1981;283:663–5.

52. Filley CM, Heaton RK, Rosenberg NL. White matter dementia in chronic toluene abuse. Neurology 1990;40:532–4.

53. Cairney S, O'Connor N, Dingwall KM, et al. A prospective study of neurocognitive changes 15 years after chronic inhalant abuse. Addiction 2013;108:1107–14.

54. Muray SB, Dwight-Johnson M, Levy MR. Mothball induced encephalopathy presenting as depression: it's all in the history. Gen Hosp Psychiatry 2010;32:341e.7–9.

55. Wu LT, Howard MO. Psychiatric disorders in inhalant users: results from the National Epidemiologic Survey on Alcohol and Related Conditions. Drug Alcohol Depend 2007;88:146–55.

56. Winek CL, Wahba WW, Rozin L. Accidental death by nitrous oxide inhalation. Forensic Sci Int 1995;73:139–41.

57. Suruda AJ, Mc Glothlin JD. Fatal abuse of nitrous oxide in the workplace. J Occup Med 1990;32:682–4.

58. Yamashita M, Matsuki A, Oyama T. Illicit use of modern volatile anesthetics. Can Anaesth Soc J 1984;31:76–9.

59. Ngai SH. Effects of anesthetics on various organs. N Engl J Med 1980;302:564–6.

60. Mayhew J. Cardiovascular collapse associated with nitrous oxide administration. Can Anaesth Soc J 1983;30:226.

61. Zainea M, Duvernoy WFC, Chauhan A, et al. Acute myocardial infarction in angiographically normal coronary arteries following induction of general anesthesia. Arch Intern Med 1994;154:2495–8.

62. Kaplan HG, Bakken J, Quadracci L, Schubach W. Hepatitis caused by halothane sniffing. Ann Intern Med 1979;90:797–8.

63. Weimann J. Toxicity of nitrous oxide. Best Pract Res Clin Anaesthesiol 2003;17:47–61.

64. Butzkueven H, King JO. Nitrous oxide myelopathy in an abuser of whipped cream bulbs. J Clin Neurosci 2000;7:73–5.

65. Miller MA, Maritnez V, McCarthy R, Patel MM. Nitrous oxide "whippit" abuse presenting as clinical B12 deficiency and ataxia. Am J Emerg Med 2004;22:124.

66. Jenkins J, Milne AC. Convulsive reaction following enflurane anesthesia. Anaesthesia 1984;39:44–5.

67. Horne MK, Waterman MR, Simon LM, et al. Methemoglobinemia from sniffing butyl nitrite. Ann Intern Med 1979;91:417–8.

68. Bradberry SM, Whittington RM, Parry DA, Vale JA. Fatal methemoglobinemia due to inhalation of isobutyl nitrite. J Toxicol Clin Toxicol 1994;32:179–84.

69. Wright RO, Lewander WJ, Woolf AD. Methemoglobinemia: etiology, pharmacology, and clinical management. Ann Emerg Med 1999;34:646–56.

70. Vignal-Clermont C, Audo I, Sahel JA, Paques M. Poppers-associated retinal toxicity. N Engl J Med 2010;363:1583–4.

71. Hoegl L, Thoma-Greber E, Poppinger J, Röcken M. Butyl nitrite-induced acrocyanosis in an HIV-infected patient. Arch Dermatol 1999;135:90–1.

72. Covalla JR, Strimlan CV, Lech JG. Severe tracheobronchitis from inhalation of an isobutyl nitrite preparation. Drug Intell Clin Pharm 1981;15:51–2.

73. Chu PL, McFarland W, Gibson S, et al. Viagra use in a community-recruited sample of men who have sex with men, San Francisco. J Acquir Immune Defic Syndr 2003;33:191–3.

74. Graves TD. Acute haemolytic anemia after inhalation of amyl nitrite. J R Soc Med 2003;96:594–5.

75. Stalnikowicz R, Amitai Y, Bentur Y. Aphrodisiac drug-induced hemolysis. J Toxicol Clin Toxicol 2004;42:313–6.

76. Ostrow DG, Beltran ED, Jospeph JG, et al. Recreational drug use and sexual behaviour in the Chicago MACS/CCS cohort of homosexually active men. J Subst Abuse 1993;5:311–25.

77. Brennan RO, Durack DT. Gay compromise syndrome. Lancet 1981;318:1338–9.

78. Konghorn S, Verachai V, Srisurapanont M, et al. Treatment of inhalant dependence and abuse. Cochrane Database Syst Rev 2010;12:CD007537.

79. Dinwiddie SH, Zorumski CF, Rubin EH. Psychiatric correlates of chronic solvent abuse. J Clin Psychiatry 1987;48:334–7.

80. Skuse D, Burrell S. A review of solvent abusers and their management by a child psychiatric out-patient service. Human Toxicol 1982;1:321–9.

81. Dinwiddie SH, Reich T, Cloninger CR. Solvent use and psychiatric comorbidity. Br J Addict 1990;85:1647–56.

12

Anabolic Steroids and Athletes

Other drugs used by athletes to enhance athletic performance include growth hormone, stimulants, erythropoietin, blood products, gonado-tropins, beta-blockers, and diuretics.

Background

Much recent media attention has focused on the use of anabolic steroids by professional athletes. However, recreational use of anabolic steroids by men wishing to increase strength and improve appearance is more common.[1] Detailed directions for obtaining and using anabolic steroids can be found on the Internet.[2] This chapter focuses on anabolic steroids, but other performance-enhancing drugs that may be used by athletes will also be discussed briefly at the end.

The anabolic or "muscle-building" effects of testosterone were first recognized in the 1930s. Initially, testosterone was used for its androgen (masculinizing) effects in the treatment of hypogonadism. Later uses included the treatment of anemia, burns, and malnutrition. However, as early as the 1940s, weightlifters started using testosterone for its anabolic (muscle building) effects to enhance athletic performance. This was followed by the synthesis of new compounds related to testosterone that are longer acting (testosterone ethanate and testosterone cypionate), orally active (methyl-testosterone and stanozolol), and more potent (nandrolone); have less conversion to estrogen, resulting in less gynecomastia (methandrostenolone); have less androgen effects (oxandrolone and oxymetholone); and are more difficult to detect by drug testing. Routes of use include injection, transdermal (as gels or creams), and oral. A list of commonly used anabolic steroids can be found in Table 12.1. By the 1970s, the use of anabolic steroids became so widespread among amateur athletes, including adolescents, that they were banned from Olympic competition in 1975.[3] They were classified as scheduled drugs by the U.S. Drug Enforcement Administration (DEA) in 1991.

Anabolic steroids promote growth of skeletal muscle and increase lean body mass.[4] They are anticatabolic and can convert a negative

TABLE 12.1 Commonly Used Anabolic Steroids

Trade Name	Generic
Injectable	
Deca-Durabolin	nandrolone decanoate
Delatestryl	testosterone enanthate
Depo-testosterone	testosterone cypionate
Durabolin	nandrolone phenylpropionate
Equipoise	boldenone undecylenate
Finajet	trenbolone acetate
Oreton	testosterone propionate
Parabolin	trenbolone
Primobolan depot	methenolone enanthate
Oral	
Anadrol	oxymetholone
Anavar	oxandrolone
Dianabol	methandrostenolone
Halotestin	fluoxymesterone
Maxibolin	ethylestrenol
Nilevar	norethandrolone
Primobolan	methenolone acetate
Proviron	mesterolone
Teslac	testolactone
Winstrol	stanozolol

(continued)

TABLE 12.1 (Continued)

Trade Name	Generic
Transdermal	
Androderm	testosterone patch
Androgel/Axiron/ Fortesta/Testim/ Vogelxo	testosterone gel
Buccal	
Striant	testosterone

nitrogen balance to a positive balance by improving utilization of dietary protein and increasing protein synthesis.[5] Oxandrolone, an oral synthetic anabolic steroid, and testosterone are prescribed for involuntary weight loss and wasting related to HIV[6,7] and to promote healing for severe burn injuries.[8] In these settings, anabolic steroids are safe to prescribe, with low abuse potential.

When used by athletes, anabolic steroids are used in cycles of weeks or months. "Stacking" (use of more than one preparation) and "pyramiding" (dosages gradually increased and then tapered) are common patterns of administration. Dosages used are much greater than those administered for therapeutic purposes, and abusers often achieve circulating androgen levels up to 100 times higher than normal levels of an adult male.[9] Some users end up using increasing amounts of anabolic steroids to get desired effects.[10]

Epidemiology

Current epidemiological data on anabolic steroid use are lacking as they are not included in any recent national household drug use surveys. A household survey on drug use conducted in 1991 estimated that there were more than one million current or former users of anabolic steroids in the United States.[11] A 2014 systematic review reported the global lifetime prevalence rate for anabolic steroid use to be 3.3% (6.44% for males and 1.6% for females).[12] Lifetime use of anabolic steroids does appear to share common characteristics with illicit substance abuse in general.[13,14] During 2013, 2.1% of 12th graders reported lifetime use of anabolic steroids and 1.5% reported past-year use.[15] In a study of high school football players, prevalence of anabolic steroid use was 6.3%.[16]

Drug Effects

Acute Effects

Acute experimental administration of single doses of testosterone to eugonadal individuals produces no acute psychoactive effect.[17] In this regard, testosterone is unlike all other drugs of abuse. How anabolic steroids produce dependence is not well understood.[18]

Chronic Effects

Testosterone is mostly bound to plasma proteins and in this form is not biologically active. The metabolites of testosterone, such as dihydroxytestosterone, are responsible for changes in intracellular protein production and the anabolic effects. With continuous use of short-acting anabolic steroids or use of a long-acting ester, total body weight increases, partly because of salt and water retention and also because of a true increase in lean body mass. Many users also take diuretics to counter the fluid retention effects of anabolic steroids.

Most studies show that body weight increases by an average of 2–5 kilograms as a result of short-term (less than 12 weeks) use of anabolic steroids.[19,20] This increase in body weight is due to an increase in muscle mass, with increases proportional to amount of anabolic steroid used and the intensity of exercise training.[21] Changes in muscle mass have been shown to result in increased strength.[22]

Many individuals who use anabolic steroids chronically feel an increased level of aggression, but the response appears to vary widely and the mechanism by which anabolic steroids may increase aggressiveness has not been established. In one study of 50 men given supraphysiological doses of testosterone over 6 weeks, 42 experienced no psychological changes, while the remaining 8 had increases in manic and aggressive symptoms.[23] Anabolic steroid use has also been associated with aggressive and violent behavior.[24] However, in one study, the association between anabolic steroid use and violent crime disappeared when accounting for other substance use, particularly amphetamines and alcohol.[25]

Acute Toxicity and Overdose

There are no reports of anabolic steroid overdose in the literature. "Steroid rage" or "roid-rage" with violence has been reported in some individuals, typically those who have been using increasing amounts of anabolic steroids over several weeks. However, as noted earlier, evidence that anabolic steroids cause aggressive or violent behavior is lacking.

Withdrawal

Despite claims of individuals developing dependence on anabolic steroids,[9,10] there is no specific classification for anabolic steroids in DSM-5.[26] Furthermore, there is no evidence of a typical withdrawal syndrome from anabolic steroids. Anecdotally, there are a variety of symptoms linked to cessation of use of anabolic steroids. These symptoms include mood swings, fatigue, restlessness, loss of appetite, insomnia, reduced sex drive, the desire to take more steroids, and depression.[10]

Assessment

There are no data to support general screening for anabolic steroid use. Specific inquiry related to use of anabolic steroids should be pursued in athletes and bodybuilders. A survey of 80 weightlifters found that 56% had never revealed their use of anabolic steroids to a physician.[27] Presence of androgen-associated side effects outlined in the next section should also raise suspicion for anabolic steroid use.

Medical Complications

The most common and almost uniformly noted medical complications of anabolic steroid use are the direct result of excess exogenous androgens. In men, this results in the suppression of endogenous androgen production with resultant testicular atrophy, decreased sperm count, and infertility.[28] Many users of anabolic steroids also inject human chorionic gonadotropin or use oral clomiphene to prevent testicular atrophy and maintain fertility. In women, excess androgen produces deeper voice, amenorrhea or dysmenorrhea, hirsutism, and clitoral hypertrophy. Excess androgens also typically cause acne and alopecia. In adolescents, excess exogenous androgens cause premature fusion of epiphyses of long bones with stunting of growth.

Pulmonary Complications

There are no direct pulmonary complications of anabolic steroid use. Anabolic steroids do not increase aerobic capacity. In a 2014 systematic review of the effects of anabolic steroids on chronic obstructive pulmonary disease, symptom scores improved with anabolic steroids, but measures of lung function did not.[29]

Cardiovascular Complications

The literature for cardiovascular complications of anabolic steroid use has been limited to case reports and small case series. Complications reported include myocardial infarction,[30,31,32,33] atrial fibrillation,[34] dilated cardiomyopathy,[35] and stroke.[36] Episodes of sudden and premature death in elite weightlifters and bodybuilders have been attributed to anabolic steroids.[37,38,39,40] However, these athletes commonly have evidence of left ventricular hypertrophy on echocardiography, even in the absence of anabolic steroid use.[41,42]

Anabolic steroids potentially increase the risk of myocardial infarction as a result of lowering levels of HDL-cholesterol and endothelial dysfunction.[43,44,45,46] Another potential factor is polycythemia leading to increased plasma viscosity, discussed in the later section on hematological complications.

Gastrointestinal Complications

Liver abnormalities are most commonly reported in association with the use of oral anabolic steroids, as these drugs require hepatic metabolism.[47,48] There are case reports of liver complications that include elevations in liver enzymes,[49] cholestasis,[50] hepatic adenomas,[51] peliosis hepatitis (formation of blood-filled sacs in the liver),[52] and hepatic carcinoma.[53,54] However, elevations in liver enzymes generally do not occur in users who do not use oral anabolic steroids.[55] Users of anabolic steroids with preexisting liver disease (i.e., related to alcohol or hepatitis C) may be especially prone to developing liver complications.

Renal Complications

Renal complications related to anabolic steroid use appear to be rare. There are two reports of renal cell carcinoma in bodybuilders using anabolic steroids.[56,57] One case report attributes the development of focal segmental glomerulosclerosis to anabolic steroid abuse.[58]

Hematological Complications

Anabolic steroids stimulate erythropoiesis and can cause polycythemia.[59] There are reports of myocardial infarction[60] and stroke[61] associated with steroid use and polycythemia; the mechanism is thought to be increased plasma viscosity.

Neuromuscular Complications

There are case reports of muscular-skeletal injury attributed to the use of anabolic steroids, including bone fractures[62] and tendon injuries.[63,64] Additionally, rhabdomyolysis has been reported in a bodybuilder using anabolic steroids.[65]

Neuropsychiatric Complications

A 2013 study of weightlifters raised the possibility that long-term high-dose exposure to anabolic steroids may contribute to cognitive deficits.[66] The most commonly reported behavioral change caused by anabolic steroids is aggression, or "roid rage."[67,68] This has been reported in women as well as in men.[69] However, as noted earlier, increased aggression does not develop in all users, and individuals who become hypomanic and aggressive do not differ at baseline from those who do not become more aggressive.[23] There are also case reports of depression[70] and suicide[71] attributed to anabolic steroid use. Many anabolic steroid users have poor self-image, much like individuals with eating disorders.[72] However, many users of anabolic steroids abuse other drugs, including alcohol, cocaine, amphetamines, marijuana, and opioids.[73] As noted earlier, studies of anabolic steroids as a trigger for violent crime are inconsistent; one study showed an increased risk independent of use of other illicit drugs,[24] and others found no increased risk.[25,74]

Treatment

There are no reports in the literature related to drug treatment specific to anabolic steroid abuse. In a survey of 175 treatment centers, only 19% of those responding had ever treated a client using anabolic steroids and almost all of these individuals also abused other drugs.[75] Patients should be clinically followed for the possible development of withdrawal symptoms such as fatigue, restlessness, or depression. Counseling needs to focus on addressing the reasons anabolic steroids were used. Most common reasons for anabolic steroid use are physical appearance, self-esteem, and athletic performance.[76] For individuals abusing other substances in addition to anabolic steroids, traditional substance abuse treatment, including 12 step self-help groups, may be helpful.

Other Drugs

Most media attention on athletes has focused on anabolic steroids, but performance-enhancing drugs include many other drugs used not only to improve strength but also to improve endurance and accuracy. The World Anti-Doping Code is the international standard for establishing the evolving list of drugs banned in international sports competitions, including the Olympics.[77] A summary of the code is found in Box 12.1. In addition to the drugs listed,

---

BOX 12.1 World Anti-Doping Code Prohibited Drug List

Prohibited at All Times

Anabolic androgenic steroids (including over the counter DHEA)
Erythropoietin
Growth hormone
Gonadotropins and their releasing factors
Corticotropins and their releasing factors
Beta-2 agonists (except if special permission to use by inhalation for asthma)
Antiestrogens (clomiphene, tamoxifen, raloxifene)
Diuretics
Blood products and blood substitutes
Drugs that enhance oxygen uptake (perfluorochemicals, efaproxiral)
Probenecid

Prohibited in Competition

Stimulants (amphetamines, modafinil, ephedrine)
Opioids (except codeine and hydrocodone)
Cannabinoids
Glucocorticoids (except topical)

beta-blockers are prohibited in some sports in which accuracy is important, including archery, curling, gymnastics, shooting, and diving.

The list of drugs has evolved over the last few years as athletes have made further attempts to gain the additional slight advantage to go from being an elite athlete to being the best. In sports such as sprinting, where the difference between winning and losing may be one-hundredth of a second, athletes have been particularly prone to using performance-enhancing drugs. In the 1980s and 1990s, many long-distance runners and cyclists started using blood products and erythropoietin to improve endurance. As more drugs were added to the banned list, athletes turned to ways to evade getting caught. Antiestrogens, gonadotropins, and clomiphene were used by male athletes to avoid the gynecomastia and infertility problems associated with anabolic steroids. Diuretics and probenecid were used to rapidly clear drugs prior to testing. Nevertheless, many drugs, including growth factors, are still difficult to detect, and as long as some athletes are so driven to do whatever it takes to win, use of performance-enhancing drugs will continue.

Although opioids are not performance-enhancing drugs, athletes are commonly prescribed opioids or take them to treat the pain of injuries. Football players have high rates of opioid use and appear to be at risk for developing problems later on.[78] Among high school athletes, participation in football and wrestling is associated with nonmedical use of prescription opioids.[79] Prescription medication misuse is covered further in Chapter 13.

Notes

1. Baker JS, Thomas NE, Davies B, Graham MR. Anabolic androgenic steroid (AAS) abuse: not only an elite performance issue? Open Sports Med J 2008;2:38–9.

2. Brennan BP, Kanayama G, Pope HG. Performance-enhancing drugs on the Web: a growing public-health issue. Am J Addict 2013;22:158–61.

3. Bahrke MS, Yesalis CE. Abuse of anabolic androgenic steroids and related substances in sport and exercise. Curr Opin Pharmacol 2004;4:614–20.

4. Bhasin S, Storer TW, Berman N, et al. The effects of supraphysiologic doses of testosterone on muscle size and strength in normal men. N Engl J Med 1996;335:1–7.

5. Sheffield-Moore M. Androgens and the control of skeletal muscle protein synthesis. Ann Med 2000;32:181–6.

6. Strawford A, Barbieri T, Van Loan M, et al. Resistance exercise and supraphysiologic androgen therapy in eugonadal men with HIV-related weight loss: a randomized controlled trial. JAMA 1999;281:1282–90.

7. Sardar P, Jha A, Roy D, et al. Therapeutic effects of nandrolone and testosterone in adult male HIV patients with AIDS wasting syndrome (AWS): a randomized, double-blind, placebo-controlled trial. HIV Clin Trials 2010;11:220–9.

8. Woerdeman J, de Ronde, W. Therapeutic effects of anabolic androgenic steroids on chronic diseases associated with muscle wasting. Expert Opin Investig Drugs 2011;20:87–97.

9. Brower KJ, Eliopulous GA, Blow FC, et al. Evidence for physical and psychological dependence on anabolic androgenic steroids in eight weight lifters. Am J Psychiatry 1990;147:510–2.

10. Kashkin KB, Kleber HD. Hooked on hormones: an anabolic steroid addiction hypothesis. JAMA 1989;262:3166–70.

11. Yesalis CE, Kennedy NJ, Kopstein AN, Bahrke MS. Anabolic-androgenic steroid use in the United States. JAMA 1993;270:1217–21.

12. Sagoe D, Molde H, Andreassen CS, et al. The global epidemiology of anabolic-androgenic steroid use: a meta-analysis and meta-regression analysis. Ann Epidemiol 2014;24:383–98.

13. Buckman JF, Yusko DA, White HR, Pandina RJ. Risk profile of male college athletes who use performance-enhancing substances. J Stud Alcohol Drugs 2009;70:919–23.

14. Hakansson A, Mickelsson K, Wallin C, Berglund M. Anabolic androgenic steroids in the general population: user characteristics and associations with substance use. Eur Addict Res 2012;18:83–90.

15. Johnston LD, O'Malley PM, Bachman JG, Schulenberg JE. Monitoring the Future National Results on Drug Use: 2012 Overview,

Key Findings on Adolescent Drug Use. Ann Arbor: Institute for Social Research, University of Michigan.

16. Stilger VG, Yesalis CE. Anabolic-androgenic steroid use among high school football players. J Commun Health 1999;24:131–45.

17. **Fingerhood MI, Sullivan JT, Testa MP, Jasinski DR. Abuse liability of testosterone. J Psychopharmacol 1997;11:65–9.** *In this study, 10 males with a history of opioid abuse, but no history of anabolic steroid abuse, received intramuscular testosterone (50, 100, and 200 mg), morphine (10 mg), or placebo for 5 consecutive days. Testosterone, unlike morphine, produced no pharmacological effects associated with other drugs of abuse.*

18. Wood RI. Reinforcing aspects of androgens. Physiol Behav 2004;83:279–89.

19. Hervey GR, Hutchinson I, Knibbs AV, et al. 'Anabolic' effects of methandienone in men undergoing athletic training. Lancet 1976;308:699–702.

20. Hervey GR, Knibbs AV, Burkinshaw L, et al. Effects of methandienone on the performance and body composition of men undergoing athletic training. Clin Sci 1981;60:457–61.

21. Bhasin S. The dose-dependent effects of testosterone on sexual function and on muscle mass and function. Mayo Clin Proc 2000;75:S70–5.

22. Giorgi A, Weatherby RP, Murphy PW. Muscular strength, body composition and health responses to the use of testosterone enanthate: a double blind study. J Sci Med Sport 1999;2:341–55.

23. **Pope HG, Kouri EM, Hudson JI. Effects of supraphysiologic doses of testosterone on mood and aggression in normal men: a randomized controlled trial. Arch Gen Psychiatry 2000;57:133–40.** *In this study, 56 men were randomized to testosterone cypionate in doses up to 600 mg/week or placebo for 6 weeks, followed by 6 weeks of no treatment, followed by 6 weeks of crossover treatment. Among 50 subjects who completed the study, 6 became mildly hypomanic and 2 became markedly hypomanic, with minimal effects in the other 42. The 8 "responders" and 42 "non-responders" did not differ on baseline demographic, psychological, or physiological measures.*

24. Beaver KM, Vaughn MG, Delisi M, Wright JP. Anabolic–androgenic steroid use and involvement in violent behavior in a nationally representative sample of young adult males in the United States. Am J Public Health 2008;98:2185–7.

25. Lundholm L, Frisell T, Lichtenstein P, Långström N. Anabolic androgenic steroids and violent offending: confounding by polysubstance abuse among 10,365 general population men. Addiction 2014;110:100–8.

26. American Psychiatric Association. *Diagnostic and Statistical Manual of Mental Disorders*, Fifth Edition (DSM-5). Arlington, VA: American Psychiatric Association; 2013.

27. Pope HG, Kanayama G, Ionescu-Pioggia, Hudson JI. Anabolic steroid users' attitudes towards physicians. Addiction 2004;99:1189–94.

28. Torres-Calleja J, Gonzalez-Unzaga M, DeCelis-Carrillo R, et al. Effect of androgenic anabolic steroids on sperm quality and serum hormone levels in adult male bodybuilders. Life Sci 2001;68:1769–74.

29. Pan L, Wang M, Xie X, et al. Effects of anabolic steroids on chronic obstructive pulmonary disease: a meta-analysis of randomised controlled trials. PLOS One 2014;9:e84855.

30. Fisher M, Appleby M, Rittoo D, Cotter L. Myocardial infarction with extensive intracoronary thrombus induced by anabolic steroids. Br J Clin Pract 1996;50:180–1.

31. Sullivan ML, Martinez CM, Gennis P, et al. The cardiac toxicity of anabolic steroids. Prog Cardiovasc Dis 1998;41:1–15.

32. Ferenchick GS, Adelman S. Myocardial infarction associated anabolic steroids use in a previously healthy 37-year-old weight lifter. Am Heart J 1992;124:507–8.

33. Palatini P, Giada F, Garavelli G, et al. Cardiovascular effects of anabolic steroids in weight-trained subjects. J Clin Pharmacol 1996;36:132–40.

34. Sullivan ML, Martinez CM, Gallagher EJ. Atrial fibrillation and anabolic steroids. J Emerg Med 1999;17:851–7.

35. Luijkx T, Velthuis BK, Backx FJ, et al. Anabolic androgenic steroid use is associated with ventricular dysfunction on cardiac MRI in strength trained athletes. Int J Cardiol 2013;167:664–8.

36. Shimada Y, Yoritaka A, Tanaka Y, et al. Cerebral infarction in a young man using high-dose anabolic steroids. J Stroke Cerebrovasc Dis 2012;21:906.e9–e11.

37. Parssinen M, Kujala U, Vartiainen E, et al. Increased premature mortality of competitive power lifters suspected to have used anabolic agents. Int J Sports Med 2000;21:225–7.

38. Far HR, Agren G, Thiblin I. Cardiac hypertrophy in deceased users of anabolic androgenic steroids: an investigation of autopsy findings. Cardiol Pathol 2012;21:312–6.

39. Luke JL, Farb A, Virmani R, et al. Sudden cardiac death during exercise in a weight lifter using anabolic androgenic steroids: pathological and toxicological findings. J Forensic Sci 1990;35:1441–7.

40. Montisci M, El Mazloum R, Cecchetto G, et al. Anabolic androgenic steroids abuse and cardiac death in athletes: morphological and toxicological findings in four fatal cases. Forensic Science Int 2012;217:e13–8.

41. Wright JN, Salem D. Sudden cardiac death and the 'athlete's heart'. Arch Intern Med 1995;155:1473–80.

42. Dickerman RD, Schaller F, McConathy WJ. Left ventricular wall thickening does occur in elite power athletes with or without anabolic steroid use. Cardiology 1998;90:145–8.

43. **Urhausen A, Torstein A, Wilfried K. Reversibility of the effects on blood cells, lipids, liver function and hormones in former anabolic-androgenic steroid abusers. J Steroid Biochem and Mol Biol 2003;84:369–75.** *This cohort study of 32 bodybuilders compared 17 current users of anabolic steroids with 15 former users (had not used anabolic steroids for at least 1 year). Mean HDL levels were 43 mg/dL in ex-users and 17 mg/dL in current users, p < 0.0001. Mean ALT and AST were 65 U/L and 38 U/L, respectively, in users and 24 U/L and 18 U/L, respectively, in ex-users, p < 0.0001.*

44. Glazer G. Atherogenic effects of anabolic steroids on serum lipid levels. Arch Intern Med 1991;151:1925–33.

45. Achar S, Rostamian A, Narayan SM. Cardiac and metabolic effects of anabolic-androgenic steroid abuse on lipids, blood pressure, left ventricular dimensions, and rhythm. Am J Cardiol 2010;106:893–901.

46. Severo CB, Ribeiro JP, Umpierre D, et al. Increased atherothrombotic markers and endothelial dysfunction in steroid users. Eur J Prev Cardiol 2013;20:195–201.

47. Soe KL, Soe M, Gluud C. Liver pathology associated with the use of anabolic-androgenic steroids. Liver 1992;12:73–9.

48. Ishak KG, Zimmerman HJ. Hepatotoxic effects of the anabolic androgenic steroids. Semin Liver Dis 1987;7:230–6.

49. Freed DL, Banks AJ, Longson D, et al. Anabolic steroids in athletics: crossover double-blind trial on weightlifters. BMJ 1975;2:471–3.

50. Elsharkawy AM, McPherson S, Masson S, et al. Cholestasis secondary to anabolic steroid use in young men. BMJ 2012;344:e468.

51. Martin NM, Abu Dayyeh BK, Chung RT. Anabolic steroid abuse causing recurrent hepatic adenomas and hemorrhage. World J Gastroenterol 2008;14:4573–5.

52. Cabasso A. Peliosis hepatis in a young adult bodybuilder. Med Sci Sports Exerc 1994;26:2–4.

53. Kosaka A, Takahashi H, Yajima Y, et al. Hepatocellular carcinoma associated with anabolic steroid therapy: report of a case and review of the Japanese literature. J Gastroenterol 1996;31:450–4.

54. Gorayski P, Thompson CH, Subhash HS, Thomas AC. Hepatocellular carcinoma associated with recreational anabolic steroid use. Br J Sports Med 2008:42:74–5.

55. Kuipers H, Wijnen JAG, Hartgens F, et al. Influence of anabolic steroids on body composition, blood pressure, lipid profile and liver function in bodybuilders. Int J Sports Med 1991;12:413–8.

56. Bryden AAG, Rothwell PJN, O'Reilly PH. Anabolic steroid abuse and renal cell carcinoma. Lancet 1995;346:1306–7.

57. Martorana G, Concetti S, Manferrari F, et al. Anabolic steroid abuse and renal cell carcinoma. Clin Urol 1999;162:2089.

58. Harrington P, Ali G, Chan A. The development of focal segmental glomerulosclerosis secondary to anabolic steroid abuse. BMJ Case Rep 2011;pii:bcr0720114531.

59. Viallard JF, Marit G, Mercie P, et al. Polycythaemia as a complication of transdermal testosterone therapy. Br J Haematol. 2000;110:237–8.

60. Stergiopoulos K, Brennan JJ, Mathews R, et al. Anabolic steroids, acute myocardial infarction and polycythemia: a case report and review of the literature. Vasc Health Risk Manag 2008;4:1475–80.

61. Harston GW, Batt F, Fan L, et al. Lacunar infarction associated with anabolic steroids and polycythemia: a case report. Case Rep Neurol 2014;6:34–7.

62. Tannenbaum SD, Rosler H. Proximal humeral fracture in weight lifter using anabolic steroids. Arch Phys Med Rehabil 1989;70:A89.

63. Seynnes OR, Kamandulis S, Kairaitis R, et al. Effect of androgenic-anabolic steroids and heavy strength training on patellar tendon morphological and mechanical properties. J Appl Physiol 2013;115:84–9.

64. Liow R, Tavares S. Bilateral rupture of the quadriceps tendon associated with anabolic steroids. Br J Sports Med 1995;29:77–9.

65. Bolgiano EB. Acute rhabdomyolysis due to body building exercise: report of a case. J Sports Med Phys Fitness 1994;34:76–8.

66. Kanayam G, Kean J, Hudson JI, Pope HG. Cognitive deficits in long-term anabolic-androgenic steroid users. Drug Alcohol Depend 2013;130:208–14.

67. Su TP, Pagliaro M, Schmidt PJ, et al. Neuropsychiatric effects of anabolic steroids in male normal volunteers. JAMA 1993;269:2760–4.

68. Thiblin I, Parlklo T. Anabolic androgenic steroids and violence. Acta Psychiatr Scand Suppl 2002;412:125–8.

69. Gruber AJ, Pope HG. Psychiatric and medical effects of anabolic-androgenic steroid use in women. Psychother Psychosom 2000;69:19–26.

70. Pope HG, Katz DL. Psychiatric and medical effects of anabolic-androgenic steroid use. A controlled study of 160 athletes. Arch Gen Psychiatry 1994;51:375–82.

71. Thiblin I, Runeson B, Rajs J. Anabolic androgenic steroids and suicide. Ann Clin Psychiatry 1999;11:223–31.

72. Bjork T, Skarberg K, Engstrom I. Eating disorders and anabolic androgenic steroids in males—similarities and differences in self-image and psychiatric symptoms. Subst Abuse Treat Prev Policy 2013;8:30.

73. Fudala PJ, Weinreb RM, Calarco JS, et al. An evaluation of anabolic-androgenic steroid users over a period of 1 year: seven case studies. Ann Clin Psychiatry 2003;15:121–30.

74. Lundholm L, Kall K, Wallin S, Thiblin I. Use of Anabolic androgenic steroids in substance abusers arrested for crime. Drug Alcohol Depend 2010;111:222–6.

75. Clancy GP, Yates WR. Anabolic steroid use among substance abusers in treatment. J Clin Psychiatry 1992;53:97–100.

76. Petersson A, Bengtsson J, Voltaire-Carlsson A, Thiblin I. Substance abusers' motives for using anabolic androgenic steroids. Drug Alcohol Depend 2010;111:170–2.

77. World Anti-Doping Agency. The World Anti-Doping Code—The 2015 Prohibited List International Standard. 2014; available at www.wada-ama.org. Accessed December 29, 2014.

78. Cottler LB, Ben Abdallah A, Cummings SM, et al. Injury, pain, and prescription opioid use among former National Football League (NFL) players. Drug Alcohol Depend 2011;116:188–94.

79. Veliz PT, Boyd C, McCabe SE. Playing through pain: sports participation and nonmedical use of opioid medications among adolescents. Am J Public Health 2013;103:e28–30.

13

Prescription and Over-the Counter Drug Misuse

Background

Prescription drug misuse is a growing problem that includes the use of prescription medications for purposes other than those intended, as well as drug diversion. A related term, *nonmedical use of a prescription drug*, is defined as "using a psychotherapeutic drug that was not prescribed for you or that you took only for the experience or feeling it caused."[1]

In the United States, during the decade of the 1990s, the nonmedical use of prescription drugs increased dramatically and has had a devastating effect on communities. Of the prescription drug classes, opioids are consistently the class with the greatest nonmedical use. How to deal with the increasing problem of prescription opioid misuse without interfering with legitimate use is a difficult problem without a clear solution.

Epidemiology

According to the 2013 National Survey on Drug Use and Health (NSDUH),[1] an estimated 2.5% of all Americans aged 12 and older used a prescription psychotherapeutic drug nonmedically in the past month; this rate has been fairly stable from 2002 through

2012. The NSDUH divides prescription psychotherapeutic drugs into four classes—past-month use was highest for pain relievers (opioids, including tramadol—1.9%), followed by tranquilizers (most benzodiazepines and muscle relaxers—0.8%), stimulants (0.5%), and sedatives (barbiturates, temazepam, halcion, and chloral hydrate—0.1%).

When past-year nonmedical users of pain relievers (opioids) were asked how they obtained the drug, most (53%) said they obtained it for free from a friend or relative, 21% obtained it directly from a doctor, and 15% reported that they bought or took it from a friend or relative. For those who obtained it for free from a friend or relative, when asked where their source obtained the drug, most (84%) obtained it from a single physician. A relatively small number of practitioners appear to be the source of most prescribed controlled substances; for example, in an analysis of the Oregon prescription drug-monitoring program, 60% of prescriptions were written by a cohort of 2,000 prescribers (4% of the total); a second cohort of 2,000 accounted for another 19% of the prescriptions.[2]

Despite the relatively stable number of people who are using prescription drugs nonmedically since 2002, the harms associated with these medications continue to grow. According to the Drug Abuse Warning Network (DAWN), an estimated 1.4 million emergency department (ED) visits in 2011 were due to misuse or abuse of prescription drugs; this is more than double the number in 2004 and higher than the rates for use of illicit drugs.[3]

Misused Prescription Drugs

Opioids and benzodiazepines are the most commonly misused controlled drugs, followed by stimulants.

Opioids

According to the NSDUH, in 2012, an estimated 37 million Americans (14% of those aged 12 or older) had ever used a "pain reliever" for nonmedical use; 4.8% reported using in the past year and 1.9% in the past month. The pain reliever category includes scheduled opioids (e.g., oxycodone, codeine, hydrocodone). It also includes tramadol (Ultram), which is an opioid-like drug; this was previously a non-scheduled drug but was reclassified as a schedule IV drug in 2014. An estimated 9.9% of the population aged 12 and older reported lifetime nonmedical use of hydrocodone products, 7.7% used propoxyphene or codeine products, 6.2% used oxycodone products, and 1.2% tramadol products. In addition, in separate a 2010 survey, an estimated 12% of the adult population in the United States reported receiving a prescription for an opioid in the past year.[4]

As the misuse of prescription opioids has garnered increasing attention, the trend of increased prescribing and misuse of prescription opioids from the early 1990s to 2010 appears to have stopped, and the rates have plateaued or decreased between 2011 and 2013.[5] However, with the decline in prescription opioid misuse, there has been an increase in heroin use as prescription opioid users are transitioning to heroin.[6]

Sedatives

The NSDUH divides this category into two groups. "Tranquilizers" includes most benzodiazepines, the muscle relaxants cyclobenzaprine and carisoprodol, the antihistamine hydroxyzine, along with buspirone and meprobamate. "Sedatives" includes barbiturates; the benzodiazepines temazepam, flurazepam, and triazolam; as well as methaqualone, chloral hydrate, and ethchlorvynol. The 2013 NSDUH estimated that 23.5 million Americans have used a tranquilizer nonmedically in their lifetime (9.0% of those aged 12 and older); 5.3 million (2.0%) have used them in the past year, and 1.7 million (0.6%) were current (past month) nonmedical users. For sedatives, 7.5 million (2.9%) have used them in their lifetime, 639,000 (0.2%) in the past year, and 251,000 (0.1%) in the past month. It should be noted that the NSDUH does not include the newer non-benzodiazepine hypnotics (zolpidem, eszopiclone, and zaleplon) in these categories.

While the rates of nonmedical use of sedatives is lower than that for opioids, DAWN reported that in 2011, a higher number of ED visits were related to misuse or abuse of antianxiety and insomnia medications (500,000) than with opioids (420,000); another 53,000 visits were due to muscle relaxants.[3] Alprazolam was the most common antianxiety and insomnia drug leading to an ED visit, followed by clonazepam, lorazepam, and zolpidem.

Specific issues related to use and misuse of sedatives are discussed further in Chapter 5.

Stimulants

In 2013, over 21 million Americans reported lifetime nonmedical use of other stimulants, including methamphetamine (8.3% of those aged 12 or older); 3.5 million had used them in the past year (1.3%), and 1.4 million in the past month (0.5%). The harms associated with these drugs appear to be lower than those of opioids and sedatives. DAWN reported 45,000 ED visits due to abuse or misuse of these drugs in 2011; this is approximately one-tenth the number associated with opioids (420,000) or sedatives (500,000).

Stimulants are further discussed in Chapter 8.

Other Prescription Drugs

Noncontrolled prescription drugs with reports of misuse include clonidine, muscle relaxants, tricyclic antidepressants, bupropion, antiemetics, gabapentinoids, and the atypical antipsychotics.

Clonidine is mostly used nonmedically by individuals with opioid dependence—some take it to alleviate withdrawal symptoms (see Chapter 6), but much of the use occurs in individuals continuing to abuse opioids[7] and among individuals receiving methadone maintenance treatment.[8] Abuse has been reported with the clonidine patch as well, with case reports of hypotension from chewing the patch.[9]

Muscle relaxants are used to take advantage of their common side effect of sedation, and all have a potential for misuse. Most reports of muscle relaxant abuse are related to carisoprodol (Soma), but others, including cyclobenzaprine (Flexeril), methocarbamol (Robaxin), and metaxalone (Skelaxin), are used nonmedically as well.

Antiemetics (promethazine and prochlorperazine) are often taken by opioid-dependent individuals to counter the nausea side effects and to potentiate the euphoric effects of opioids.[10] They should be used with caution among individuals with a history of opioid dependence.

Individuals with substance use disorders commonly have sleep problems and depression and may receive prescriptions for tricyclic antidepressants. Most reports of misuse and intoxication from these drugs have been related to amitriptyline (Elavil).[11] Patients on methadone maintenance may be particularly susceptible.[12,13]

The antidepressant bupropion has some stimulant-like effects.[14] There are reports of use of this drug by the intranasal route,[15] and this may be complicated by seizures.[16] There have also been reports of intravenous use of bupropion.[17]

The gabapentinoids gabapentin and pregabalin appear to have some potential for misuse, particularly pregabalin, which has quicker absorption and higher potency.[18]

The atypical antipsychotics, particularly quetiapine (Seroquel), are also misused.[19] In a survey of addiction treatment inpatients in New York City, 17% reported misuse of atypical antipsychotics in the past; quetiapine was most commonly reported, followed by risperidone (Risperdal) and aripiprazole (Abilify).[20] There is also a report of intranasal use of quetiapine among prisoners in Los Angeles[21] and one case report of quetiapine dependence and withdrawal.[22]

Misused Over-the-Counter Drugs

Most of the recent attention related to misuse of over-the-counter drugs has focused on the use of pseudoephedrine to manufacture methamphetamine. Many pharmacies have restricted sales of pseudoephedrine and taken bottles off open shelves. Dimethylamylamine is another stimulant that is available in some over-the-counter dietary supplements and has been reported to have abuse potential.[23]

The over-the-counter drugs most commonly misused are dextromethorphan-containing cough syrups or tablets and the antihistamines diphenhydramine (Benadryl) and dimenhydrinate (Dramamine).

Dextramethorphan (DXM or DM) is an antitussive found in a number of cold medicines. Dextromethorphan abuse appears to be most common among male adolescents.[24] After ingesting large amounts (8 ounces or more) of dextromethorphan containing cough syrup, individuals may experience symptoms similar to those of the dissociative anesthetics ketamine and phencyclidine, including euphoria, disorientation, and hallucinations.[25] Withdrawal symptoms may develop in some individuals and consist of insomnia and dysphoria. Symptoms of overdose include altered mental status, ataxia, and nystagmus; deaths from overdose have been reported.[26] Dissociative anesthetics are covered further in Chapter 9.

Dimenhydrinate, therapeutically used for motion sickness, is composed of diphenhydramine, plus the methylxanthine, 8-chlorotheophylline. Dimenhydrinate can cause euphoria, visual and tactile hallucinations, and sedation.[27,28] The antimuscarinic properties of diphenhydramine become more prominent at high doses, and these properties cause hallucinations and euphoria and are likely responsible for misuse potential.[29] There are also some reports of misuse of diphenhydramine (Benadryl), an antihistamine that is available over the counter.[30]

Assessment

Identification of individuals with a prescription drug use disorder is complicated by the fact that the practitioners who are evaluating these patients are often themselves the source of the problem medication. Patients who are obtaining the medication through "legitimate" means may perceive their use as therapeutic even when there is a problem. Moreover, even if they are aware of a problem, they may be less likely to be open about it for fear of being cut off from the drug they are dependent on. Therefore, clinicians must be vigilant and rely on other signs and indications to determine if there is a problem. It is often impossible to prove that a patient has a prescription drug use disorder, and clinicians must weigh potential benefits and risks and rely on their clinical judgment.

Risk Factors and Markers of Misuse

The most consistent risk factor for misuse of prescription drugs is a personal history of substance use disorders,[31] including tobacco use.[32] Additional risk factors that have been identified include a family history of substance use disorders,[31] psychiatric illness,[33] and history of incarceration.[34]

A study of patients in an urban primary care clinic who were taking analgesics for chronic pain[35] found that

- 18% met criteria for lifetime prescription drug use disorder.
- 25% met criteria for another lifetime substance use disorder diagnosis.
- Of those with a prescription drug use disorder, 90% also had another substance use disorder.

In this study, other risk factors associated with a prescription drug use disorder included history of incarceration, greater limitations from pain, smoking, family history of substance use disorder, white race, male gender, and history of post-traumatic stress disorder. The investigators also found that all patients with a prescription drug use disorder had at least two risk factors, and of those with six or more risk factors, over 90% had a prescription drug use disorder.[36]

An evaluation of the NSDUH 2002–2004 surveys found that nonmedical use of prescription opioids in the previous year was associated with panic, depressive, and social phobic/agoraphobic symptoms. Of those with nonmedical use, 13% met criteria for a substance use disorder.[34] Another study of veterans referred for behavioral health evaluation by their primary care physicians found that younger age, depressive symptoms, smoking, illicit drug use, and chronic pain were associated with nonmedical use of prescription drugs.[36]

Aberrant Drug-Related Behaviors

There are a number of behaviors that may be suggestive of misuse of prescription drugs; these are referred to as "aberrant drug-related behaviors" (ADRBs) but may also be referred to as "aberrant drug-taking behaviors" or "aberrant medication-taking behaviors." ADRBs are a spectrum of patient behaviors that may reflect misuse.[37] A pattern of ADRBs, or severe or persistent ADRB, should trigger further evaluation for misuse or a substance use disorder.

Some examples of ADRBs include the following:

- Requests for early refills or running out of medication early
- Reporting lost or stolen medication
- Obtaining prescription medications from multiple clinicians
- Taking more medication than prescribed or recommended
- Obtaining medications from others
- Using medication for the purpose of affecting one's mood
- Illicit drug use or nonmedical use of other prescription drugs
- Illegal activities, such as forging prescriptions or diversion of medication

These behaviors in and of themselves do not necessarily indicate misuse or a substance use disorder, and not all of these behaviors are equally concerning. For example, forging a prescription is probably more indicative of a problem than asking for an early refill. When evaluating patients who exhibit these behaviors, clinicians must rely on their clinical judgment. Strategies for addressing these behaviors are discussed at the end of this chapter.

Screening Instruments

There are a number of instruments that have been developed for the identification of prescription drug misuse among persons being prescribed opioids for chronic pain. They generally use a combination of risk factors and ADRBs discussed earlier. These screening instruments include the following:

- The Prescription Drug Use Questionnaire (PDUQ).[38] This is a 42-item questionnaire designed to screen for substance use disorders among patients prescribed opioids for chronic pain. A 31-item version that can be completed by patients (PDUQp) has also been developed.[39]
- The Screener and Opioid Assessment for Patients with Pain (SOAPP).[40] This is a 14-item self-report screening tool designed to assess the risk of aberrant drug-related behaviors among patients with chronic pain who are prescribed opioids. A 24-item revised version (SOAPP-R)[41,42] has also been developed.
- The Current Opioid Misuse Measure (COMM).[43] This 17-item questionnaire is designed to screen for opioid medication misuse among patients prescribed opioids for chronic pain.
- The Addiction Behaviors Checklist (ABC) is a 20-item checklist designed to identify individuals with addiction among those who are receiving opioids for chronic pain.[44]
- The Prescription Opioid Misuse Index (POMI) is an 8-item questionnaire designed to identify individuals prescribed opioids who are misusing the medication.[45]

A 2009 systematic review of risk stratification instruments concluded that the evidence for prediction and identification was limited, and that there is a need for high-quality, prospective studies evaluating these instruments.[46]

Medical Complications

The most serious complication of prescription drug misuse is overdose. While prescription opioids are generally thought to be relatively safe when used as directed, there is some evidence of other potential harms. In an analysis of Medicare claims data, in comparison with older adults who were prescribed nonsteroidal anti-inflammatory drugs (NSAIDs), those prescribed opioids had significantly higher rates of cardiovascular events, fractures, hospitalizations, and death; their risk for gastrointestinal bleeding was not any lower.[47]

Overdose

Prescription drug overdose, particularly opioid overdose, is a growing problem.[48] As opioid prescribing has increased, morbidity and mortality from opioid overdose has increased substantially in the United States.[49] In 2011, an estimated 488,000 ED visits in the United States involved the nonmedical use of opioid analgesics.[3]

The problem of increased overdose morbidity and mortality is complex and multifactorial. A study of unintentional prescription medication overdose deaths in West Virginia (a state that had a 550% increase in unintentional poisoning deaths from 1999 to 2004) found that 63% of unintentional prescription medication overdose deaths in 2006 were associated with diversion of prescription medications and that 21% were associated with doctor shopping (defined as having five more clinicians prescribing controlled substances in the prior year). The majority of cases involved opioids (93%), but other potentially contributing substances were present in 79%. Additionally, among those who died, 78% had a history of substance abuse.[50]

The dose of opioids prescribed is another important factor in the risk of overdose.[51] A study of over 9,000 health maintenance organization patients found that, in comparison to patients receiving 1–20 mg/day of morphine equivalents, those receiving 50–99 mg of morphine equivalents per day had a 3.7-fold increase in overdose risk, and those receiving 100 mg or more morphine equivalents per day had a 8.9-fold increase in overdose risk. Patients who had recently received sedative-hypnotic medications were also at increased risk.[52] The type of opioid also plays a role in the risk of overdose; long-acting opioids,[53] particularly methadone[54] prescribed for chronic pain, are associated with a higher risk of fatal overdose than that of other opioids.

Strategies to Address Prescription Drug Misuse

In this section, we will discuss some strategies to address prescription drug misuse. The discussion will focus on opioids, because this class is responsible for most of the problem, but the principles also apply to prescription sedatives and stimulants. When thinking of strategies to address prescription drug misuse, there are four overlapping populations to consider:

1. Those who are not taking controlled substances (either prescribed or nonmedically)
2. Those who are taking these medications therapeutically
3. Those who have a prescription drug use disorder
4. Those who are diverting prescription drugs

Primary Prevention

For those who are not taking controlled substances, our goal should be to avoid them developing a prescription drug use disorder (PDUD). The simplest way to do this is to avoid exposure to these drugs. Increasingly, individuals with opioid use disorders are introduced to opioids through prescriptions rather than recreational use. Therefore, medications with abuse liability should not be prescribed unless they are indicated, and patients should be counseled on their risks. While studies suggest that a minority of individuals who are exposed to these drugs will develop a PDUD, initiation of these drugs will lead to some becoming persistent users[55,56] and others to developing a PDUD.[57] Why some individuals who are exposed become addicted but most others do not is not completely understood, but is probably at least partly mediated by differences in the subjective effects of opioids.[58]

While opioids may be indicated for treatment of acute severe pain, they are not indicated for treatment of mild or moderate pain. Studies have shown that 400 mg of ibuprofen is a more effective analgesic than 5 mg of oxycodone after minor surgery or dental procedures.[59] NSAIDs have also been shown to be more effective than opioids for the treatment of acute renal colic.[60] When treating individuals with chronic pain, it is important to keep in mind that the efficacy of opioids for chronic pain has not been established[61,62] and is modest at best.[63] In fact, there is evidence that taking opioids chronically decreases pain tolerance[64] and that these changes may persist long after an individual is off of opioids.[65]

Secondary Prevention

When prescribing controlled substances, particularly opioids for chronic pain, we must balance benefit and risk. Available data suggest that the rates of opioid use disorders among chronic pain patients on long-term opioid therapy ranges from 3% to 20%, depending on the patient population and how the problem is defined.[66] There are a number of strategies to reduce opioid misuse and the harms associated with it, including development and dissemination of treatment guidelines, limiting the dosage of medication, pharmaceutical strategies, and monitoring strategies.

Guidelines

Several organizations have developed guidelines for the use of prescription analgesics for the treatment of pain. The Federation of State Medical Boards of the United States released its "Model Policy for the Use of Controlled Substances for the Treatment of Pain" in 2004 to serve as a guide for state medical boards and other health regulatory agencies and to encourage them to adopt policies that promote the appropriate treatment of pain.[67]

The American Pain Society and the American Academy of Pain Medicine commissioned a systematic review on the use of chronic opioid therapy for chronic noncancer pain and an expert panel to review the evidence and develop clinical guidelines, which were published in 2009.[68] The authors acknowledge that the evidence for most of these recommendations is weak, and note that more prospective studies are needed to address the appropriate initiation and monitoring of chronic opioid therapy for chronic noncancer pain. A full review of their recommendations is beyond the scope of this chapter; a summary of certain key recommendations is as follows:

- Conduct a history and physical, including risk factors for prescription drug misuse.
- Perform appropriate diagnostic testing.
- Consider and weigh potential benefits and risks, and document this prior to initiating chronic opioid therapy and on an ongoing basis.
- Obtain informed consent and consider a written treatment agreement or treatment plan.
- Therapy should be individualized.
- Methadone must be used with extreme caution, given its complicated pharmacokinetic and pharmacodynamic properties.
- Perform ongoing periodic assessment. Consider urine drug testing or other information to confirm adherence to the treatment plan. Strongly consider consultation with an addiction or mental health expert for those with a history of substance use disorders, mental illness, or serious ADRBs.
- Taper or discontinue opioids in patients who demonstrate repeated ADRBs or diversion, experience no progress toward therapeutic goals, or have intolerable side effects.

Limiting Dosage

Another strategy to decrease the harm associated with opioids is to limit the dose that is prescribed. As noted earlier, studies have found an association between the dosage and overdose risk. This has led some to recommend limiting the dose prescribed; for example, Washington state guidelines disseminated in 2007 recommend that the "total daily dose of opioids should not be increased above 120 mg oral MED [morphine equivalent daily] without either the patient demonstrating improvement in function and pain or first obtaining a consultation from a practitioner qualified in chronic pain management."[69] In analyses of individuals covered by the Washington State Worker's Compensation Fund, these guidelines appear to have had an effect on prescribing practices.[70] However, the guidelines have not led to a significant reduction in the rate of opioid overdoses; most overdoses occurred among individuals who were prescribed doses lower than 120 mg MED or were not being prescribed opioids.[71]

Pharmaceutical Strategies

A number of strategies have been developed by the pharmaceutical industry to reduce the risk of misuse of opioid medications. One strategy is to provide a gradual onset and sustained delivery of medication into the bloodstream or central nervous system. Drug formulations with gradual onset are generally associated with reduced abuse liability, when compared with rapid-onset or immediate-release formulations. However, sustained-release formulations do not necessarily ensure low abuse liability if users can circumvent the intended slow-release feature. Such tampering was noted with the original formulation of extended-release oxycodone (OxyContin); by crushing or dissolving the tablet, the entire dose intended for slow release was immediately available and used as a bolus by oral, intranasal, or injection routes. A reformulation of the extended-release oxycodone has made it more difficult to manipulate the drug and has resulted in less misuse.[72] Another example is the fentanyl transdermal system; the diversion or misuse of this is generally thought to be uncommon, but there have been reports of individuals swallowing or chewing the patch,[73] or extracting the fentanyl from the patch for intravenous use.[74]

Another way to discourage misuse of opioids is to combine them with an opioid antagonist. For example, adding the opioid antagonist naloxone would deter abuse by injection or intranasal use (but not by other routes); this is done with sublingual and buccal formulations of buprenorphine (Suboxone, Zubsolv) and a formulation of extended-release oxycodone (Targiniq ER). There is also a formulation of extended-release morphine with sequestered naltrexone (Embeda) that is released if the tablet is chewed or crushed.

Monitoring Strategies

When opioids are prescribed for chronic pain, particularly for individuals at risk for a prescription drug use disorder, it is recommended that they be monitored closely. Two strategies mentioned earlier and that are frequently employed in the monitoring of patients on prescribed chronic opioid therapy are the use of written treatment agreements and urine drug testing (UDT), although there is no strong evidence to support their use.[75] Another measure that can help identify individuals who are misusing prescription drugs is prescription drug monitoring programs (PDMPs).

Urine Drug Testing

Despite the lack of evidence, many experts recommend the use of UDT to monitor patients who are prescribed opioids, particularly those at high risk for misuse and those who exhibit ADRBs. UDT can be used to verify that the patient is taking the prescribed medication and not taking other illicit or nonprescribed substances. As with any test, it is important to be aware of the performance characteristics of the test—that is, what the test tells you and what it cannot tell you. It is also important to interpret the results in the context of other factors. Urine drug testing is covered in more detail in Chapter 2.

It is important to realize that many urine drug test panels are designed to identify illicit drugs, not prescription drugs. Most standard panels test for the presence of opiates, which include morphine, heroin (which is metabolized to morphine), and codeine. Hydrocodone and hydromorphone are metabolites of codeine and morphine and are generally detected with the opiate test, but at a somewhat lower sensitivity. Oxycodone and its metabolite, oxymorphone, are generally not detected with the opiate test, but they may trigger a positive result at high concentrations.[76] Methadone, buprenorphine, and fentanyl do not trigger a positive opiate test result and specific tests are needed to detect their presence. Another factor to consider when using UDT is the possibility of false-positive results. A number of substances may trigger positive enzyme-linked immunoassay (EIA) results; this is covered further in Chapter 2.

Drug testing should be done in an open manner. Telling a patient prior to prescribing a controlled substance that drug testing is routine can help reduce the stigma. When an unexpected result occurs (either positive or negative), this should lead to a nonjudgmental discussion with the patient about the results. If there is suspicion of a false-positive result, gas chromatography/mass spectrometry (GC/MS) testing can be performed to confirm the EIA results. The clinician should express her or his concerns over the results and always do what he or she believes is best for the patient. If a test is unexpectedly negative for a prescribed medication, one strategy is to ask the patient to return with the medication for a pill count to make sure the patient is not diverting the medication, although the person may circumvent this by "pill renting."[77]

Patient Agreements

Patient agreements (sometimes referred to as "pain contracts") are written documents that outline the goals and expectations prior to the prescribing of controlled substances. Box 13.1 shows a sample agreement. The general components of an agreement include outlining the goals of treatment, warning the patient of the risks, and advising the patient on aberrant behaviors. While these agreements have not been shown to prevent or reduce misuse, their use is recommended in expert guidelines.

BOX 13.1 Sample Controlled Substances Agreement

1. I understand that the aim of pain/anxiety management is to improve my quality of life and increase the amount of activity I can perform.
2. I understand that it is unlikely that all of my pain/anxiety will be relieved.
3. I agree to pursue non-medication therapies that may improve my pain/anxiety.
4. I understand that opioid pain and benzodiazepine anxiety medications used over long periods of time cause dependence and if stopped abruptly may result in withdrawal symptoms.
5. I understand that these medications can be dangerous if taken more than prescribed or if taken with alcohol or other medications, particularly sedatives.
6. I agree to have only one provider prescribe my pain/anxiety medications. I will notify my provider or the clinic if I am prescribed medications by other providers or clinics.
7. I agree to always take my pain/anxiety medication as prescribed. Any changes in dose must be made by agreement with my provider.
8. I am responsible for the safekeeping of these medications and for my prescriptions lasting the appropriate amount of time. I understand I may not receive additional medication ahead of time.
9. I understand that I may be asked to provide urine samples for testing to verify that I am taking the prescribed medication and not misusing other medications. I also agree to bring in my pill bottles for a pill count when requested.

_____
Patient Signature/Date

_____
Provider Signature

Prescription Drug Monitoring Programs

Prescription drug monitoring programs provide clinicians access to records of controlled substance prescriptions in order to guard against doctor shopping. Most states in the United States have PDMPs, but the programs vary from state to state and are evolving over time. While these programs are theoretically a useful tool to reduce misuse and overdose, there are a number of limitations. One is that clinicians do not consistently use these programs. Some programs are not user-friendly or up to date. The programs are state-based and individuals can circumvent them by crossing state borders. Finally, these programs only identify a minority of individuals who are using prescription drugs nonmedically; most obtain the drugs from family or friends or from a single clinician.

A study of U.S. data from 1999–2005 found that states with PDMPs did not have lower rates of drug overdose mortality or opioid consumption.[78] In Florida, however, which had high rates of prescription drug overdose deaths, a number of state policy changes, including establishment of a PDMP in 2011, was associated with a decline in overdose deaths.[79]

Addressing Aberrant Drug-Related Behaviors and Prescription Opioid Misuse

When treating patients, we must always balance benefit and risk and be prepared to change the therapeutic plan when the risks outweigh the benefits, even if the patient does not agree with this decision. It is important to keep in mind that opioids are effective for the treatment of acute pain; their effectiveness for treatment of chronic pain has not been established and they carry serious risks.

The basic approach to dealing with ADRBs is to match the response to the behavior. For example, if the patient does not understand that he or she should not to be obtaining opioids concurrently from more than one provider, then patient education is an appropriate response; this can be documented in a treatment agreement. If the patient is running out of medication early because the pain is inadequately controlled, then it would be best to adjust the treatment plan accordingly or refer the patient to a specialist. For more serious behaviors, such as forging prescriptions, diverting medication, or overdose, discontinuation of the opioids is generally most appropriate. Other strategies to deal with ADRBs include closer monitoring with urine drug testing or pill counts, providing smaller quantities of medication and seeing the patient more frequently, or referral to a pain management specialist.

Patients who have a prescription opioid use disorder should be offered treatment; simply cutting them off from the medications is not a solution for their problem. Often, the most difficult task is getting patients to acknowledge that they have a problem. It is best to approach the patient in a supportive and nonjudgmental manner. Treatment may include medically supervised withdrawal or taper from opioids, which can be followed by any of a number of forms of non-pharmacological treatment (e.g., 12-step groups, group or individual therapy, residential treatment). For patients with opioid dependence, medication-assisted treatments with methadone (in a supervised program) or office-based buprenorphine are important therapeutic options, particularly for those who have chronic pain.[80] The treatment of opioid use disorders is covered in more detail in Chapter 6.

Notes

1. Substance Abuse and Mental Health Services Administration. *Results from the 2013 National Survey on Drug Use and Health: National Findings*, NSDUH Series H-48, HHS Publication No. (SMA) 14-4863. Rockville, MD: Substance Abuse and Mental Health Services Administration; 2014.

2. Oregon Health Authority. Oregon Prescription Drug Monitoring Program: 2012 Annual Report to the PDMP Advisory Commission. 2013. http://www.orpdmp.com/orpdmpfiles/PDF_Files/Reports/PDMP-AC_AnnualReport_2012.pdf. Accessed November 10, 2014.

3. Substance Abuse and Mental Health Services Administration, Center for Behavioral Health Statistics and Quality. *The DAWN*

Report: Highlights of the 2011 Drug Abuse Warning Network (DAWN) Findings on Drug-Related Emergency Department Visits. Rockville, MD.

4. Sites BD, Beach ML, Davis MA. Increases in the use of prescription opioid analgesics and the lack of improvement in disability metrics among users. Reg Anesth Pain Med 2014;39:6–12.

5. Dart RC, Surratt HL, Cicero TJ, et al. Trends in opioid analgesic abuse and mortality in the United States. N Engl J Med 2015;372:241–8.

6. Cicero TJ, Ellis MS, Surratt HL, Kurtz SP. The changing face of heroin use in the United States: a retrospective analysis of the past 50 years. JAMA Psychiatry 2014;71:821–5.

7. Dennison SJ. Clonidine abuse among opiate addicts. Psychiatr Q 2001;72:191–5.

8. Beuger M, Tommasello A, Schwartz R, Clinton M. Clonidine use and abuse among methadone program applicants and patients. J Subst Abuse Treat 1998;15:589–93.

9. Rapko DA, Rastegar DA. Intentional clonidine patch ingestion by 3 adults in a detoxification unit. Arch Intern Med 2003;163:367–8.

10. Shapiro BJ, Lynch KL, Toochinda T, et al. Promethazine misuse among methadone maintenance patients and community based injection drug users. J Addict Med 2013;7:96–101.

11. Prahlow JA, Landrum JE. Amitriptyline abuse and misuse. Am J Forensic Med Pathol 2005;26:86–8.

12. Cohen MJ, Hanbury R, Stimmel B. Abuse of amitriptyline. JAMA 1978;240:1372–3.

13. Peles E1, Schreiber S, Adelson M. Tricyclic antidepressants abuse, with or without benzodiazepines abuse, in former heroin addicts currently in methadone maintenance treatment (MMT). Eur Neuropsychopharmacol 2008;18:188–93.

14. Mori T, Shibasaki M, Ogawa Y, et al. Comparison of the behavioral effects of bupropion and psychostimulants. Eur J Pharmacol 2013;718:370–5.

15. Hillard WT, Barloon L, Farley P, et al. Bupropion diversion and misuse in the correctional facility. J Correct Health Care 2013;19:211–7.

16. Lewis JC, Sutter ME, Albertson TE, et al. An 11-year review of bupropion insufflation exposures in adults reported to the California Poison Control System. Clin Toxicol (Phila) 2014;52:969–72.

17. Oppek K, Koller G, Zwergal A, Pogarell O. Intravenous administration and abuse of bupropion: a case report and review of the literature. J Addict Med 2014;8:290–3.

18. Schifano F. Misuse and abuse of pregabalin and gabapentin: cause for concern? CNS Drugs 2014;28:491–6.

19. Klein-Schwartz W, Schwartz EK, Anderson BD. Evaluation of quetiapine abuse and misuse reported to poison centers. J Addict Med 2014;8:195–8.

20. Malekshahi T, Tioleco N, Ahmed N, et al. Misuse of atypical antipsychotics in conjunction with alcohol and other drugs of abuse. J Subst Abus Treat 2015;48:8–12.

21. Pierre JH, Shnayder I, Wirshing DA, Wirshing WC. Intranasal quetiapine abuse. Am J Psychiatry 2004;161:1718.

22. Yargic I, Caferov C. Quetiapine dependence and withdrawal: a case report. Subst Abus 2011;32:168–9.

23. Dolan SB, Gatch MB. Abuse liability of the dietary supplement dimethylamylamine. Drug Alcohol Depend 2015;146:97–102.

24. Wilson MD, Ferguson RW, Mazer ME, Litovitz TL. Monitoring trends in dextromethorphan abuse using the National Poison Data System: 2000–2010. Clin Toxicol (Phila) 2011;49:409–15.

25. Reissig CJ, Carter LP, Johnson MW, et al. High doses of dextromethorphan, an NMDA antagonist, produce effects similar to classic hallucinogens. Psychopharmacology (Berl) 2013;223:1–15.

26. Logan BK, Goldfogel G, Hamilton R, Kuhlman J. Five deaths resulting from abuse of dextromethorphan sold over the Internet. J Anal Toxicol 2009;33:99–103.

27. Malcolm R, Miller WC. Dimenhydrinate (Dramamine) abuse: hallucinogenic experiences with a proprietary antihistamine. Am J Psychiatry 1972;128:1012–3.

28. Halpert AG, Olmstead MC, Beninger RJ. Mechanisms and abuse liability of the anti-histamine dimenhydrinate. Neurosci Biobehav Rev 2002;26:61–7.

29. Dilsaver SC. Antimuscarinic agents as substances of abuse: a review. J Clin Psychopharmacol 1988;8:14–22.

30. Thomas A, Nailur DG, Jones N, Deslandes PN. Diphenhydramine abuse and detoxification: a brief review and case report. J Psychopharmacol 2009;23:101–5.

31. McCabe SE, Cranford JA, West BT. Trends in prescription drug abuse and dependence, co-occurrence with other substance use disorders, and treatment utilization: results from two national surveys. Addict Behav 2008;33:1297–305.

32. Zale EL, Dorfman ML, Hooten WM, et al. Tobacco smoking, nicotine dependence, and patterns of prescription opioid misuse: results from a nationally representative sample. Nicotine Tob Res 2014;pii:ntu227.

33. Becker WC, Sullivan LE, Tetrault JM, et al. Non-medical use, abuse and dependence on prescription opioids among U.S. adults: psychiatric, medical and substance use correlates. Drug Alcohol Depend 2008;94:38–47.

34. Huang B, Dawson DA, Stinson FS, et al. Prevalence, correlates, and comorbidity of nonmedical prescription drug use and drug use disorders in the United States: results of the National Epidemiologic Survey on Alcohol and Related Conditions. J Clin Psychiatry 2006;67:1062–73.

35. Liebschutz JM, Saitz R, Weiss RD, et al. Clinical factors associated with prescription drug use disorder in urban primary care patients with chronic pain. J Pain. 2010;11:1047–55.

36. Becker WC, Fiellin DA, Gallagher RM, et al. The association between chronic pain and prescription drug abuse in veterans. Pain Med 2009;10:531–6.

37. Kirsh KL, Whitcomb LA, Donaghy K, et al. Abuse and addiction issues in medically ill patients with pain: attempts at clarification of terms and empirical study. Clin J Pain 2002;18(4 Suppl):S52–60.

38. Compton P, Darakjian J, Miotto K. Screening for addiction in patients with chronic pain and "problematic" substance use: evaluation of a pilot assessment tool. J Pain Symptom Manage 1998;16:355–63.

39. Compton PA, Wu SM. Schieffer B, et al. Introduction of a self-report version of the Prescription Drug Use Questionnaire and relationship to medication agreement non-compliance. J Pain Symptom Manage 2008;38:383–95.

40. Butler SF, Budman SH, Fernandez K, Jamison RN. Validation of a screener and opioid assessment measure for patients with chronic pain. Pain 2004;112:65–75.

41. Butler SF, Fernandez K, Benoit C, et al. Validation of the revised Screener and Opioid Assessment for Patients with Pain (SOAPP-R). J Pain 2008;9:360–72.

42. Butler SF, Budman SH, Fernandez KC, et al. Cross-validation of a Screener to Predict Opioid Misuse in Chronic Pain Patients (SOAP-R). J Addict Med 2009;3:66–73.

43. Butler SF, Budman SH, Fernandez KC, et al. Development and validation of the Current Opioid Misuse Measure. Pain 2007;130:144–56.

44. Wu SM, Compton P, Bolus R, et al. The addiction behaviors checklist: validation of a new clinician-based measure of inappropriate opioid use in chronic pain. J Pain Symptom Manage 2006;32:342–51.

45. Knisely JS, Wunsch MJ, Cropsey KL, Campbell ED. Prescription Opioid Misuse Index: a brief questionnaire to assess misuse. J Subst Abuse Treat 2008;35:380–6.

46. Chou R, Fanciullo GJ, Fine PG, et al. Opioids for chronic non-cancer pain: prediction and identification of aberrant drug-related behaviors: a review of the evidence for an American Pain Society and American Academy of Pain Medicine clinical practice guideline. J Pain 2009;10:131–46.

47. Solomon DH, Rassen JA, Glynn RJ, et al. The comparative safety of analgesics in older adults with arthritis. Arch Intern Med 2010;170:1968–76.

48. **Jones CM, Mack KA, Paulozzi LJ. Pharmaceutical overdose death, United States, 2010. JAMA 2013;309:657–59.** *In this analysis of death certificate data, there were 38,329 drug overdose deaths reported, 58% involving prescription drugs. Of the deaths that involved prescription drugs, 74% were unintentional. The most commonly used medications were opioids (75%), followed by benzodiazepines (29%), antidepressants (18%), and antiepileptic/antiparkinsonism drugs (8%).*

49. Centers for Disease Control and Prevention (CDC). Vital signs: overdoses of prescription opioid pain relievers-United States, 1999–2008. MMWR Morbid Mortal Wkly Rep 2011;60:1487–92.

50. Hall AJ, Logan JE, Toblin RL, et al. Patterns of abuse among unintentional pharmaceutical overdose fatalities. JAMA 2008;300:2613–20.

51. Bohnert AS, Valenstein M, Bair MJ, et al. Association between opioid prescribing patterns and opioid overdose-related deaths. JAMA 2011;305:1315–21.

52. Dunn KM, Saunders KW, Rutter CM, et al. Opioid prescriptions for chronic pain and overdose: a cohort study. Ann Intern Med 2010;152:85–92.

53. Miller M, Barber CW, Leatherman S, et al. Prescription opioid duration of action and risk of unintentional overdose among patients receiving opioid therapy. JAMA Intern Med 2015;175:608–15.

54. Ray WA, Chung CP, Murray KT, et al. Out-of-hospital mortality among patients receiving methadone for noncancer pain. JAMA Intern Med 2015;175(3):420–7.

55. Alam A, Gomes T, Zheng H, et al. Long-term analgesic use after low-risk surgery: a retrospective cohort study. Arch Intern Med 2012;172:425–30.

56. Clarke H, Soneji N, Ko DT, et al. Rates and risk factors for prolonged opioid use after major surgery: population based cohort study. BMJ 2014;348:1251.

57. Fishbain DA, Cole B, Lewis J, et al. What percentage of chronic non-malignant pain patients exposed to chronic opioid analgesic therapy develop abuse/addiction and/or aberrant drug-related behaviors? A structured evidence-based review. Pain Med 2008;9:444–59.

58. Bieber CM, Fernandez K, Borsook D, et al. Retrospective accounts of initial subjective effects of opioids in patients treated for pain who do or do not develop addiction: a pilot case-control study. Exp Clin Psychopharmacol 2008;16:429–34.

59. Singla N, Pong A, Newman K, et al. Combination oxycodone 5 mg/ibuprofen 400 mg for the treatment of pain after abdominal or pelvic surgery in women: a randomized, double-blind, placebo- and active-controlled parallel group study. Clin Ther 2005;27:45–57.

60. Holdgate A, Pollock T. Systematic review of the relative efficacy of non-steroidal anti-inflammatory drugs and opioids in the treatment of acute renal colic. BMJ 2004;328:1401.

61. Chaparro LE, Furlan AD, Deshpande A, et al. Opioids compared to placebo or other treatments for chronic low-back pain. Cochrane Database Syst Rev 2013;8:CD004959.

62. Chou R, Deyo R, Devine B, et al. The Effectiveness and Risks of Long-Term Opioid Treatment of Chronic Pain. Evidence Report/Technology Assessment No. 218. (Prepared by the Pacific Northwest Evidence-based Practice Center under Contract No. 290-2012-00014-I.) AHRQ Publication No. 14-E005-EF. Rockville, MD: Agency for Healthcare Research and Quality; September 2014.

63. **Roth SH, Fleischmann RM, Burch FX, et al. Around-the-clock, controlled release oxycodone therapy for osteoarthritis-related**

pain: placebo-controlled trial and long-term evaluation. **Arch Intern Med 2000;160:853–60.** *In this study of 133 subjects with osteoarthritis pain, 20 mg of controlled-release oxycodone twice daily reduced the mean pain intensity score from 2.5 to 1.7 (on a 3-point scale).*

64. Zhang Y, Ahmed S, Vo T, et al. Increased pain sensitivity in chronic pain subjects on opioid therapy: a cross-sectional study using quantitative sensory testing. Pain Med 2014; doi: 10.1111/pme.12606.

65. Wachholtz A, Gonzalez G. Co-morbid pain and opioid addiction: long term effect of opioid maintenance on acute pain. Drug Alcohol Depend 2014;145:142–9.

66. Fishbain DA, Cole B, Lewis J, et al. What percentage of chronic non-malignant pain patients exposed to chronic opioid analgesic therapy develop abuse/addiction and/or aberrant drug-related behaviors? A structured evidence-based review. Pain Med 2008;9:444–59.

67. Model policy for the use of controlled substances for the treatment of pain. Federation of State Medical Boards of the United States, Inc. www.fsmb.org/pdf/2004_grpol_Controlled_Substances.pdf, Accessed November 10, 2014.

68. Chou R, Fanciullo GJ, Fine PG, et al. Clinical guidelines for the use of chronic opioid therapy in chronic noncancer pain. J Pain 2009;10:113–30.

69. Agency Medical Directors Group. Interagency Guideline on Opioid Dosing for Chronic Non-cancer Pain: An educational aid to improve care and safety with opioid therapy. 2010; http://www.agencymeddirectors.wa.gov/files/opioidgdline.pdf. Accessed November 6, 2014.

70. Garg RK1, Fulton-Kehoe D, Turner JA, et al. Changes in opioid prescribing for Washington workers' compensation claimants after implementation of an opioid dosing guideline for chronic noncancer pain: 2004 to 2010. J Pain 2013;14:1620–8.

71. Fulton-Kehoe D, Garg RK, Turner JA, et al. Opioid poisonings and opioid adverse effects in workers in Washington State. Am J Ind Med 2013;56:1452–62.

72. Havens JR, Leukefeld CG, DeVaugh-Geiss AM, et al. The impact of a reformulation of extended-release oxycodone designed to deter abuse in a sample of prescription opioid abusers. Drug Alcohol Depend 2014;139:9–17.

73. Nevin J. Drug update: Fentanyl patch abuse. Emerg Med Serv 2004;33:24–5.

74. Tharp AM, Winecker RE, Winston DC. Fatal intravenous fentanyl abuse: four cases involving extraction of fentanyl from transdermal patches. Am J Forensic Med Pathol 2004;25:178–81.

75. Starrels JL, Becker WC, Alford DP, et al. Systematic review: treatment agreements and urine drug testing to reduce opioid misuse in patients with chronic pain. Ann Intern Med 2010;152:712–20.

76. Milone MC. Laboratory testing for prescription opioids. J Med Toxicol 2012;8:408–16.

77. Viscomi CM, Covington M, Christenson C. Pill counts and pill rental: unintended entrepreneurial opportunities. Clin J Pain 2013;29:623–4.

78. Paulozzi LJ, Kilbourne EM, Desai HA. Prescription drug monitoring programs and death rates from drug overdose. Pain Med 2011;12:747–54.

79. Johnson H, Paulozzi L, Porucznik C, et al. Decline in drug overdose deaths after state policy changes—Florida, 2010–2012. MMWR Morbid Mortal Wkly Rep 2014;63:569–74.

80. Roux P, Sullivan MA, Cohen J, et al. Burpenorphine/naloxone as a promising therapeutic option for opioid abusing patients with chronic pain: reduction of pain, opioid withdrawal symptoms, and abuse liability of oral oxycodone. Pain 2013;154:1442–8.

14

Medical Care for Patients with Substance Use Disorders

Background

Substance use disorders are chronic conditions that are associated with medical complications. Moreover, there are special challenges in providing this care to this population. In this chapter, we will discuss some of these issues. We begin by discussing the role of primary care clinicians in the identification and treatment of substance use disorders. We then cover the medical complications of injection drug use; complications associated with specific substances are addressed in the individual chapters on those substances. We then discuss issues that arise in caring for individuals on opioid agonist treatment and treating pain in individuals who have opioid use disorders.

Primary Care and Substance Use Disorders

Substance use disorders are common and associated with significant morbidity and mortality. Primary care clinicians are on the front line of identifying these individuals and engaging them in treatment. Substance use disorders have traditionally been viewed as the domain of mental health specialists, but they have much in common with other chronic medical conditions that primary care clinicians routinely treat, such as type II diabetes mellitus: both have behavioral, environmental, and genetic factors that contribute to the illness and both can be treated with a combination of behavioral counseling and medications. Like diabetes, there is no "cure" for substance use disorders, but with proper treatment and support, primary care clinicians can help patients lead healthier and more productive lives.

More than two thirds of individuals with addiction see a primary care clinician within a 6-month time frame.[1] Thus, these clinicians have the opportunity to recognize, diagnose, and help most individuals with addiction. Unfortunately, many clinicians avoid issues related to addiction and often do not recognize this problem in their patients.[2,3] This may be because they find it easier not to address substance use disorders, they do not feel comfortable discussing the topic, they do not know how to help, or they have a perception that little can be done. However, the primary care setting offers a safe place for patients and clinicians to explore addiction problems, build rapport, develop treatment plans, and work together toward long-term recovery.

Providing primary care to individuals with substance use disorders has a positive impact on their health.[4,5] Integrating treatment of substance use disorders into primary care services can provide additional benefits.[6,7] For example, in one clinical trial, medically ill patients with alcohol dependence were randomly assigned to standard treatment (primary care plus a referral for alcoholism treatment) or integrated outpatient treatment (IOT).[8] IOT patients saw primary care practitioners in a general outpatient medical setting on a monthly basis (or more often if needed) and were questioned and counseled on their alcohol use by their primary care practitioner. Patients assigned to IOT were more likely to be abstinent after 2 years of follow-up. In another study, patients with alcohol dependence were randomly assigned to receive treatment either in their primary care clinic or at a specialty clinic; those assigned to primary care treatment were more likely to engage in care and had greater reductions in heavy drinking.[9]

The approval of buprenorphine for office-based treatment for opioid use disorders has given primary care physicians the opportunity to provide an effective treatment within their regular practice. Numerous studies have shown the effectiveness of buprenorphine in office-based practice and show that many patients do well with routine medical management and do not require additional services. In addition to facilitating substance use disorder treatment,[10] providing buprenorphine in a primary care setting helps engage patients in medical care[11,12] and is highly valued by patients.[13] Nonetheless, many physicians are reluctant to prescribe buprenorphine, even after receiving training. Perceived barriers include lack of mental health and psychosocial support, time constraints, lack of confidence, resistance from practice partners, and lack of institutional support.[14]

Despite the high prevalence and significant health impact, primary care practitioners receive relatively little training in the treatment of substance use disorders[15,16] and trainees often have negative attitudes toward patients with substance use disorders and their prospects for rehabilitation.[17,18,19] Some experts have called for integrating addiction medicine into primary care graduate medical education;[20] it remains to be seen if these calls are heeded.

Medical Complications of Injection Drug Use

Many of the medical complications that individuals with substance use disorders acquire are due to the use of needles to administer the drug. According to the 2006–2008 National Survey on Drug Use and Health (NSDUH), an estimated 425,000 Americans had used a needle to inject an illicit drug in the past year (0.2% of those aged 12 and older); 13% of them reported using a needle that had previously been used by someone else.[21] Injection drug use is risky; in a cohort of injection drug users in Scotland followed from 1980 to 2001, the average annual mortality was 2.3%. Overdose was the primary cause of death early on and was overtaken by the complications of human immunodeficiency virus (HIV) infection in the late 1980s. Mortality from HIV declined after 1996 and hepatitis C subsequently became a significant cause of mortality.[22]

Other than conventional treatment for substance use disorders, there are a number of specific measures that may help reduce the risks of injection drug use. One is the provision of supervised injecting facilities where users can inject illicit drugs under medical supervision. These facilities can provide clean needles to prevent transmissible diseases and offer treatment in the event of overdose. While there is some concern that supervised injecting facilities may encourage such drug use and discourage users from obtaining treatment, they may actually facilitate entry into treatment; observational data indicate that individuals who use these facilities are more likely to start treatment.[23] Another measure that may help reduce the risks of injection drug use is the provision of clean needles and syringes through needle-exchange programs. Studies suggest that these programs can reduce the risk of transmissible infections, particularly HIV and hepatitis C.[24]

Infectious Complications

Injection drug users are at risk for infectious complications, particularly those associated with sharing needles. Hepatitis C, hepatitis B, and HIV infection are spread through this route. Other infectious complications (e.g., cellulitis and endocarditis) will be covered in the subsequent organ system-based sections.

Hepatitis B

Epidemiological studies indicate that injection drug users are at high risk for acquiring the hepatitis B virus (HBV); in one study of users in Baltimore, 80% were HBV seropositive, and this was associated with needle-sharing and duration of use, but not high-risk sexual behavior.[25] Most who acquire hepatitis B have a clinical illness with nausea, vomiting, and jaundice that resolves within a few weeks. In contrast to hepatitis C, only a minority develop persistent infection and remain infectious to others; in one case series, this occurred in about 2% of drug users with acute hepatitis B.[26] Detection of hepatitis B surface antigen (HBsAg) generally identifies those who are chronically infected. However, a number of studies have found evidence of occult hepatitis B infection (defined as negative HBsAg and detectable serum HBV DNA) among hepatitis C–infected injection drug users.[27] This has been associated with the presence of anti-hepatitis B core antibody and more severe liver disease.[28,29]

Needle-exchange programs appear to reduce the risk of hepatitis B transmission.[30] All drug users who are not hepatitis B infected or are immune (i.e., do not have positive hepatitis B surface antigen or surface antibody) should be offered hepatitis B vaccine.

Hepatitis C

Hepatitis C virus (HCV) infection is common among injection drug users. In a nationally representative household survey in the United States, 58% of those who had used injection drugs at some time had antibodies to HCV; injection drug use accounted for about half of all infections.[31] In this same study, adults who reported lifetime non-injection illicit drug use (except marijuana) had an infection rate of 3.5%, compared with 0.7% among those who had never used illicit drugs (or had used only marijuana). HCV can be found in nasal secretions, so sharing of implements for snorting is a potential route of transmission.[32] The rates of HCV infection are even higher in drug treatment settings; in one study of subjects in a detoxification program, 71% of the heroin users had HCV antibodies.[33]

Acute hepatitis C is usually asymptomatic, but some individuals do develop an acute self-limited illness with jaundice. This is actually a good prognostic sign, as those with symptomatic acute hepatitis C are more likely to clear the virus.[34] Overall, about 80% become chronically infected; those who do clear the virus spontaneously can be reinfected but are at lower risk than others.[35] HCV carriers are generally asymptomatic but may develop complications such as essential mixed cryoglobulinemia, which can lead to systemic vasculitis, peripheral neuropathy, and glomerulonephritis.[36] Over the long term, chronic HCV infection can lead to cirrhosis and hepatocellular carcinoma. In one cohort of 1,667 anti-HCV positive injection drug users who had used for a median of 14 years at entry, the rate of end-stage liver disease was 3 per 1,000 person-years. However, liver disease accounted for a relatively small proportion of the deaths in this cohort; only 9% were due to liver disease, while 40% were due to complications of HIV, 19% due to overdose, and 12% due to bacterial infections.[37] In another cohort of injection drug users in Norway who were hepatitis C antibody positive, opioid overdose was the most common cause of death, and those who were RNA positive (had chronic infection) did not have a significantly higher overall mortality than those who were RNA negative (spontaneously cleared the infection). However, when the analysis was limited to those over 50, the RNA-positive subjects had a significantly higher liver-related mortality.[38] This finding suggests that we should be targeting those over age 50 for treatment.

For many years, the only treatment for HCV was a combination of interferon and ribavirin, but this had limited efficacy and high rates of side effects. With the introduction of direct-acting antivirals, the current standard treatment for HCV is rapidly evolving.[39] The newer treatments are more effective and have fewer side effects, but they are also very expensive. The treatment regimens and duration vary depending on the genotype.

Those who do have a sustained response are still at risk for reacquiring the infection if they share needles again. Although it is generally recommended that individuals with HCV abstain from alcohol, drinking does not appear to significantly impair their response to HCV therapy[40] and should not be considered a contraindication to treatment.

For those who develop liver failure from HCV, liver transplantation is the only treatment option. While almost all programs consider active drug use a contraindication for transplantation, many also exclude those on methadone maintenance treatment.[41] However, one study of 36 liver transplant recipients on methadone maintenance (followed for an average of 4 years) reported outcomes comparable to the national average; all of these subjects were abstinent from alcohol and illicit drugs for at least 6 months prior to transplantation.[42]

Needle-exchange programs and opioid agonist treatment have been shown to reduce HCV transmission.[43,44] The risk of transmission may also be reduced by cleaning syringes and needles with bleach.[45]

HIV Infection

In the United States, injection drug use has been an important route of transmission of HIV infection. Of the estimated 1,148,200 Americans living with HIV infection in 2009, 183,400 (16%) had injection drug use as their main risk factor and another 60,200 (5%) had injection drug use and male-to-male sexual contact as their main risk factors.[46] The proportion of new infections through injection drug use has been declining; it was estimated that 8% of new infections in 2010 were due to transmission by this route.[47] Although a minority of individuals are infected through injection drug use, illicit drug use is common among those with HIV, with an estimated 64% reporting lifetime use.[48]

The acquisition of HIV infection is usually followed by a mild to severe flu-like illness that has been called the "acute retroviral syndrome." The most common signs and symptoms of primary HIV infection are fever, malaise, myalgia, pharyngitis, and rash. The syndrome is nonspecific and cannot be differentiated from other acute viral illnesses on the basis of signs or symptoms alone.[49] Patients commonly do not seek medical attention and even when they do, primary HIV infection is often not recognized. HIV antibody is negative during this phase of the illness, but acute infection can be diagnosed by measurement of the plasma mRNA level (viral load), which is very high.

The acute phase of HIV infection is followed by a prolonged asymptomatic phase that generally lasts several years. During this phase, there is a gradual decline in immunity and infected persons are at higher risk for community-acquired pneumonia and tuberculosis, but not the opportunistic infections that are seen in immune-compromised hosts. The final phase of this illness, the acquired immunodeficiency syndrome (AIDS), is when the immune system is so impaired that the host is at risk for opportunistic infections. This stage is generally defined as a CD4 count below 200 or the presence of an opportunistic infection (for example, *Pneumocystis* pneumonia). Injection drug users do not appear to be at any higher risk for progression to AIDS than non-users,[50] but they are at high risk for other infections, particularly pneumonia and endocarditis.[51]

The introduction in 1996 of potent three-drug combinations of antiretroviral medications (combined antiretroviral therapy, or cART) has dramatically improved survival and quality of life for those who have access to these medications.[52] Studies have shown that success rates with cART (as defined by complete suppression of HIV) are poorer with injection drug users than with others; this is due to poorer adherence to these unforgiving regimens.[53] However, drug use is not a contraindication to therapy, and injection drug users have been found to have survival rates comparable to those of others after starting cART.[54] For those who are opioid dependent, engagement in opioid agonist treatment has been associated with increased initiation and better adherence to cART.[55]

Needle-exchange programs appear to reduce the risk of HIV transmission,[56] and some have advocated that physicians write prescriptions for needles and syringes for injection drug users who would not otherwise have access to them. Opioid agonist treatment has also been shown to reduce the risk of HIV infection among injection drug users, most of the evidence coming from methadone maintenance programs.[57] Another strategy that would likely reduce transmission in this population is a "test and treat" strategy in which drug users are tested frequently and started on treatment soon after diagnosis.[58]

Syphilis and Other STDs

Although injection drug use does not directly cause sexually transmitted diseases (STDs), these infections are a concern among this population because of an association between injection drug use and risky behaviors, such as having multiple partners, commercial sex work, or exchanging sex for drugs or money. This appears to be particularly a concern for those who use the stimulants cocaine and methamphetamine.[59]

A number of studies indicate that injection drug users are at increased risk for syphilis,[60] particularly those who trade sex for money or drugs.[61] Injection drug use also appears to be associated with an increased risk of other STDs, such as gonorrhea[62] and chlamydia.[63] It is probably prudent to routinely test injection drug users for these STDs (i.e., serum RPR/VDRL and urine, endocervical or endourethral specimen for gonorrhea and chlamydia). At the very minimum, these individuals should be questioned about their sexual practices and those who engage in high-risk sexual behavior, tested (and counseled).

Cutaneous Complications

Injection drug users are at high risk for developing skin and soft tissue infections. In one community-based study of injection drug users in San Francisco, 32% reporting having an abscess or cellulitis; many of them had treated themselves by lancing the abscess or taking antibiotics they had purchased on the street. In this study, subcutaneous or intramuscular injection ("skin-popping") and less experience with use were associated with these infections.[64] In a case-control study of injection drug users, development of an abscess that required drainage was associated with skin-popping and use of speedballs (heroin and cocaine mixture); cleaning the skin with alcohol appeared to have a protective effect.[65] Many injection drug users treat themselves with antibiotics they purchase on the street. As a result, they are at increased risk of carrying—and being infected with—antibiotic-resistant organisms.[66] For those who have recurrent soft tissue infections, intranasal mupirocin may help eradicate carriage of *Staphylococcus aureus* and prevent further infections, though this has not been demonstrated in a clinical trial.[67]

While the treatment of cellulitis and abscesses is relatively straightforward, injection drug users are also at risk for necrotizing soft tissue infections that require much more aggressive surgical management and may be difficult to recognize on clinical exam. A study of patients treated at San Francisco General Hospital over 5 years reported that among 3,560 injection drug users who underwent incision and drainage of an abscess, 30 (0.8%) were found to have necrotizing soft tissue infections and required wide debridement or amputation—20% of them died.[68]

Injection drug users are also at risk for developing chronic wounds in the upper or lower extremities. Treatment requires cessation of the drug use and (often prolonged) wound care; skin grafting may be helpful in some cases.

Neuromuscular Complications

Botulism

Although botulism is generally a foodborne illness, the organism can also be introduced through subcutaneous injection and has been seen in injection drug users.[69] The organism *C. botulinum* produces an endotoxin that blocks transmission at the neuromuscular junction, leading to descending paralysis and even death. Treatment is generally supportive; botulinum antitoxin may be beneficial.

Tetanus

Tetanus is caused by toxin-producing anaerobic bacteria *Clostridium tetani*, which can result in localized or generalized muscles spasms. The spores of this organism are present in soil and can enter the body through cutaneous wounds. One of the first (if not *the* first) descriptions of intravenous drug use in the medical literature was an 1876 report of a woman who developed tetanus as a result.[70] While tetanus is quite rare in the United States (about 40 cases/year), injection drug users have been noted to be at risk and in one study accounted for 15% of the cases.[71] Tetanus can be prevented by immunization; the disease is generally seen in those who have not been adequately vaccinated.

Pulmonary Complications

Injection drug users who inject talc-containing crushed tablets are at risk for pulmonary granulomatosis, which may lead to pulmonary hypertension[72] and chronic obstructive lung disease.[73] This complication has been generally (but not exclusively) associated with intravenous methylphenidate (Ritalin) use.

Injection heroin users have been noted to sometimes develop noncardiogenic pulmonary edema, generally in the setting of overdose. In one series, of 1,278 heroin overdoses treated at one hospital, 27 (2.1%) developed pulmonary edema as a complication and 9 required mechanical ventilation; most recovered within 24 hours.[74] In addition, users who inject into their neck are at risk for pneumothorax.[75]

Cardiovascular Complications

Endocarditis

Endocarditis is one of the most serious complications of injection drug use. In one prospective study of 2,529 injection drug users, the incidence of endocarditis was 7 cases/1,000 person-years and was higher among women and those with HIV infection or a history of previous endocarditis.[76] Cocaine use in particular appears to increase the risk of this complication.[77] Endocarditis is a concern when evaluating an injection drug user with an acute febrile illness. Unfortunately, clinical history, examination, and routine laboratory tests may not be reliable for ruling out this potentially lethal complication and one must rely on blood cultures.[78,79] A 2014 study found that tachycardia, cardiac murmur, and absence of skin infection were the best predictors of endocarditis among injection drug users with a fever. The authors suggested that a clinical prediction rule using these three may be useful for ruling out endocarditis.[80]

Staph. aureus is by far the most common organism (about 70% of cases), followed by streptococci (8%).[81] The tricuspid valve is infected in about 50% of these cases, followed by the aortic valve (25%) and mitral valve (20%). Endocarditis may be complicated by septic emboli to the lungs (in right-sided infections) or to the brain, extremities, kidneys, or viscera (in left-sided cases). Persons with endocarditis may also develop osteomyelitis or septic arthritis; the pain from these complications may be the presenting symptom of this illness.[82] The risk of mortality is increased with large vegetations (>2.0 cm),[83] aortic valve involvement,[84] and severe immunosuppression due to HIV infection (i.e., CD4 count <200 cells/mm^3).[85]

The standard treatment for endocarditis is 2–6 weeks of intravenous antibiotics, the type of antibiotic and duration depending on the organism, location, and presence of other complications. Oral antibiotics may be an option in some right-sided cases if intravenous treatment is not feasible.[86] Surgery is generally indicated for severe valvular insufficiency, persistent systemic embolization, or persistent sepsis from a ring or myocardial abscess. In one series of surgical treatment for 80 injection drug users with endocarditis, 30-day surgical mortality was 7.5% and 5-year survival was 70%.[87]

Simple measures, such as cleaning the skin, may reduce the risk of endocarditis in injection drug users.[88] Of course, the most effective prevention measure is effective addiction treatment.

Vascular Complications

Injection drug users are also at risk for endovascular complications in locations other than the cardiac valves. These include venous thrombosis,[89] septic thrombophlebitis, or infected pseudoaneurysms.[90] Injection drug users may also develop arterial thrombosis and upper extremity ischemia from inadvertent injection into an artery.[91]

Renal Complications

In the 1970s and 1980s, an association was observed between injection heroin use and nephrotic syndrome ("heroin-nephropathy"), sometimes leading to end-stage renal disease. These patients were generally African-American men and pathological evaluation revealed sclerosing glomerulonephritis.[92] The etiology of this condition has never been clearly established and may well have been due to an adulterant mixed with the heroin. It appears that the problem has declined since then[93] but may still account for some new cases of end-stage renal disease.[94] Hepatitis C may also be responsible for some of the renal disease seen in injection drug users.[95]

Injection drug users who inject into their subcutaneous tissues, generally when veins are no longer accessible ("skin-poppers"), can develop chronic skin infections or wounds that may lead to amyloidosis and renal failure.[96] In addition, those who suffer an overdose may develop renal failure due to rhabdomyolysis and myoglobinuria.[97]

Medical Care of Patients on Opioid Agonist Treatment

Opioid agonist treatment (OAT) has become a common treatment modality for opioid dependence. In a 2008 survey, there were approximately 250,000 Americans receiving methadone from 1,100 treatment programs,[98] while in the same year, there were approximately 16,000 physicians certified to prescribe buprenorphine and 500,000 patients receiving the medication.[99] Some individuals remain on this treatment for years and even decades. There are a number of special issues that arise in caring for individuals on OAT that we will address in this section. These include long-term medical complications, drug interactions, pain management, and treatment of hospitalized patients on OAT.

Medical Complications

Opioids are associated with relatively few long-term sequelae. Patients on stable doses of opioids generally develop a tolerance to the side effects, particularly sedation and respiratory depression. However, there are a number of medical complications that are particularly problematic for patients who are on long-term methadone maintenance; these include constipation, hypogonadism, prolonged QT interval, and cognitive impairment. Constipation is briefly discussed in Chapter 6, on opioids.

Hypogonadism

Experimental and clinical studies have shown that opioids can produce hypogonadotropic hypogonadism; it appears to do this via suppression of gonadotropin-releasing hormone (GnRH).[100] This results in low testosterone levels, impotence, and osteoporosis in men, and amenorrhea or irregular menstrual cycles and infertility in women. Hypogonadism is commonly seen among individuals on methadone and appears to be dose-dependent.[101] In contrast, buprenorphine appears to have less of an effect; in one study, men on buprenorphine (8–20 mg/day) had testosterone levels that were significantly higher than those of individuals on methadone and comparable to levels of healthy controls.[102] In another study, 28% of the men on buprenorphine had low testosterone levels compared to 65% of the men receiving methadone.[103] In a study of women started on transdermal buprenorphine, subjects did not experience significant changes in sex hormones.[104]

QT Prolongation

Methadone is associated with a dose-dependent prolongation of the QT interval.[105] This has been attributed to blockade of the cardiac potassium ion (hERG) channel, resulting in prolongation of cardiac repolarization. Methadone is a chiral mixture of (R,S) methadone; the opioid effect is primarily from the (R)-methadone, while (S)-methadone blocks the hERG channels more potently. In one study, substitution of (R,S)-methadone with (R)-methadone resulted in a significant reduction of the QTc interval.[106]

Prolonged QT does not appear to be a common problem, but it has been linked with reports of syncope and arrhythmia—specifically, torsades de pointes.[107,108,109] In a series of 167 hospitalized patients who were on methadone, 16% had a prolonged QT (QTc >0.50 sec) and 6 (3.6%) had presented with torsades de pointes; their QTc ranged from 0.43 to 0.75 sec and their methadone dose ranged from 40 to 200 mg/day.[110] In an analysis of a national adverse event registry in the United States, the mean number of monthly reports of QTc prolongation or torsade de pointes from 1997 to 2011 rose from 0.3 to 3.5. The median methadone dose was 150 mg/day (range 90–360 mg/day) and concomitant medications most commonly reported were antiretroviral drugs and benzodiazepines.[111]

While there is some evidence to suggest an increased risk of sudden cardiac death associated with methadone use,[112] the absolute risk appears to be low and is probably lower than the risk of fatal overdose for individuals who are not in treatment. In a cohort of 138 subjects on methadone maintenance, 3 (2.2%) had a prolonged QTc >0.50 seconds and 19 (14%) had a mildly prolonged QTc between 0.45 and 0.49 seconds; all of them were on doses over 120 mg/day. However, the authors found no correlation between the QTc and methadone dose or serum levels, and no subjects had cardiac problems over 2 years of follow-up.[113] Another cohort study in Norway reported that among 173 patients on methadone maintenance, 8 (4.6%) had a QTc >0.50 seconds, 26 (15%) >0.47 seconds, and 50 (29%) >0.45 seconds. The authors found a relationship between methadone dose and QTc length, and all of those with a QTc >0.50 seconds were on doses exceeding 120 mg/day. Using a national death certificate registry, they estimated that the maximum mortality attributable to QTc prolongation was 0.06 per 100 patient-years.[114]

A number of other factors may increase the risk of arrhythmia. The use of cocaine may trigger torsades in some individuals on methadone.[115] There is also evidence that protease inhibitors, used for the treatment of HIV infection, may also prolong the QT interval and there are case reports of torsades de pointes associated with their use. This risk may be increased by concurrent use of methadone.[116] There are case reports of prolonged QT and ventricular arrhythmias associated with ritonavir-boosted atazanavir and methadone; discontinuation of atazanavir resulted in a reduction of the QT interval.[117] Concurrent use of benzodiazepines may also increase QTc intervals. In a study of 512 individuals initiating methadone maintenance, baseline benzodiazepine use was not associated with QTc intervals, but after initiation of methadone, QTc intervals were significantly longer among those who tested positive for benzodiazepines.[118] Coadministration of other drugs that can prolong QT intervals may also increase the risk, including the antidepressants citalopram, escitalopram, and amitriptyline;[119] the antifungal fluconazole;[120] and macrolide antibiotics.[121]

There are fewer data on the effect of other opioids on QT interval. Buprenorphine has not been found to be associated with QT prolongation,[114,122] even among patients on antiretroviral treatment.[123] One study of eight chronic pain patients on morphine who were switched to methadone (daily doses ranging from 30 to 85 mg/day) reported that the mean QTc increased from 0.416 to 0.436 seconds, suggesting that morphine has less effect on QTc than methadone (or no effect at all).[124] Another study of 100 patients with chronic pain found that methadone and oxycodone were associated with prolonged QT interval in a dose-dependent fashion, but morphine and tramadol were not. These researchers also reported that oxycodone was capable of inhibiting hERG channels in vitro, albeit with low affinity.[125]

Cognitive Impairment

Another possible complication of opioid agonist treatment is cognitive impairment and psychomotor slowing. When looking at this issue, one must be careful to tease out the contribution of other drugs, particularly alcohol, benzodiazepines, and cannabinoids. A study of subjects on methadone maintenance (mean dose of 67 mg) found significantly impaired performance on cognitive tests compared with that of healthy, non-drug-using controls; psychomotor slowing appeared to be the most prominent impairment.[126] A follow-up study of abstinent individuals with prior opioid abuse found that their performance fell in between that of individuals on methadone and of controls without a history of opioid abuse, suggesting that the observed impairments on methadone are not entirely due to the effects of prior drug use.[127] Studies suggest that buprenorphine has minimal cognitive effects[128] and is associated with less cognitive impairment and psychomotor slowing than methadone.[129]

There are mixed data on the effect of opioid agonist treatment on driving ability. A study of simulated driving performance of individuals on methadone and buprenorphine maintenance found no impairment when compared with non-drug-using controls; however, the methadone doses in this study were relatively modest (mean 48 mg).[130] Other studies have reported that buprenorphine is not associated with significant impairment in driving ability[131] and is associated with less impairment than that from methadone in a "driving-relevant psychomotor battery" of tests.[132] A study in France, however, found that individuals receiving methadone or buprenorphine were at increased risk of being responsible for traffic crashes resulting in injuries, although this could at least partly be due to risky behaviors and use of other substance use (especially alcohol and benzodiazepines).[133]

Drug Interactions with Methadone

Clinicians who care for patients on methadone maintenance must be aware of possible drug interactions. The most obvious of these is the use of other opioids or opioid antagonists. Box 14.1 lists some

BOX 14.1 Drugs That May Interact with Methadone

Drugs That May Increase Methadone Effects/Levels

Antibiotics

Ciprofloxacin (Cipro)
Macrolide antibiotics—erythromycin, clarithromycin (Biaxin), azithromycin (Zithromax)

Antifungal agents

Azoles—fluconazole (Diflucan), itraconazole (Sporanox), ketoconazole (Nizoral)

Antidepressants

Fluvoxamine (Luvox)
Paroxetine (Paxil)
Sertraline (Zoloft)

Others

Cimetidine (Tagamet)

Drugs That May Decrease Methadone Effects/Levels

Antibiotics

Rifampin (Rifadin, Rimactane)
Rifapentine (Priftin)

Antiretroviral agents

Efavirenz (Sustiva)
Fosamprenavir (Lexiva)
Nevirapine (Viramune)
Nelfinavir (Viracept)
Ritonavir (Norvir, Kaletra)

Antiepileptic agents

Carbamazepine (Carbatrol, Tegretol)
Fosphenytoin (Cerebyx)
Phenytoin (Dilantin, Phenytek)
Phenobarbital

Opioid antagonists/partial agonists

Buprenorphine (Buprenex, Subutex, Suboxone)
Pentazocine (Talwin)
Naloxone (Narcan)
Naltrexone (Revia)
Nalmefene (Revex)

Other agents

Ammonium Chloride
Metyrapone
Risperidone (Risperdal)
St. John's wort

Brand names are in parentheses. These interactions are not always clinically significant; see text for more details.

other drugs that may affect the serum levels or drug effects of methadone. Methadone is metabolized by the cytochrome P450 system; the isoenzymes CYP3A4, CYP2C8, and CYP2D6 appear to be most important in this process.[134] However, there is a great deal of genetic variation in the p450 activity that leads to variations in drug effects and the impact of drug–drug interactions.[135] Nevertheless, inhibitors of these enzymes may increase methadone levels, and inducers of these enzymes will tend to lower levels. In many cases, these interactions produce only modest changes and are not clinically significant. However, in other cases, individuals may experience withdrawal symptoms or toxicity and dose modification may be necessary.

In practice, these drug interactions are particularly important for HIV-infected persons on methadone who require antiretroviral treatment. The non-nucleoside reverse transcriptase inhibitors (NNRTIs) efavirenz[136] and nevirapine[137] lower methadone levels and may precipitate withdrawal symptoms. A number of protease inhibitors have also been shown to reduce serum methadone levels, including ritonavir, lopinavir/ritonavir (Kaletra),[138] nelfinavir, and fosamprenavir,[139] but the changes are mild and generally not clinically significant.[140]

The antimicrobial rifampin, which is frequently used for treatment of tuberculosis, has also been reported to lower methadone levels and precipitate withdrawal symptoms;[141] however, a related agent, rifabutin, does not seem to have this effect.[142] In addition, a number of antiepileptic drugs (phenytoin,[143] phenobarbital,[144] and carbamazepine[145]) reduce methadone levels and have been reported to cause withdrawal symptoms. Fosphenytoin, which is a prodrug of phenytoin, probably has a similar effect. St. John's wort, a popular herbal over-the-counter remedy for depression, is known to be a potent inducer of CYP3A4 and has been reported to decrease methadone levels and precipitate withdrawal.[146] Finally, the antipsychotic risperidone has been reported to have caused withdrawal in two individuals on methadone maintenance.[147]

By contrast, a number of drugs may *increase* methadone levels, by inhibiting its metabolism. This effect, which is generally mild and of limited clinical significance, has been noted with the SSRI antidepressants sertraline[148] and paroxetine,[149] but appears to be most significant with fluvoxamine.[150] In contrast, another SSRI, fluoxetine, does not appear to have any effect on methadone levels.[151] The azole antifungal agents (ketoconazole, fluconazole, itraconazole, and voriconazole) are cytochrome p450 inhibitors[152] and may increase methadone levels. Studies of the pharmacokinetics of methadone in volunteers who were given fluconazole[153] or voriconazole[154] have found increased methadone levels, but there was no evidence of clinical toxicity or overdose. The macrolide antibiotics (especially erythromycin) are also P450 inhibitors and may increase methadone levels. However, we have not been able to find any reports on the clinical significance of this interaction for patients on methadone and have not observed any ill effects with the use of clarithromycin or azithromycin in this population. Finally, the antibiotic ciprofloxacin has been reported (in one case) to have led to clinically significant opioid toxicity in an individual on chronic methadone.[155]

While there is no medication that is absolutely contraindicated for an individual on methadone—except the opioid antagonists (naltrexone, nalmefene, and naloxone), outside of the setting of overdose—practitioners should remain vigilant for possible interactions and coordinate care with the patient's methadone program when there is a potential for interaction. Measuring trough serum methadone levels may be helpful in determining whether a dose adjustment is needed, especially when a patient reports continued withdrawal symptoms despite a dose increase. However, methadone levels may not always correlate with its therapeutic effect; one study found no correlation between trough levels of methadone (or its metabolite) and withdrawal symptoms or illicit heroin use,[156] while another study suggested that a level of 100 ng/mL is generally adequate.[157]

There are a number of other medications that do not interact directly with methadone metabolism but should be avoided in patients on methadone maintenance. First and foremost among these are the benzodiazepines, which enhance the effects (and toxicity) of methadone and are frequently misused by individuals on methadone maintenance.[158] There may be some individuals who have an anxiety disorder or another condition that requires chronic benzodiazepine use, but it is probably best that this only be prescribed after a careful assessment and under the close supervision of a mental health professional. Clonidine is also misused by individuals on methadone and should be avoided, even for those who have hypertension. The antiemetics promethazine (Phenergan) and prochlorperazine (Compazine) potentiate the sedative effects of methadone and should also be avoided.

Drug Interactions with Buprenorphine

Buprenorphine, like methadone, is metabolized by the cytochrome P450 enzymes in the liver.[159] Therefore, there is a theoretical potential for interactions with medications that induce or suppress these enzymes, but little is known regarding the clinical significance of these interactions. Pharmacokinetic studies have found interactions with antiretroviral medications—an increase in buprenorphine levels when coadministered with the ritonavir[160] and decreased levels with efavirenz[161]—but neither appeared to be clinically significant. However, there have been reports of buprenorphine toxicity (primarily drowsiness and dizziness) when coadministered with the antiretrovirals atazanavir and ritonavir.[162]

Treating Pain

The approach to the treatment of pain in patients on methadone maintenance is generally the same as with other patients, with a few caveats. In general, practitioners should avoid prescribing opioids, particularly for patients with chronic pain, since there is a substantial risk of misuse or diversion. Chronic severe pain is a common problem among clients on methadone programs and many of them take prescribed opioids in addition to their methadone.[163] There is evidence that use of chronic opioids may induce hyperalgesia and relative pain intolerance.[164] In general, it is best to focus on nonpharmacological treatments and non-opioid analgesics for treatment of chronic pain. If these are not effective, an increase in methadone dosage may help, particularly if the program allows clients to split their dose (i.e., divide it into two or three doses). Many programs are willing to work with primary care practitioners to help their clients and will allow take-home dosages if the client has been compliant with the treatment program.

Caring for Hospitalized Patients on Opioid Agonist Treatment

A number of issues may arise in the management of patients on methadone or buprenorphine who are hospitalized or require surgery, particularly the issue of treating acute pain.[165] In general, patients on methadone who require surgery or hospitalization should be continued on their regular dose after this has been confirmed by their program. If this cannot be confirmed, a dose of 30 mg of methadone can be given; this is generally sufficient to avoid significant withdrawal with minimal overdose risk. Individuals on methadone can be given supplemental opioid analgesics, if necessary. However, their methadone dose should not be altered without coordinating changes with their treatment program. Patients on methadone have high tolerance to opioids and generally require higher than usual doses at more frequent intervals; their usual methadone dose will not provide them with analgesia. Buprenorphine and pentazocine should be avoided in patients on methadone because they may precipitate withdrawal syndrome due to their antagonistic effects.

For patients on methadone maintenance who are unable to take oral medications (for example, in the postoperative period), there are a few options. One option is to use patient-controlled analgesia (PCA) and to set the basal rate to give (over 24 hours) an amount of morphine or hydromorphone that is equivalent to their daily methadone dose.[166] Methadone can be given parenterally; two-thirds of the regular daily dose can be given intramuscularly in two divided doses.[167] For example, someone on 100 mg per day of methadone could instead be given 30 mg intramuscularly twice daily. There are some positive reports of use of intravenous methadone in PCA.[168] This may simplify the estimation of a safe and effective basal rate, but these studies were not done on patients who were on methadone maintenance and the experience with this practice is fairly limited.

The treatment of patients on buprenorphine maintenance is somewhat more complex. Buprenorphine has analgesic effects, but these are limited by its partial agonist properties and it will tend to block the effect of other opioids because of its high affinity for opioid receptors and long duration of action. Therefore, one must decide whether to continue the buprenorphine or stop it altogether. In our experience, for patients who are undergoing minor procedures or are expected to have mild-moderate pain of limited duration, one can continue buprenorphine and supplement it with non-opioid analgesics or a limited course of opioid analgesics.

For individuals who are having major surgical procedures or who are hospitalized and are expected to have severe pain over an extended period of time, another option is to stop the buprenorphine and provide full opioid agonists for pain until the patient has recovered and then transition back to buprenorphine. One way of doing this is to replace the buprenorphine with a standing dose of 20–40 mg of methadone daily and supplement that with short-acting opioids as needed.[169] As with patients on methadone, one should expect that the patient will need higher doses than are typically given; this should not be misinterpreted as drug seeking. The data on the clinical effects of continuing or stopping buprenorphine are limited; in one observational study, individuals who had their buprenorphine stopped postoperatively required higher doses of opioid analgesics than those for patients who had it continued.[170]

Treating Pain in Opioid-Dependent Patients

Treating pain in opioid-dependent patients—whether on opioid maintenance treatment or not—is a difficult task for even the most experienced clinicians. On the one hand, clinicians should be conscious of the fact that there is a risk of misuse or diversion of the medication and that individuals with a substance use disorder will often go to great lengths to obtain these drugs. On the other hand, it is wrong to make someone needlessly suffer because of his or her addiction. Clinicians should resist the temptation to punish individuals for their addiction by denying them adequate palliative treatment. It is important to remember that withholding opioid analgesics from someone who is opioid dependent will not cure them of their addiction, and giving them opioids will not necessarily make their addiction worse.

In general, the best policy is to give the patient the benefit of the doubt and aim to effectively treat the pain, but be vigilant for signs of misuse and be ready to act when a patient shows these signs. As with other patients, depending on the nature of the problem, it may be appropriate to begin treatment with opioids, or to start with other agents and then move on to opioids if they are not effective. In the inpatient setting, the dosage can be titrated quickly and the patient's response assessed. However, in the ambulatory setting, assessment of response is more difficult, and diversion or misuse is more of a concern. When prescribing opioids to someone with active opioid use disorder or who is in recovery, it is important to be honest and up front about your concerns and to understand the patient's goals and be clear about your expectations at the beginning of treatment. A treatment agreement may be a useful tool to document this discussion (see Chapter 13, Box 13.1). It is generally prudent to give limited amounts of medication for shorter periods of time and assess these patients more frequently. As with other patients, providers should be on the lookout for signs of prescription drug misuse; urine drug testing may be helpful in this setting. This problem is discussed further in Chapter 13.

For individuals with an active opioid use disorder and acute pain (an acute fracture, for example), intravenous administration of an opioid such as morphine would be appropriate. PCA is often very effective. Given their high tolerance to opioids, opioid-dependent individuals with acute pain generally require higher doses of medication than others and will be less susceptible to the side effects. If the pain is expected to last more than a few days, it would be appropriate to begin a long-acting opioid. In general, it is best to minimize the use of as-needed medication and to rely more on long-acting medication or standing doses of medications to provide better symptom control and avoid a focus on immediate relief. The patient should always be included in the decision-making process and be informed of any changes in advance.

Buprenorphine is generally not the best choice for treatment of severe acute pain, but it may be used in some situations where withdrawal from opioids or detoxification is a concurrent goal—for example, an opioid-dependent individual with an abscess or cellulitis who wishes to stop using opioids. A 4 mg sublingual dose of buprenorphine is roughly equivalent to 10 mg of morphine. In cases where the patient is experiencing severe pain or where withdrawal from opioids is not a goal (for example, someone on methadone maintenance), buprenorphine would *not* be the treatment of choice.

Treating opioid-dependent individuals who have chronic pain is a more difficult task. One strategy is to enroll them in a methadone maintenance program so that they can receive opioids in a controlled and supervised manner. Methadone is generally not effective for 24 hours as an analgesic, so this may need to be supplemented by other medications. Those who earn take-home dosages can split their dose to get a more even analgesic effect. Buprenorphine also has analgesic effect; some studies have reported buprenorphine to be effective for the treatment of chronic pain[171] and suggest that this may be a good option, especially when addiction is a problem or concern.[172] Of note, any physician with a DEA license can prescribe buprenorphine for pain, and there is no limit on the number of patients they can treat for this indication. This is in contrast to the prescribing of buprenorphine for opioid use disorder, which requires a special license and a limit on the number of patients treated.

Notes

1. American Society of Addiction Medicine. Public policy statement on screening for addiction in primary care settings. http://www.asam.org/advocacy/find-a-policy-statement/view-policy-statement/public-policy-statements/2011/12/16/screening-for-addiction-in-primary-care-settings

2. Coulehan JL, Zettler-Segal M, Block M, et al. Recognition of alcoholism and substance abuse in primary care patients. Arch Intern Med 1987;147:349–52.

3. Ray MK, Beach BC, Nicolaidis C, et al. Patient and provider comfort discussing substance use. Fam Med 2013;45:109–17.

4. **Laine C, Hauck WW, Gourevitch MN, et al. Regular outpatient medical and drug abuse care and subsequent hospitalization of persons who use illicit drugs. JAMA 2001;285:2355–62.** *Among Medicaid recipients in New York who were drug users, the adjusted odds of hospitalization were about 20–30% lower among those with regular medical care or drug abuse care (or both).*

5. Saitz R, Horton NJ, Larson MJ, et al. Primary medical care and reductions in addiction severity: a prospective cohort study. Addiction 2005;100:70–8.

6. Saitz R, Horton NJ, Cheng DM, Samet JH. Alcohol counseling reflects higher quality of primary care. J Gen Intern Med 2008; 23:1482–1486.

7. **Weisner C, Mertens J, Parthasarathy S, et al. Integrating primary medical care with addiction treatment: a randomized controlled trial. JAMA 2001;286:1715–23.** *Adults (n = 654) with substance abuse/dependence were randomized to integrated or independent medical and addiction care; 592 (91%) completed 6-month follow-up. Overall, both groups had comparable improvements in addiction outcomes. Among those with substance abuse–related medical conditions, integrated care was associated with improved odds of achieving abstinence.*

8. **Willenbring ML, Olson DH. A randomized trial of integrated outpatient treatment for medically ill alcoholic men. Arch Intern Med 1999;159:1946–52.** *There were 105 participants in this trial. After 2 years, 74% of the surviving IOT patients were abstinent compared with 47% of those receiving the standard care. Mortality was also lower in the IOT group (30% vs. 18%), but this difference was not statistically significant. There was no difference in hospitalization rate.*

9. **Oslin DW, Lynch KG, Maisto SG, et al. A randomized clinical trial of alcohol care management delivered in Department of Veterans Affairs primary care clinics versus specialty addiction treatment. J Gen Intern Med 2014;29:162–8.** *In this 26-week trial, 163 alcohol-dependent subjects were randomly assigned to receive primary care–based alcohol care management (ACM) or referral to specialty outpatient treatment. ACM included a behavioral health provider who met weekly with subjects for motivational interviewing and promoted the use of naltrexone pharmacotherapy.*

10. Lucas GM, Chaudhry A, Hsu J, et al. Clinic-based treatment of opioid-dependent HIV-infected patients versus referral to an opioid treatment program: a randomized trial. Ann Intern Med 2010;152:704–11.

11. Rowe TA, Jacapraro JS, Rastegar DA. Entry into primary care-based buprenorphine treatment is associated with identification and treatment of other chronic medical problems. Addict Sci Clin Pract 2012;7:22.

12. Altice FL, Bruce RD, Lucas GM, et al. HIV treatment outcomes among HIV-infected, opioid-dependent patients receiving buprenorphine/

naloxone treatment within HIV clinical care settings: results from a multisite study. J Acquir Immune Defic Syndr 2011;56(Suppl 1):S22–32.

13. Drainoni ML, Farrell C, Sorensen-Alawad A, et al. Patient perspectives of an integrated program of medical care and substance use treatment. AIDS Patient Care STDS 2014;28:1–11.

14. Hutchinson E, Catlin M, Andrilla CHA, et al. Barriers to primary care physicians prescribing buprenorphine. Ann Fam Med 2014;12:128–33.

15. Fleming MF, Manwell LB, Kraus M, et al. Who teaches residents about the prevention and treatment of substance abuse disorders? A national survey. J Fam Pract 1999;48:725–9.

16. Isaacson JH, Fleming M, Kraus M, et al. A national survey of training in substance use disorders in residency programs. J Study Alcohol 2000;61:912–5.

17. Geller G, Levine DM, Mamon JA, et al. Knowledge, attitudes and reported practices of medical students and house staff regarding the diagnosis and treatment of alcoholism. JAMA 1989;261:115–20.

18. Miller NS, Sheppard LM, Colenda CC, Magen J. Why physicians are unprepared to treat patients who have alcohol- and drug-related problems. Acad Med 2001;76:410–8.

19. Saitz R, Friedmann PD, Sullivan LM, et al. Professional satisfaction experienced when caring for substance abusing patients. J Gen Intern Med 2002;17:373–6.

20. O'Connor PG, Nyquist JG, McLellan AT. Integrating addiction medicine into graduate medical education in primary care: the time has come. Ann Intern Med 2011;154:56–9.

21. Substance Abuse and Mental Health Services Administration, Office of Applied Studies. *The NSDUH Report: Injection Drug Use and Related Risk Behaviors*. Rockville, MD; October 29, 2009.

22. Copeland L, Budd J, Robertson JR, Elton RA. Changing patterns in causes of death in a cohort of injecting drug users, 1980–2001. Arch Intern Med 2004;164:1214–20.

23. Wood E, Tyndall MW, Zhang R, et al. Attendance at supervised injecting facilities and use of detoxification services. N Engl J Med 2006;354:2512–3.

24. Des Jarlais DC, Marmor M, Paone D, et al. HIV incidence among injecting drug users in New York City syringe-exchange programmes. Lancet 1996;348:987–91.

25. Levine OS, Vlahov D, Koehler J, et al. Seroepidemiology of hepatitis B virus in a population of injection drug users. Association with drug injection patterns. Am J Epidemiol 1995;142:331–41.

26. Gjeruldsen SR, Myrang B, Opjordsmoen S. A 25-year follow-up study of drug addicts hospitalised for acute hepatitis: present and past morbidity. Eur Addict Res 2003;9:80–6.

27. Torbenson M, Kannangai R, Astemborski J, et al. High prevalence of occult hepatitis B in Baltimore injection drug users. Hepatology 2004;39:51–7.

28. Cacciola I, Pollicino T, Squadrito G, et al. Occult hepatitis B virus infection in patients with chronic hepatitis C liver disease. N Engl J Med 1999;341:22–6.

29. El-Sherif A, Abou-Shady M, Abou-Zeid H, et al. Antibody to hepatitis B core antigen as a screening test for occult hepatitis B virus infection in Egyptian chronic hepatitis C patients. J Gastroenterol 2009;44:359–64.

30. Hagan H, DesJarlais DC, Friedman SR, et al. Reduced risk of hepatitis B and hepatitis C among injection drug users in the Tacoma syringe exchange program. Am J Public Health 1995;85:1531–7.

31. Armstrong GL, Wasley A, Simard EP, et al. The prevalence of hepatitis C virus infection in the United States, 1999 through 2002. Ann Intern Med 2006;144:705–14.

32. McMahon JM, Simm M, Milano D, Clatts M. Detection of hepatitis C virus in the nasal secretions of an intranasal drug-user. Ann Clin Microbiol Anitmicrob 2004;3:6.

33. Fingerhood MI, Jasinski DR, Sullivan JT. Prevalence of hepatitis C in a chemically dependent population. Arch Intern Med 1993;153:2025–30.

34. Gerlach JT, Diepolder HM, Zachoval R, et al. Acute hepatitis C: high rate of both spontaneous clearance and treatment-induced viral clearance. Gastroenterology 2003;125:80–8.

35. Mehta SH, Cox A, Hoover DR, et al. Protection against persistence of hepatitis C. Lancet 2002;359:1478–83.

36. Gumber SC, Chopra S. Hepatitis C: a multifaceted disease. Review of extrahepatic manifestations. Ann Intern Med 1995;123:615–20.

37. Thomas DL, Astemborski J, Rai RM, et al. The natural history of hepatitis C: host, viral, and environmental factors. JAMA 2000;284:450–6.

38. Kielland KB, Skaug K, Amundsen EJ, Dalgard O. All-cause and liver-related mortality in hepatitis C infected drug users followed for 33 years: a controlled study. J Hepatol 2013;58:31–7.

39. Kohli A, Shaffer A, Sherman A, Kottilil S. Treatment of hepatitis C: a systematic review. JAMA 2014;312:631–40.

40. Bruggmann P, Dampz M, Gerlach T, et al. Treatment outcome in relation to alcohol consumption during hepatitis C treatment: analysis of the Swiss Hepatitis C Cohort Study. Drug Alcohol Depend 2010;100:167–71.

41. Jiao M, Greanya ED, Haque M, et al. Methadone maintenance in liver transplantation. Prog Transplant 2010;20:209–14.

42. Liu LU, Schiano TD, Lau N, et al. Survival and risk of recidivism in methadone-dependent patients undergoing liver transplantation. Am J Transplant 2003;3:1273–7.

43. Turner KM, Hutchinson S, Vickerman P, et al. The impact of needle and syringe provision and opiate substitution therapy on the incidence of HCV in injecting drug users. Addiction 2011;106:1978–88.

44. Tsui JI, Evans JL, Lum PJ, et al. Association of opioid agonist therapy with lower incidence of hepatitis C virus infection in young adult injection drug users. JAMA Intern Med 2014;174:1974–81.

45. Kapadia F, Vlahov D, DesJarlais DC, et al. Does bleach disinfection of syringes protect against hepatitis C infection among young adult injection drug users? Epidemiology 2002:13:738–41.

46. Centers for Disease Control and Prevention. Monitoring selected national HIV prevention objectives by using HIV surveillance data—United States and 6 U.S. dependent areas—2010. HIV Surveillance Supplemental Report 2012;17(No. 3, part A).

47. Centers for Disease Control and Prevention. Estimated HIV incidence in the United States, 2007–2010. HIV Surveillance Supplemental Report 2012;17(No 4).

48. Substance Abuse and Mental Health Services Administration, Center for Behavioral Health Statistics and Quality. The NSDUH Report: HIV/AIDS and Substance Use. Rockville, MD; December 1, 2010.

49. Daar ES, Little S, Pitt J, et al. Diagnosis of primary HIV-1 infection. Ann Intern Med 2001;135:25–9.

50. Chaisson RE, Kerully JC, Moore RD. Race, sex, drug use, and the risk of progression of human immunodeficiency virus disease. N Engl J Med 1995;333:751–6.

51. Selwyn PA, Alcabes P, Hartel D, et al. Clinical manifestations and predictors of disease progression in drug users with human immunodeficiency virus infection. N Engl J Med 1992;327:1697–709.

52. Detels R, Muñoz A, McFarlane G, et al. Effectiveness of potent antiretroviral therapy on time to AIDS and death in men with known HIV infection duration. JAMA 1998;280:1497–503.

53. Wood E, Montaner JS, Yip B, et al. Adherence and plasma HIV RNA responses to highly active antiretroviral therapy among HIV-1 infected injection drug users. CMAJ 2003;169:656–61.

54. Wood E, Hogg RS, Dias Lima V, et al. Highly active antiretroviral therapy and survival in HIV-infected drug users. JAMA 2008;300:550–4.

55. Uhlmann S, Milloy MJ, Kerr T, et al. Methadone maintenance therapy promotes initiation of antiretroviral therapy among injection drug users. Addiction 2010;105:901–13.

56. Hurley SF, Jolley DJ, Kaldor JM. Effectiveness of needle-exchange programmes for prevention of HIV infection. Lancet 1997;349:1797–800.

57. MacArthur GJ, Minozzi S, Martin N, et al. HIV infection incidence is reduced 54% in people with injection drug use who receive opioid agonist treatment. BMJ 2012;345:e5945.

58. de Vos AS, Prins M, Coutinho RA, et al. Treatment as prevention among injection drug users; extrapolating from the Amsterdam cohort study. AIDS 2014;28:911–8.

59. Hudgins R, McCusker J, Stoddard A. Cocaine use and risky injection and sexual behaviors. Drug Alcohol Depend 1995;37:7–14.

60. Gourevitch MN, Hartel D, Schoenbaum EE, et al. A prospective study of syphilis and HIV infection among injection drug users receiving methadone in the Bronx, NY. Am J Public Health 1996;86:1112–5.

61. López-Zetina J, Ford W, Weber M, et al. Predictors of syphilis seroreactivity and prevalence of HIV among street recruited injection drug users in Los Angeles County, 1994-6. Sex Transm Infect 2000;76:462–9.

62. Upchurch DM, Brady WE, Reichart CA, Hook EW III. Behavioral contributions to acquisition of gonorrhea in patients attending an inner city sexually transmitted disease clinic. J Infect Dis 1990;161:938–41.

63. Latka M, Ahern J, Garfein RS, et al. Prevalence, incidence, and correlates of chlamydia and gonorrhea among young adult injection drug users. J Subst Abuse 2001;13:73–88.

64. Binswanger IA, Kral AH, Blumenthal RN, et al. High prevalence of abscesses and cellulitis among community-recruited injection drug users in San Francisco. Clin Infect Dis 2000;30:579–81.

65. Murphy EL, DeVita D, Liu H, et al. Risk factors for skin and soft-tissue abscesses among injection drug users: a case control study. Clin Infect Dis 2001;33:35–40.

66. Charlebois ED, Bangsberg DR, Moss NJ, et al. Population-based community prevalence of methicillin-resistant *Staphylococcus aureus* in the urban poor of San Francisco. Clin Infect Dis 2002;34:425–33.

67. Kluytmans JA, Wertheim HF. Nasal carriage of *Staphylococcus aureus* and prevention of nosocomial infections. Infection 2005;33:3–8.

68. Callahan TE, Schecter WP, Horn JK. Necrotizing soft tissue infection masquerading as cutaneous abscess following illicit drug injection. Arch Surg 1998;133:812–9.

69. Merrison AF, Chidley KE, Dunnett J, Sieradzan KA. Wound botulism associated with subcutaneous drug use. BMJ 2002;325:1020–1.

70. Anonymous. Tetanus after hypodermic injection of morphia. Lancet 1876;108:873.

71. Pascual FB, McGinley EL, Zanardi LR, et al. Tetanus surveillance—United States 1998–200. MMWR Morbid Mortal Wklt Rep 2003:52(SS08):1–8.

72. Arnett EN, Battle WE, Russo JV, Roberts WC. Intravenous injection of talc-containing drugs intended for oral use. A cause of pulmonary granulomatosis and pulmonary hypertension. Am J Med 1976;60:711–8.

73. Sherman CB, Hudson LD, Pierson DJ. Severe precocious emphysema in intravenous methylphenidate (Ritalin) abusers. Chest 1987;92:1085–7.

74. Sporer KA, Dorn E. Heroin-related noncardiogenic pulmonary edema: a case series. Chest 2001;120:1628–32.

75. Lewis JW, Groux N, Elliot JP, et al. Complications of attempted central venous injections performed by drug abusers. Chest 1980;78:613–7.

76. Wilson LE, Thomas DL, Astemborski J, et al. Prospective study of infective endocarditis among injection drug users. J Infect Dis 2002;185:1761–6.

77. Chambers HF, Morris DL, Täuber MG, Modin G. Cocaine use and the risk for endocarditis in intravenous drug users. Ann Intern Med 1987;106:833–6.

78. Marantz PR, Linzer M, Feiner CL, et al. Inability to predict diagnosis in febrile drug abusers. Ann Intern Med 1987;106:823–8.

79. Samet JH, Shevitz A, Fowle J, Singer DE. Hospitalization decision in febrile intravenous drug users. Am J Med 1990;89:53–7.

80. **Chung-Esaki H, Rodriguez RM, Alter H, Cisse B. Validation of a prediction rule for endocarditis in febrile injection drug users. Am J Emerg Med 2014;32:412–6.** *Of 249 subjects presenting to two emergency departments, 18 (7%) had endocarditis. Among those who had none of the three criteria (no murmur, no tachycardia, but presenting with a skin infection), none had endocarditis.*

81. Moreillon P, Que Y. Infective endocarditis. Lancet 2004;363:139–49.

82. Sapico FL, Liquete JA, Sarma RJ. Bone and joint infections in patients with infective endocarditis: review of a 4-year experience. Clin Infect Dis 1996;22:783–7.

83. Hecht SR, Berger M. Right-sided endocarditis in intravenous drug users: prognostic features in 102 episodes. Ann Intern Med 1992;117:560–6.

84. Matthew J, Addai T, Anand A, et al. Clinical features, site of involvement, bacteriologic findings, and outcome of infective endocarditis in intravenous drug users. Arch Intern Med 1995;155:1641–8.

85. Ribera E, Miró J, Cortés E, et al. Influence of human immunodeficiency virus 1 infection and degree of immunosuppression in the clinical characteristics and outcome of infective endocarditis in intravenous drug users. Arch Intern Med 1998;158:2043–50.

86. Heldman AW, Hartert TV, Ray SC, et al. Oral antibiotic treatment of right-sided staphylococcal endocarditis in injection drug users: prospective randomized comparison with parenteral therapy. Am J Med 1996;101:68–76.

87. Mathew J, Abreo G, Namburi K, et al. Results of surgical treatment for infective endocarditis in intravenous drug users. Chest 1995;106:73–7.

88. Vlahov D, Sullivan M, Astemborski J, Nelson KE. Bacterial infections and skin cleaning prior injections among intravenous drug users. Public Health Rep 1992;107:595–8.

89. Lisse JR, Davis CP, Thurmond-Anderle ME. Upper extremity deep venous thrombosis: increased prevalence due to cocaine abuse. Am J Med 1989;87:457–8.

90. Johnson JE, Lucas CE, Ledgerwood AM, Jacobs LA. Infected pseudoaneurysm. A complication of drug addiction. Arch Surg 1984;119:1097–8.

91. Charney MA, Stern PJ. Digital ischemia in clandestine intravenous drug users. J Hand Surg (Am) 1991;16:308–10.

92. Cunningham EE, Brentjens JR, Zielezny MA, et al. Heroin nephropathy. A clinicopathologic and epidemiologic study. Am J Med 1980;68:47–53.

93. Friedman EA, Tao TK. Disappearance of uremia due to heroin-associated nephropathy. Am J Kidney Dis 1995;25:689–93.

94. Perneger TV, Klag MJ, Whelton PK. Recreational drug use: a neglected risk factor for end-stage renal disease. Am J Kidney Dis 2001;38:49–56.

95. do Sameiro Faria M, Sampaio S, Faria V, Carvalho E. Nephropathy associated with heroin abuse in Caucasian patients. Nephrol Dial Transplant 2003;18:2308–13.

96. Neugarten J, Gallo GR, Buxbaum J, et al. Amyloidosis in subcutaneous heroin abusers ("skin poppers' amyloidosis"). Am J Med 1986;81:635–40.

97. Rice EK, Isbel NM, Becker GJ, et al. Heroin overdose and myoglobinuric acute renal failure. J Clin Nephrol 2000;54:449–54.

98. Substance Abuse and Mental Health Services Administration, Medication-Assisted Treatment for Opioid Addiction: 2010 State Profiles, Substance Abuse and Mental Health Services Administration, 2011.

99. Clark HW. The state of buprenorphine treatment. Buprenorphine in the treatment of Opioid Addiction: Reassessment 2010. http://buprenorphine.samhsa.gov/bwns/2010_presentations_pdf/01_Clark_508.pdf. Accessed November 9, 2014.

100. Abs R, Verhelst J, Maeyaert J, et al. Endocrine consequences of long-term intrathecal administration of opioids. J Clin Endocrin Metab 2000;85:2215–22.

101. Mendelson JH, Mendelson JE, Patch VD. Plasma testosterone levels in heroin addiction and during methadone maintenance. J Pharmacol Exp Ther 1975;192:211–7.

102. Bliesener N, Albrecht S, Schwager A, et al. Plasma testosterone and sexual function in men receiving buprenorphine maintenance for opioid dependence. J Clin Endocrinol Metab 2005;90:203–6.

103. Hallinan R1, Byrne A, Agho K, et al. Hypogonadism in men receiving methadone and buprenorphine maintenance treatment. Int J Androl 2009;32:131-9.

104. Aurilio C, Ceccarelli I, Pota V, et al. Endocrine and behavioural effects of transdermal buprenorphine in pain-suffering women of different reproductive ages. Endocr J 2011;58:1071-8.

105. Martell BA, Arnsten JH, Krantz MJ, Gourevitch MN. Impact of methadone treatment on cardiac repolarization and conduction in opioid users. Am J Cardiol 2005;95:915-8.

106. Ansermot N, Albayrak Ö, Schläpfer J, et al. Substitution of (R,S)—methadone by (R)—methadone: impact on QTc interval. Arch Intern Med 2010;170:529-36.

107. Krantz MJ, Lewkowiez L, Hays H, et al. Torsades de pointes associated with very-high-dose methadone. Ann Intern Med 2002;137:501-4.

108. Krantz MJ, Kutinsky IB, Robertson AD, Mehler PS. Dose-related effects of methadone on QT prolongation in a series of patients with torsades de pointes. Pharmacotherapy 2003;23:802-5.

109. Gil M, Sal M, Anguera I, et al. QT prolongation and torsades de pointes in patients infected with human immunodeficiency virus and treated with methadone. Am J Cardiol 2003;92:995-7.

110. Ehret GB, Voide C, Gex-Fabry M, et al. Drug-induced long QT syndrome in injection drug users receiving methadone: high frequency in hospitalized patients and risk factors. Arch Intern Med 2006;166:1280-7.

111. Kao D, Bartelson RB, Khatri V, et al. Trends in reporting methadone-associated cardiac arrhythmia, 1997–2011: an analysis of registry data. Ann Intern Med 2013;158:735-40.

112. **Chugh SS**, Socoteanu C, **Reiner K**, et al. **A community-based evaluation of sudden cardiac death associated with therapeutic levels of methadone. Am J Med 2008;121:66-71.** *Over a 4-year period in Portland, Oregon, 22 sudden cardiac deaths associated with therapeutic levels of methadone were identified. These subjects, compared with 106 consecutive controls, were less likely to have cardiac abnormalities (23% vs. 60%) on autopsy.*

113. Peles E, Bodner G, Kreek MJ, et al. Corrected-QT intervals as related to methadone dose and serum level in methadone maintenance treatment (MMT) patients—a cross-sectional study. Addiction 2007;102:289-300.

114. Anchersen K, Clausen T, Gossop M, et al. Prevalence and clinical relevance of corrected QT interval prolongation during methadone and buprenorphine treatment: a mortality assessment study. Addiction 2009;104:993–9.

115. Krantz MJ, Rowan SB, Mehler PS. Cocaine-related torsade de pointes in a methadone maintenance patient. J Addict Dis 2005;24:53–60.

116. Anson BD, Weaver JGR, Ackerman MJ, et al. Blockade of HERG channels by HIV protease inhibitors. Lancet 2005;365:682–6.

117. Gallagher DP, Kieran J, Sheehan G, et al. Ritonavir-boosted atazanavir, methadone, and ventricular tachycardia: 2 case reports. Clin Infect Dis 2008;47:e36–8.

118. Peles E, Linzy S, Kreek MJ, Adelson M. Prospective study of QTc changes among former opiate addicts since admission to methadone maintenance treatment. J Addict Med 2013;7:428–38.

119. Castro VM, Clements CC, Murphy SN, et al. QT interval and antidepressant use: a cross-sectional study of electronic health records. BMJ 2103;346:f288.

120. Han S, Zhang Y, Chen Q, et al. Fluconazole inhibits hERG K(+) channel by direct block and disruption of protein trafficking. Eur J Pharmacol 2011;650:138–44.

121. Winton JC, Twilla JD. Sudden cardiac arrest in a patient on chronic methadone after the addition of azithromycin. Am J Med Sci 2013;345:160–2.

122. Wedam EF, Bigelow GE, Johnson RE, et al. QT-interval effects of methadone, levomethadyl and buprenorphine in a randomized trial. Arch Intern Med 2007;167:2469–75.

123. Baker JR, Best AM, Pade PA, McCance-Katz EF. Effect of buprenorphine and antiretroviral agents on the QT interval in opioid-dependent patients. Ann Pharmacother 2006;40:392–6.

124. Fredheim OM, Borchgrevink PC, Hergrenaes L, et al. Opioid switching from morphine to methadone causes a minor but not clinically significant increase in QTc time: a prospective 9-month follow-up study. J Pain Symptom Manage 2006;32:180–5.

125. Fanoe S, Jensen GB, Sjøgren P, Korsgaard MP, Grunnet M. Oxycodone is associated with dose-dependent QTc prolongation in patients and low-affinity inhibiting of hERG activity in vitro. Br J Clin Pharmacol 2009;67:172–9.

126. Mintzer MZ, Stitzer ML. Cognitive impairment in methadone maintenance patients. Drug Alcohol Depend 2002;67:41–51.

127. Mintzer MZ, Copersino ML, Stitzer ML. Opioid abuse and cognitive performance. Drug Alcohol Depend 2005;78:225–30.

128. Mintzer MZ, Correia CJ, Strain EC. A dose-effect study of repeated administration of buprenorphine/naloxone on performance in opioid-dependent volunteers. Drug Alcohol Depend 2004;74:205–9.

129. Rapelli P, Fabritius C, Alho H, et al. Methadone vs. buprenorphine/naloxone during early opioid substitution treatment: a naturalistic comparison of cognitive performance relative to health controls. BMC Clin Pharmacol 2007;7:5.

130. Lenné MG, Dietze P, Rumbold GR, et al. The effects of the opioid pharmacotherapies methadone, LAAM and buprenorphine, alone and in combination with alcohol, on simulated driving. Drug Alcohol Depend 2003;72:271–8.

131. Shmygalev S, Damm M, Weckbecker K, et al. The impact of long-term maintenance treatment with buprenorphine on complex psychomotor and cognitive function. Drug Alcohol Depend 2011;117:190–7.

132. Soyka M, Hock B, Kagerer S, et al. Less impairment on one portion of a driving-relevant psychomotor battery in buprenorphine-maintained than in methadone-maintained patients: results of a randomized clinical trial. J Clin Psychopharmacol 2005;25:490–3.

133. Corsenac P, Lagarde E, Gadegbeku B, et al. Road traffic crashes and prescribed methadone and buprenorphine: a French registry-based case-control study. Drug Alcohol Depend 2012;123:91–7.

134. Wang JS, DeVane CL. Involvement of CYP3A4, CYP2C8 and CYP2D6 in the metabolism of (R)- and (S)-methadone in vitro. Drug Metab Dispos 2003;31:742–7.

135. Rogers JF, Nafziger AN, Bertino JS. Pharmacogenetics affects dosing, efficacy, and toxicity of cytochrome p450-metabolized drugs. Am J Med 2002;113:746–50.

136. **Clarke SM, Mulcahy FM, Tija J, et al. Pharmacokinetics of methadone in HIV-positive patients receiving the non-nulceoside reverse transcriptase inhibitor efavirenz. Br J Clin Pharmacol 2001;51:213–7.** *In 11 patients, the mean methadone area under the curve (AUC) was reduced by >50% after starting efavirenz; 9 reported withdrawal symptoms. The mean methadone dose increase required was 22% (15–30 mg/day).*

137. **Clarke SM, Mulcahy FM, Tija J, et al. Pharmacokinetic interactions of nevirapine and methadone and guidelines for use of nevirapine to treat injection drug users. Clin Infect Dis 2001;33:1595–7.** *In 8 subjects, the mean methadone area under the curve (AUC) was reduced by >50% after starting nevirapine; 6 reported withdrawal symptoms; the mean methadone dose increase required was 16%.*

138. McCance-Katz EF, Rainey PM, Friedland G, Jatlow P. The protease inhibitor lopinavir-ritonavir may produce opiate withdrawal in methadone-maintained patients. Clin Infect Dis 2003;37:476–82.

139. Cao YJ, Smith PF, Wire MB, et al. Pharmacokinetics and pharmacodynamics of methadone enantiomers after coadministration with fosamprenavir-ritonavir in opioid-dependent subjects. Pharmacotherapy 2008;28:863–74.

140. Clarke S, Mulcahy F, Bergin C, et al. Absence of opioid withdrawal symptoms in patients receiving methadone and the protease inhibitor lopinavir-ritonavir. Clin Infect Dis 2002;34:1143–5.

141. **Kreek MJ, Garfield JW, Gutjahr CL, Giusti LM. Rifampin-induced methadone withdrawal. N Engl J Med 1976;294:1104–6.** *Among 86 patients with tuberculosis on methadone maintenance, 30 received rifampin and 21 (70%) developed withdrawal symptoms. None of the 56 who received regimens that did not include rifampin developed withdrawal symptoms.*

142. Brown LS, Sawyer RC, Li R, et al. Lack of pharmacologic interaction between rifabutin and methadone in HIV-infected former injecting drug users. Drug Alcohol Depend 1996;43:71–7.

143. Tong TG, Pond SM, Kreek MJ, et al. Phenytoin-induced methadone withdrawal. Ann Intern Med 1981;94:349–51.

144. Liu SJ, Wang RI. Case report of barbituate-induced enhancement of methadone metabolism and withdrawal syndrome. Am J Psychiatry 1984;141:1287–8.

145. Kuhn KL, Halikas JA, Kemp KD. Carbamazepine treatment of cocaine dependence in methadone maintenance patients with dual opiate-cocaine addiction. NIDA Res Monogr 1989;95:316–7.

146. Eich-Hochli D, Oppliger R, Golay KP, et al. Methadone maintenance treatment and St. John's Wort—a case report. Pharmacopsychiatry 2003;36:35–7.

147. Wines JD Jr, Weiss RD. Opioid withdrawal during risperidone treatment. J Clin Psychopharmacol 1999;19:265–7.

148. Hamilton SP, Nunes EV, Janal M, Weber L. The effect of sertraline on methadone plasma levels in methadone-maintenance patients. Am J Addict 2000;9:63–9. *Depressed patients on methadone (n = 31) were randomly assigned to sertraline or placebo and followed for 12 weeks. Those on sertraline had an increase in serum methadone levels during the first 6 weeks; this declined toward baseline during the second 6 weeks. None had signs or symptoms of toxicity.*

149. Begre S, von Bardeleben U, Ladewig D, et al. Paroxetine increases steady-state concentrations of (R)-methadone in CYP2D6 extensive but not poor metabolizers. J Clin Psychopharmacol 2002;22:211–5.

150. Alderman CP, Frith PA. Fluvoxamine-methadone interaction. Aust NZ J Psychiatry 1999;33:99–101.

151. Batki SL, Manfredi LB, Jacob P III, Jones RT. Fluoxetine for cocaine dependence in methadone maintenance: quantitative plasma and urine cocaine/benzoylecgonine concentrations. J Clin Psychopharmacol 1994;13:243–50.

152. Venkatakrishnan K, von Moltke LL, Greenblatt DJ. Effects of the antifungal agents on oxidative drug metabolism: clinical relevance. Clin Pharmacokinet 2000;38:111–80.

153. Cobb MN, Desai J, Brown LS, et al. The effect of fluconazole on the clinical pharmacokinetics of methadone. Clin Pharmacol Ther 1998;63:655–62.

154. Liu P, Foster G, Labadie R, et al. Pharmacokinetic interaction between voriconazole and methadone at steady state in patients on methadone therapy. Antimicrob Agents Chemother 2007;51:110–8.

155. Herrlin K, Segerdahl M, Gustafsson LL, Kalso E. Methadone, ciprofloxacin, and adverse drug reactions. Lancet 2000;356:2069–70.

156. Torrens M, Castillo C, San L, et al. Plasma methadone concentrations as an indicator of opioid withdrawal symptoms and heroin use in a methadone maintenance program. Drug Alcohol Depend 1998;52:193–200.

157. Bell J, Seres V, Bowron P, et al. The use of serum methadone levels in patients receiving methadone maintenance. Clin Pharmacol Ther 1988;43:623–9.

158. Iguchi MY, Handelsman L, Bickel WK, Griffiths RR. Benzodiazepine and sedative use/abuse by methadone maintenance clients. Drug Alcohol Depend 1993;32:257–66. *Clients in methadone*

programs in Baltimore, Philadelphia, and New York City (n = 547) were asked about sedative use; overall, 84% reported using these agents at one time and 50% reported using in the last 6 months. Among the benzodiazepines, diazepam, lorazepam, and alprazolam were frequently used to get a high or sold for money.

159. Bruce RD, McCance-Katz E, Kharasch ED, et al. Pharmacokinetic interactions between buprenorphine and antiretroviral medications. Clin Infect Dis 2006;43(Suppl 4):S216–3.

160. McCance-Katz EF, Moody DE, Smith PF, et al. Interactions between buprenorphine and antiretrovirals. II. The protease inhibitors nelfinavir, lopinavir/ritonavir, and ritonavir. Clin Infect Dis 2006;43(Suppl 4):S235–46.

161. McCance-Katz EF, Moody DE, Morse GD, et al. Interactions between buprenorphine and antiretrovirals. I. The nonnucleoside reverse-transcriptase inhibitors efavirenz and delavirdine. Clin Infect Dis 2006;43(Suppl 4):S224–34.

162. Bruce RD, Altice FL. Three case reports of a clinical pharmacokinetic interaction with buprenorphine and atazanavir plus ritonavir. AIDS 2006;20:783–4.

163. Rosenblum A, Joseph H, Fong C, et al. Prevalence and characteristics of chronic pain among chemically dependent patients in methadone maintenance and residential treatment facilities. JAMA 2003;289:2370–8.

164. Zhang Y, Ahmed S, Vo T, et al. Increased pain sensitivity in chronic pain subjects on opioid therapy: a cross-sectional study using quantitative sensory testing. Pain Med 2014; doi: 10.1111/pme.12606.

165. Alford DP, Compton P, Samet JH. Acute pain management for patients receiving maintenance methadone or buprenorphine treatment. Ann Intern Med 2006;144:127–34.

166. Peng PHW, Tumber PS, Gourlay D. Review article: perioperative pain management of patients on methadone therapy. Can J Anesth 2005;52:513–23.

167. Fultz JM, Senay EC. Guidelines for the management of hospitalized narcotic addicts. Ann Intern Med 1975;82:815–8.

168. Santiago-Palma J, Khojainova N, Kornick C, et al. Intravenous methadone in the management of chronic cancer pain: safe and effective starting doses when substituting methadone for fentanyl. Cancer 2001;92:1919–25.

169. Alford DP, Compton P, Samet JH. Acute pain management for patients receiving maintenance methadone or buprenorphine therapy. Ann Intern Med 2006;144:127–34.

170. MacIntyre PE, Russell RA, Usher KA, et al. Pain relief and opioid requirements in the first 24 hours after surgery in patients taking buprenorphine and methadone opioid substitution therapy. Anesth Intensive Care 2013;41:222–30.

171. Daitch J, Frey ME, Silver D, et al. Conversion of chronic pain patients from full-opioid agonists to sublingual buprenorphine. Pain Physician 2012;15(3 Suppl):ES59–66.

172. Malinhoff HL, Barkin RL, Wilson G. Sublingual buprenorphine is effective in the treatment of chronic pain syndrome. Am J Therapeut 2005;12:379–84.

15

Psychiatric Co-occurring Disorders

Kenneth B. Stoller

pharmacotherapies, psychotherapeutic approaches are a mainstay of treatment.

Psychotic Disorders   456

Schizophrenia is particularly disabling and associated with an increased risk for substance use disorders, particularly nicotine. Antipsychotic medications can be effective, but persistent negative symptoms warrant comprehensive, supportive approaches with sufficient ancillary services.

Personality Disorders   459

Those with personality disorders, especially borderline and antisocial personality disorders, have high rates of substance use disorders and can be a challenge to treat. A strong team-based approach, psychosocial treatments, and sometimes medications can improve outcomes.

Attention Deficit/Hyperactivity Disorder (ADHD)   462

Those with ADHD are at increased risk for substance use disorders. Impairing symptoms of inattention and impulsivity may persist into adulthood, complicating engagement with and outcomes of substance use disorder treatment. Medications can be helpful, but care must be taken when considering prescribing of stimulants.

Background

Psychiatric and substance use disorders are common and, not surprisingly, are often found concurrently in individuals seeking care. Having one of these classes of disorders increases risk for development of the other, and the presence of one complicates the treatment and course of the other. Individuals with co-occurring psychiatric and substance use disorders have been referred to as "dual-diagnosed." However, that term oversimplifies this multimorbid population, as there is also overrepresentation of chronic somatic illnesses, including human immunodeficiency virus (HIV), chronic obstructive pulmonary disease (COPD), diabetes, and hepatitis, as well as chronic pain syndrome, and a host of psycho-social struggles.

This chapter will provide a brief review of the association between psychiatric and substance use symptomology and diagnosis. It will also address the various ways that the presence of co-occurring disorders can affect outcomes of psychiatric and substance use disorder treatment, and discuss strategies that may assist in maximizing treatment engagement and effectiveness. It is beyond the scope of this handbook to provide a thorough guide to the diagnosis and management of a broad range of psychiatric disorders. Nor does it provide a detailed review of the relative efficacy of particular medications used for the treatment of psychiatric disorders. The interested reader can refer to more detailed discussions of such topics in any one of several excellent general psychiatric textbooks.[1,2] The Substance Abuse and Mental Health Services Administration has also issued treatment guidelines for individuals with co-occurring substance use and mental disorders; this Treatment Improvement Protocol (TIP 42)[3] is a useful resource for those who would like to explore these issues in more depth. It can be obtained free of charge through their website (www.store.samhsa.gov).

Epidemiology

A number of studies have shown that individuals with a history of psychiatric disorders have higher rates of substance use disorder. Conversely, individuals with substance use disorder are at increased risk of having psychiatric disorders. It should be noted that much of the data comes from treatment-seeking populations, and this may result in an overestimate of the actual prevalence of co-occurring disorders and their association. Nonetheless, these associations have been observed in large epidemiological studies such as the Epidemiologic Catchment Area (ECA) study,[4] conducted in the United States between 1980 and 1984. In that study, among individuals with a psychiatric disorder, the odds ratio (OR) of having any substance use disorder was 2.7; conversely, among those with one or more substance use disorders, the odds ratio for having a psychiatric disorder was 3.0. This association between substance use disorders and psychiatric disorders was observed for all major substances of abuse and all major categories of psychiatric diagnoses. Table 15.1 provides data from this study on the lifetime prevalence rates of a number of psychiatric disorders, and the OR of substance use disorder associated with each. The 2013 National Survey of Drug Use and Health (NSDUH)[5] reported that, in the past year, 18.5% of adults aged 18 or older had a mental illness; 4.2% were characterized as having had a serious mental illness; and 3.9% had serious thoughts of suicide; 7.7 million (17.6%) of the 43.8 million adults with any

TABLE 15.1 Lifetime Prevalence of Alcohol or Illicit Drug Use Disorder (Abuse or Dependence) among Persons with Psychiatric Disorders

Psychiatric Disorder	Overall Lifetime Prevalence of Disorder	Lifetime Prevalence of Substance Abuse or Dependence	Odds Ratio*
Schizophrenia	1.5%	47.0%	4.6
Antisocial personality disorder	2.6%	83.6%	29.6
Anxiety disorders	14.6%	23.7%	1.7
Obsessive-compulsive disorder	2.5%	32.8%	2.5
Affective (mood) disorders	8.3%	32.0%	2.6
Any (non–substance use) psychiatric disorder	16.2%	28.9%	2.7

*Odds of substance abuse or dependence among those with the psychiatric disorder (compared with those without the disorder).

Source: Regier DA, Farmer ME, Rae DS, et al. Comorbidity of mental disorders with alcohol and other drug abuse. Results from the Epidemiologic Catchment Area (ECA) Study. JAMA 1990;264(19):2511–8.

mental illness also had a substance use disorder, compared to 10.5% of those without any mental illness. Studies from other countries have also found an association between substance use disorders and psychiatric disorders.[6]

Although these studies did not include it in their analyses, nicotine addiction is also associated with psychiatric disorders. In one study, among individuals with nicotine dependence, the 12-month prevalence of mood disorder was 21% (OR: 3.3), of anxiety disorder 22% (OR: 2.7), and of personality disorder 32% (OR: 3.3).[7]

Assessment

The assessment and diagnosis of psychiatric disorders among patients in or entering addiction treatment can be a complex undertaking. There is no universally accepted assessment strategy; methods are varied, as are the time frames for completion. The gold standard is a full clinical evaluation by a trained expert in psychiatric assessment; however, this may not be practical for all patients in all settings. Fortunately, there are several well-studied instruments for general psychiatric assessments that may be used, ranging from self-assessment questionnaires completed by the patient to instruments implemented by a trained professional. Self-rated questionnaires are more easily performed in nonpsychiatric settings and require less effort by staff. Although they can characterize psychiatric symptomology, they cannot be relied on to produce definitive psychiatric diagnoses. A commonly used example of a general psychiatric symptom questionnaire is the Symptom Checklist-90-R (SCL-90),[8] which provides useful information about reported psychological distress across specific domains such as depression or anxiety. There are also tools that may be used for assessment of more specific common psychiatric symptomology. The Patient Health Questionnaire is another general screening tool for psychiatric symptomology, but its length makes it less practical to use in clinical settings. The module for depression (PHQ-9)[9] is the most common screening tool for depression. It rates the frequency of symptoms factoring into a severity index and includes a question regarding suicidal ideation. A two-question version can be used as an initial depression screening. The Beck Depression Inventory[10] is another rapidly administered questionnaire that rates depressive features over the prior week. In regard to structured interviews, the Structured Clinical Interview for DSM-IV (SCID) is a semi-structured interview that produces Axis I and Axis II disorders based on DSM criteria.[11,12] It can be used to assess for mood, psychotic, anxiety, eating, and personality disorders, in addition to substance use disorders. A new version for DSM-5 is forthcoming. Interviewers should be well trained to enable them to ask the given interview questions and then reword the questions if needed to clarify responses. The Diagnostic Interview Schedule (DIS)[13] is a structured interview that also produces diagnoses based on DSM criteria. It requires less training than the SCID, since there are specific instructions that must be adhered to regarding how questions are asked.

Independent versus Induced Psychiatric Disorder

The symptom clusters associated with substance intoxication, withdrawal, and chronic use can overlap remarkably with the symptoms of some non–substance use psychiatric disorders. Isolated or syndromal affective dysfunction (depression or euphoria), severe anxiety, psychosis (hallucinations, delusions, or thought disorder), cognitive changes, and maladaptive behavioral tendencies are hallmark features of common psychiatric disorders such as major depressive, bipolar, adjustment, generalized anxiety, delirium, and personality disorders. In order to predict the course of symptoms and embark on an effective treatment course, it is critical to discern whether the presenting problems are most consistent with an etiology related to substance use disorder, independent psychiatric disorder, or a combination thereof.

Before suggesting evaluation strategies, it is worthwhile mentioning that in the medical literature, the terms *primary* versus *secondary* psychiatric syndrome are frequently cited, rather than *independent* versus *induced*. This is problematic, as this language can imply a temporal relationship between the onset of psychiatric and substance use disorders, rather than indicating etiology. Psychiatric disorder and substance use disorder can each emerge at various ages, even in childhood. The clinician should not assume that the "primary" (first-occurring) disorder is the primary cause of all subsequent symptomology.

The most helpful tool in discerning whether a patient's psychiatric symptom cluster is most consistent with an independent psychiatric disorder or is induced by substance use is a careful past and present history, attending meticulously to the time course of substance use and psychiatric symptoms.[14,15] In a substance-induced psychiatric disorder, there is evidence that the onset or the decline of psychiatric symptoms are, over time, preceded by changes (initiation, cessation, increase, or decrease) in substance use. Conversely, the presence of episodic symptomology that has no relation to changes in substance use lends itself to a formulation of an independent psychiatric disorder. An exception is when ongoing substance use leads to the gradual development of persistent symptoms, such in the case of alcoholic hallucinosis. While it is possible for an individual with prior history of an independent psychiatric disorder to later have an episode that clearly appears to have been preceded by changes in substance use, a simpler way to formulate that presentation is as a recurrence of the independent psychiatric disorder, triggered by recent changes in substance use. The therapeutic approach to that episode can be individualized (whether or not to employ psychopharmacology or psychotherapy or both) on the basis of factors such as symptom severity, as well as prior remission with abstinence versus need for targeted psychiatric treatment. Table 15.2 provides general guidance related to the determination of independent versus substance-induced psychiatric disorder. In either case, psychiatric symptoms must be recognized, acknowledged, and attended to, particularly if thoughts of harm to self or others are present.

Other Assessment Considerations

It is critical to recognize that patients with substance use disorders are also at elevated risk for (somatic) medical conditions—acute

TABLE 15.2 Symptom Time Course Patterns Suggestive of Independent versus Substance-Induced Psychiatric Disorder

Suggestive of IndependentPsychiatric Disorder	Suggestive of Substance-Induced Psychiatric Disorder
First episode occurred prior to onset of substance use	All episodes with symptom onset/offset following changes in substance use
Clear episodes during periods of extended substance abstinence	No episodes during extended periods of substance abstinence
Symptoms continue for more than 1–2 weeks after substance cessation	Symptoms primarily remit within 1–2 weeks after substance cessation
Prior documented episodes of clear independent psychiatric disorder with good response to medication	No prior episodes of clear independent psychiatric disorder with good response to medication

or chronic. These conditions, in turn, can present in such a way that symptoms are confused for those present in psychiatric disorders. For example, patients presenting with new hallucinations (especially visual), confusion, psychomotor slowing, or acute agitation may be exhibiting signs of delirium caused by potentially dangerous medical problems, such as an opportunistic infection in an HIV-infected individual or hepatic encephalopathy associated with end-stage liver disease. Depressed mood, as another example, can be the presenting symptom of medical diseases, such as hypothyroidism or Parkinson's disease. A thorough medical evaluation with consideration of potentially reversible somatic conditions as the possible cause of the presenting symptoms is an essential prerequisite to making a definitive determination that the etiology is related to a psychiatric disorder, whether independent or substance induced.

In terms of potential for suicide, risk is increased if the patient has had any prior suicide attempts, has had high suicidal preoccupation and intent, or has formulated a plan. The availability of lethal means, such as firearms, would be particularly concerning. Risk is also increased if there is a family history of completed suicide, active mental illness, current negative life events, serious medical illness, and, of course, active substance abuse. Similarly, for patients with possible homicidal ideation, the provider should assess whether there is an identifiable person threatened, whether the threatened person is aware, current access to weapons, and past history of violence toward others. Each of these factors should be weighed when determining the current danger to self and others, and what actions may need to be taken to mitigate that risk.

General Treatment Strategies

Patients identified as having co-occurring psychiatric and substance use disorders comprise a group at risk of poor addiction treatment performance.[16,17,18,19] They may require treatment for their psychiatric condition in order to reduce distress and morbidity associated with the disorder, and thereby enhance the potential for more positive addiction treatment engagement and outcome. However, as indicated earlier, symptoms present early in treatment may abate along with, or shortly after, stabilization of substance use. Therefore, it is important for the provider to stress the need of the patient to abstain from substance use in order to determine the appropriate diagnosis and ultimate need for specific treatment(s).

Pharmacotherapy

If the patient continues to exhibit continued significant psychiatric symptomology even after 2 or more weeks of substance abstinence, referral for psychiatric evaluation, and possible pharmacotherapy, is indicated. A meta-analysis of studies between 1970 and 2003 concluded that the diagnosis of depression was best determined after at least 1 week of abstinence.[20] Prescribing a psychotropic medication immediately after treatment presentation may reinforce the patient's problematic belief that an independent depression or anxiety is the primary cause of their substance use, minimize the importance of focusing on addiction recovery, and justify the patient's self-medicating in the future. Also, as symptoms decline over time, it may be unclear to future care providers whether the improvement was due to the pharmacological treatment of an independent disorder or whether it was the result of other factors such as cessation of drug use, stabilized environment, and reduced situational stress. The medication will therefore be more likely to be continued, potentially with no benefit, and carrying with it possible adverse effects. Additionally, a determination of an independent psychiatric disorder may be falsely "confirmed" on the basis of the apparent "medication response." An exception to this approach of delaying consideration of pharmacotherapy may be taken when past records, a meticulous timeline of symptoms and substance use, and outside informants provide a clear history of independent psychiatric disorder, and especially if there has been a clear response to specific medications or other specialized treatments previously. For these patients, beginning targeted psychiatric treatment concurrently while addressing addictive disorders can help improve the morale of the patient and provide for an earlier onset of effect from psychiatric treatments that may take several weeks before emergence of significant clinical effect.

Once a decision to start pharmacotherapy is made, the choice of agent should be determined with some consideration of abuse potential. The use of sedatives such as benzodiazepines should be avoided for considerations such as diversion, misuse, need for escalating dose, withdrawal potential, toxicity, and reduced ability to monitor for illicit sedative use. In addition, sedated patients are less able to process information and participate in meaningful recovery activities such as employment, school, counseling, and prosocial activities. In rare situations where prescribing more highly abusable medications such as benzodiazepines appears unavoidable, it is best to consider safeguards such as limiting the duration of treatment, using low doses, writing short prescriptions, performing medication checks (such as pill counts), and recruiting the assistance of family to monitor medication administration, storage, and effects. Finally, the regular use of prescription drug monitoring programs (PDMPs) is highly encouraged for any provider of services for patients with substance use disorders. This topic is covered further in Chapter 13.

Psychosocial Treatment

In addition to psychopharmacological approaches, counseling and psychotherapy can be helpful. Factors such as severity of illness, treatment setting, and expertise of the provider determine whether such services would best be arranged through referral to a community mental health center. Many studies have demonstrated the efficacy of individual and group-based psychotherapy for improving addiction treatment and psychiatric outcomes in this population.[21,22] However, the delivery of these verbal therapies can be thwarted by a number of factors, including limited insurance coverage, stigma related to psychiatric diagnosis and treatment, and poor adherence to scheduled sessions. Whenever possible, treatment models and structures should be employed that reinforce adherence to verbal therapies, such as co-located psychiatric treatment, close collaboration between providers, or behavioral contingencies. This can enhance outcome by increasing the effective "dose" of verbal therapies actually delivered.[23,24]

Care Coordination

When separate providers deliver addiction and psychiatric treatment services, close coordination of care is of paramount importance. Individuals with co-occurring addictive and psychiatric disorders are vulnerable to confusion about treatment recommendations and requirements, poor motivation for interventions that are not directly reinforcing, and especially in personality-disordered patients, engaging in splitting behaviors. Ongoing communication between providers, patients, and their families can help clarify understanding of the treatment plan and reduce the impact of splitting behaviors. Making adherence to verbal therapies a condition for provision of ongoing essential pharmacological treatments, especially those that are more reinforcing such as buprenorphine or methadone, has been shown in a number of studies to improve adherence and treatment outcome.[25,26]

Other Treatment Considerations

For patients with severe psychiatric symptomology that presents clear danger to the patient or others (such as suicidal or homicidal ideation) or that interferes with the patient's ability to engage meaningfully in treatment (such as psychosis), an inpatient psychiatric admission may be warranted. Relatedly, some patients exhibiting psychiatric symptoms are unable to achieve substance abstinence within 1–2 weeks. They may continue to have positive drug tests, report ongoing use of large amounts of substances, continue high-risk behaviors, and repeatedly present for care in an intoxicated or withdrawal state. These patients have elevated ongoing risk factors on multiple ASAM Criteria dimensions and may require a residential level of care.[27] Admission of such patients to a residential unit can be quite helpful, by facilitating initial abstinence and to sort out whether the symptoms are consistent with an independent disorder. Finally, ongoing work on aspects of the patient's recovery foundation, including optimizing somatic medical care, addressing chronic pain, improving sleep and diet, building a social support network, and beginning to engage in productive, spiritual and recreational activities, can also impact recovery from psychiatric disorders in very powerful ways.

Mood Disorders

Depression

Common independent mood disorders among substance-addicted patients include major depression, bipolar disorder, and dysthymic disorder. Of these, major depression is the most prevalent disorder in the general population, and substance-addicted populations carry even higher rates. In a study of individuals presenting for outpatient treatment of major depression, 27.3% were nicotine dependent, 6.1% abused or were dependent on alcohol, and 4.6% abused or were dependent on other drugs; overall, 33% had a current substance use disorder and 60% had had one at some point during their lifetime.[28] Conversely, in a study of 747 individuals entering a substance abuse treatment program, 29% had depression, in contrast to just 3% of matched controls.[29] In the Epidemiological Catchment Area study,[4] affective disorders were found to be associated with increased lifetime risk of abuse of alcohol (OR: 1.9), cocaine (OR: 5.9), opiates (OR: 5.0), amphetamines (OR: 5.7), barbiturates (OR: 6.6), and hallucinogens (OR: 5.9). Of the affective disorders, individuals with bipolar disorders had a particularly high risk of substance use disorders (OR: 6.6 vs. 1.9 for those with major depression). That said, there is considerable variability in rates of major depression reported in studies of individuals with substance use disorders. For example, among patients with opioid dependence, the lifetime rate of major depression has been reported as low as 16% and as high as 54%, while the prevalence of current major depression ranges from 0% to 26%.[30] The lack of a standard accepted time frame for evaluation accounts for a large degree of the variability in rates of depression among newly admitted patients to substance abuse treatment.

Higher rates of depressive disorder may be accounted for in part by individuals out of treatment or, among addiction patient populations, those with very recent admission. Often, depression symptomology among these groups eventually reveals itself to be substance induced or an adjustment disorder in the setting of recent stressors. Frequently, low mood is associated not just with the direct effects of the abused substance or related withdrawal; low mood may also be connected meaningfully with substance use—related to guilt and shame associated with failure to control use and with addiction-related behaviors (e.g., crime or failure to meet responsibilities). Low mood can improve remarkably within days of drug abstinence and early engagement in addiction treatment and supportive counseling.

Features of major depression include low mood; diminished pleasure, interest, or energy; changes in appetite or sleep; physical or mental agitation or slowness; and thoughts of death or suicide. The presence of current major depression has been found to be associated with poorer addiction treatment outcome in a variety of settings.[17,31,32,33] Similarly, but not as thoroughly studied, symptoms of dysthymia—chronic low-grade depressive symptoms that may persist well after initiation of addiction treatment—can adversely affect prognosis. Alcohol use is associated with symptoms of depression and anxiety,[34] and some features can persist for many weeks after initiation of abstinence. A severe depressive syndrome can occur for several days after a cocaine or amphetamine binge and supportive treatments are indicated. Regular marijuana users report elevated rates of depression, in addition to impairments in cognitive function. Since addiction treatment alone is often associated with improvement in symptoms,[35,36] aggressive treatment of the substance use disorder is key.

A number of studies have addressed pharmacological treatment of depression in patients with substance use disorders. In general, treatment benefits the patient, and outcomes are no different than those found in the general population. Moreover, a recently published study demonstrated that retention in substance abuse treatment is higher when an antidepressant is prescribed to individuals with co-occurring depression.[37] Tricyclic antidepressants (TCAs) have been the most studied agents and have generally been found to have high efficacy, along with other noradrenergic or mixed-action antidepressants.[20,38] When taken at bedtime, the potential for sedation with a TCA can enhance adherence. The presence of a therapeutic window in relation to serum levels helps the prescriber optimize care; the efficacy of TCAs in the treatment of chronic pain is another positive feature. On the other hand, adverse effects (such as dry mouth, constipation, or orthostatic hypotension), drug interactions, and toxicity potential in case of overdose are factors that limit the use of TCAs. Some of the most used antidepressants currently include the selective serotonin reuptake inhibitors (SSRIs), for which studies of efficacy seem less consistently positive. However, good tolerability and favorable safety profiles have made SSRIs common first-line treatments. Monoamine oxidase inhibitors (MAOIs) are not recommended for this population because of their severe and potentially fatal interactions with many prescribed and over-the-counter medications, alcoholic beverages, drugs of abuse, and foods. Medications that may be used to augment antidepressant effects include lithium, atypical antipsychotics, and antiepileptics drugs. Alone or in combination with medications, verbal psychotherapies are also effective treatments for depression. A recent study demonstrated that for patients with severe, non-chronic major depression, a combination of cognitive-behavioral therapy (CBT) and optimized antidepressant medication was more effective than treatment with medication alone.[39]

Bipolar Disorder

Bipolar disorder is characterized by distinct periods of mania (in bipolar I) or hypomania (in bipolar II), typically alternating with periods of depression. Symptoms of mania may include elevated self-attitude, decreased need for sleep, hypertalkativeness, racing thoughts, distractibility, psychomotor agitation, and risky behavior.[40] A number of studies indicate that persons with concurrent bipolar disorder and substance use problems often suffer more severe episodes of mania[41] and take longer for symptoms to remit.[42] They tend to have a more severe disease course, are more likely to require hospitalization,[43] and are at higher risk for suicide attempts.[44] In the ECA study, individuals with bipolar disorder had an increased lifetime risk of alcohol abuse or dependence (43.6%; OR: 5.1) and of illicit substance use disorder (33.6%; OR: 8.3).[4] In a study of 288 outpatients with bipolar disorder, a lifetime history of substance use disorder was highest for alcohol (33%), followed by marijuana (16%), non-cocaine stimulants (9%), cocaine (9%), opiates (7%), and hallucinogens (6%).[45] It should be noted that the self-report of a past diagnosis of bipolar disorder is very common among those presenting for addiction treatment; however, this is not uncommonly due to misinterpretation of the effects of drug or alcohol use, such as irritability, impulsivity, mood lability, and insomnia.

Treatment can be challenging for patients with bipolar disorder and, in particular, those with co-occurring substance use disorders. Three troublesome features of bipolar disorder are euphoria, poor insight, and disinhibition. Mania and hypomania, especially the latter, can at times be experienced as pleasurable or otherwise desirable due to increased productivity, creativity, and feelings of competence and well-being. Impaired insight makes it difficult for the treatment provider to persuade the patient to continue taking medications that may reverse these features. Disinhibition makes it difficult for the individual to resist urges to use alcohol and drugs despite knowledge of potential negative consequences. The engagement of family and other supports, delivery of rehabilitative services that enhance self-management skills, and an integrated or closely coordinated care structure can be useful. One small controlled study of patients with bipolar disorder and substance use disorder reported that integrated group therapy was associated with significant improvements in addiction outcomes.[46]

The foundation of pharmacological treatment of bipolar disorder is mood stabilizers and, in particular, lithium and antiepileptic drugs such as divalproex sodium. Carbamazepine can be effective as well, but care must be taken in patients on methadone maintenance because of hepatic induction of methadone metabolism resulting in precipitated opioid withdrawal. Lamotrigine is another antiepileptic approved by the FDA for the maintenance treatment of adults with bipolar disorder and is especially helpful for the depression of bipolar depression. However, its use has been limited by safety concerns, including boosting the effect of central nervous system depressants and the potential for development of a potentially dangerous rash, including Stevens-Johnson's syndrome. A number of second-generation antipsychotic (neuroleptic) medications (e.g., aripiprazole, quetiapine, risperidone, olanzapine, ziprasidone) may be used, typically in combination with lithium or valproate. These are particularly helpful in patients with concomitant psychotic features (hallucinations, delusions, thought disorder).

Given the chronic, severe, and disabling course often seen in bipolar disorder, and the risk of continued substance use and poor adherence to treatments, an integrated, behavioral approach is recommended. Cognitive-behavioral therapy can be effective, as can other verbal therapies such as integrated group therapy—a validated group-based approach specifically designed for patients with substance use disorders receiving pharmacotherapy for co-occurring bipolar disorder.[47] Engagement of family, wrap-around services such as psychosocial rehabilitation, and consistent emphasis on the need to promote recovery from both substance use and bipolar disorders are important.

Anxiety and Trauma-Related Disorders

Anxiety Disorders

Anxiety disorders are characterized by persistent and excessive anxiety and worry. They include disorders such as specific phobia, panic, and generalized anxiety—conditions commonly seen in patients with substance use disorders. Post-traumatic stress disorder (PTSD) and obsessive-compulsive disorder (OCD) are also strongly associated with symptoms of anxiety, but are now included in separate categories in DSM-5. As with other psychiatric disorders, anxiety disorders are associated with substance use disorders. In the ECA study, the lifetime prevalence of anxiety disorders was 14.6%, of whom 23.7% had a lifetime diagnosis of a substance use disorder (OR: 1.7).[4] The National Epidemiologic Survey on Alcohol and Related Conditions found a 17.7% 12-month prevalence of any anxiety disorder, the highest prevalence being for specific phobia (10.5%), then social phobia (4.7%), and generalized anxiety disorder (4.2%).[48] The prevalence of OCD is relatively low, with most studies finding lifetime rates of less than 2%.[14,49]

Regarding evaluation and treatment, the same general principle applies here as with mood disorders: in the absence of clear determination of independent anxiety disorder, a period of abstinence is essential to rule out substance-induced symptomology and the need for targeted treatments. Anxiety symptoms are a common complaint among individuals with active or recent substance use, especially those with alcohol or sedative use disorder. Such symptoms can have a protracted course and may complicate attempts to initiate and sustain abstinence. For this reason and the potential morbidity from acute alcohol or sedative withdrawal, a period of observation and evaluation in an inpatient or residential setting can be useful. In addition, medical conditions and chaotic psychosocial situations can be important contributors to current anxiety complaints. The use of cognitive-behavioral and problem-oriented strategies can help patients learn to cope with life stressors without self-medicating. Additionally, for individuals with independent mood disorder, treating it aggressively is essential if anxiety appears to primarily co-occur with affective episodes. In general, benzodiazepines should be avoided, but when they are absolutely necessary, their use should be short term and monitored by a responsible family member. An SSRI or tricyclic agent is typically the better choice. Buspirone has weaker efficacy but is well tolerated. Emerging evidence suggests that gabapentin can be safely and effectively used to reduce symptoms of agitation, anxiety, and insomnia among patients undergoing or recently completing alcohol or sedative detoxification.[50,51]

Post-Traumatic Stress Disorder (PTSD)

PTSD is characterized by exposure to actual or threatened traumatic event(s); recurrent intrusive experiences such as nightmares, memories, or flashbacks; persistent distress at exposure to cues resembling the traumatic event; avoidance of associated stimuli; negative alterations in cognition or mood; and increased arousal such as irritability, increased startle, or sleep disturbance.[40] PTSD is one of the most commonly reported anxiety-related disorders among patients with substance use disorder. The National Comorbidity Survey found that the prevalence of PTSD in the general population was 7.8% and that those individuals, were 2–4 times more likely to have substance use disorders than those without PTSD.[52] Prevalence rates of up to 50% have been reported among patients in addiction treatment.[53] One study of cocaine-dependent outpatients demonstrated that 30% of the women and 15% of the men met criteria for PTSD.[54] A report on cocaine or opiate abusers reported lifetime rates of 8.3%.[55] For new admissions to opioid treatment (methadone) programs, rates range as high as 29% and as low as 4%.[56] The high degree of variability is likely due to a lack of standardized methods of assessment and inconsistent administration techniques. Regardless, psychiatric distress and drug use severity are elevated when PTSD is not treated.[57,58] An overview of treatment-related issues follows, but for comprehensive information, a new SAMHSA Treatment Improvement Protocol (TIP 57: Center for Substance Abuse Treatment)[59] is an excellent resource.

A number of treatment approaches may be effective in the prevention and treatment of PTSD. A study of acute trauma survivors demonstrated that those assigned to a "stepped collaborative care" model including case management, and psychiatric care if needed, had decreased risk of developing PTSD and alcohol use disorders over 12 months.[60] Cognitive-behavioral therapy has been shown to be effective for patients with co-occurring post-traumatic stress and substance use disorders. Of CBT approaches, exposure-based therapy is the primary therapeutic approach for treating PTSD. In exposure therapy, the patient is gradually exposed to fear-eliciting cues (typically imagined) in such a way that traumatic outcome is avoided; this results in gradual abatement of anxiety associated with similar cues in the real world. One study of 18 incarcerated women with PTSD and substance abuse reported improvement in PTSD symptoms and substance use after 12 weeks of twice-weekly CBT sessions.[61] Another study evaluating two different CBT approaches—one integrated model specifically for this population ("Seeking Safety"), and the other a more general addiction relapse prevention approach—demonstrated significant and equal improvements in both groups compared to treatment as usual.[62] In terms of pharmacotherapy, two medications, both SSRIs, are approved for the treatment of PTSD—sertraline and paroxetine; and the mixed-action antidepressant venlafaxine appears to be effective as well.[63,64] Although data are more limited regarding the pharmacological treatment of PTSD among individuals with substance use disorders, these medications have been shown to improve symptoms and quality of life in general populations with PTSD. Recent research has also found prazosin, an adrenergic alpha-1 antagonist that reduces central nervous system autonomic activity, to hold promise in decreasing nightmares and flashbacks associated with PTSD—symptoms that often do not respond to SSRIs.[65,66]

Psychotic Disorders

The psychotic disorders include schizophrenia as well as schizotypal, delusional, brief psychotic, schizophreniform and schizoaffective disorders. They share the common feature of problematic thinking, most often delusions (fixed, false, idiosyncratic beliefs) or hallucinations (perceptions without a stimulus). It is important to note that psychotic features can be present during severe episodes of other disorders such as major depression or bipolar disorder; in that context, the hallucinations or delusions tend to be mood-congruent and limited to periods of severe affective instability. A general awareness of psychotic-symptom recognition, evaluation, and management is important for any addiction medicine practitioner. For example, marijuana use appears to be increasing in the context of the recent push to medicalize, decriminalize, and legalize its use. Although it remains unclear whether early marijuana use is an independent cause of psychosis, research has demonstrated an association between its use and earlier-onset psychosis.[67] Another recent study demonstrated that among individuals with schizophrenia, those who had used cannabis had a longer duration of first hospitalization, had a higher readmission rate, and were more likely to be hospitalized for more than 2 years.[68] Because schizophrenia is by far the most common and disabling of the psychotic disorders, the remainder of this section will be dedicated to discussion of that condition.

Schizophrenia

Schizophrenia is a severe and disabling brain disorder that often follows a chronic, debilitating course. It is characterized by hallucinations, delusions, disorganized speech and behavior, and "negative symptoms," such as anhedonia, affective blunting, alogism, avolition/apathy, and attentional deficits (the 5 A's). Schizophrenia occurs in about 1% of the general population, and there is evidence of increasing use, through the years, of alcohol and drugs by persons with schizophrenia (from 14–22% in the 1960s and 1970s to 25–50% in the 1990s).[69] Diagnosis of schizophrenia among populations of substance users can be more straightforward and reliable than for substance-independent anxiety or mood disorders, as patients often have a clear history supporting the diagnosis, with a "life break" onset of symptoms during adolescence or early adulthood, followed by escalating symptoms and declining functioning over time.

There is evidence that among patients requiring hospitalization for psychotic illnesses, those with substance use disorders respond at least as well as those who do not. A study of 83 hospitalized psychotic patients (mostly with schizophrenia) found that those reporting substance abuse had less severe psychopathology by the time of discharge.[70] Despite this observation, the outpatient care for patients with schizophrenia can produce a number of challenges. Negative symptoms of schizophrenia such as apathy and avolition, especially when combined with paranoia, can impair motivation and intent to engage in treatment. The social disconnectedness so often present in this population makes development of an effective therapeutic alliance, and improving engagement in community-based prosocial activities, particularly difficult. Persons with schizophrenia are also at higher risk of violent behavior (to self or others) and are vulnerable to homelessness, inadequate somatic health care, poor nutrition, poverty, and victimization. For this reason, it follows that a treatment approach that is specialized, comprehensive, supportive, and adequately staffed is critical. Access to ancillary services such as supportive housing, psychosocial rehabilitation, and occupational therapy can be particularly helpful. One randomized controlled trial of an integrative approach (motivational interviewing, CBT, and family intervention) for patients with co-occurring schizophrenia and substance use disorders demonstrated better functioning and reduced relapse rates in the intervention arm.[71]

There is no clear pattern of drug choice among patients with schizophrenia—substance use decisions tend to be based mostly on availability. That said, nicotine might be an exception to the rule, as it is by far the most commonly used substance among people with schizophrenia. About 60–95% of patients in addiction treatment are regular users of tobacco, and about 40–50% are heavy smokers (more than 25 cigarettes per day).[72,73] People with schizophrenia sometimes smoke in part to self-medicate their symptoms, yet unfortunately it can interfere with the response to antipsychotic drugs, requiring higher doses of antipsychotic medication.[74] Because psychotic symptoms may worsen with nicotine withdrawal, smoking cessation can be difficult, and patient status should be closely monitored during planned quit attempts.

For patients with severe opioid use disorder, methadone and buprenorphine have been reported to impart some antipsychotic effects.[75,76,77] For this reason, and the disincentive to abruptly self-discontinue dosing, these medication-assisted therapies can be particularly useful for patients with co-occurring opioid use disorder and schizophrenia. In terms of setting, the regular contact and treatment structure inherent to opioid treatment programs can be particularly helpful—especially if the program offers integrated wrap-around services to benefit such patients.

In terms of pharmacotherapies, the antipsychotic medications (neuroleptics) are first-line treatments. Long-acting injectable preparations are available for some medications and can help to address the problem of medication nonadherence, as can directly observed pharmacotherapy—for example, at a methadone dispensary or by mobile treatment-unit staff. Care must be taken to monitor for side effects, such as metabolic syndrome and tardive dyskinesia, and for at-risk patients (e.g., those on high-dose methadone), QTc interval prolongation.[78]

Personality Disorders

The way individuals process their external and internal environment, how they feel about themselves and others, and how they tend to behave as a function of those thoughts and feelings in the setting of a variety of situations—their personality—can at times adversely affect how individuals function in multiple aspects of life. The person with a personality disorder suffers from persistent, inflexible, and long-standing (at least back to early adulthood) maladaptive behavioral patterns that cause significant functional impairment or internal distress. The personality disorders have been divided into three "clusters."[40] Cluster A (the "odd, eccentric" cluster) includes paranoid, schizoid, and schizotypal personality disorders. Cluster B (the "dramatic, emotional, erratic" cluster) includes antisocial, borderline, histrionic, and narcissistic personality disorders. Cluster C (the "anxious, fearful" cluster) includes avoidant, dependent, and obsessive-compulsive personality disorders. Although these disorders are often discussed as if they were each separate entities, in clinical practice, patients may meet criteria for more than one, and often have features of many. Data from the 2001–2002 National Epidemiologic Survey on Alcohol and Related Condition suggest that the approximately 15% of U.S. adults have a personality disorder.[48]

Personality disorders should not be diagnosed on the basis of evidence only present during periods of active substance use or withdrawal because of the shared features of personality disorders and substance use disorders and their effects on cognition, affect, and behavior. Diagnosis of personality disorder should be based on enduring traits and behavioral patterns that span periods of extended abstinence or that predate onset of substance use. It is clear, though, that personality disorders are strongly associated with substance use disorders.[4] Substance use disorders are most strongly associated with the cluster B borderline and antisocial personality disorders (APD). Borderline personality disorder is characterized by unstable mood and self-image, unstable and intense interpersonal relationships, and recurrent self-injurious behavior or threats. Antisocial personality disorder is characterized by a history of behavior that disregards and violates the rights of others, beginning by the age of 15, including failure to conform to social norms, deceitfulness, impulsivity, aggressiveness, irresponsibility, and lack of remorse. These individuals (like many persons with other personality disorders) often have parasitic relationships and feel that others, not they, are the cause of their problems. Fortunately, longitudinal studies tend to support the notion that features of personality disorder often decline over the course of the lifetime; in the case of APD, it has been observed that criminality in particular tends to begin to decline by the age of 27—a phenomenon that has been termed "antisocial burnout."[79] A study of new admissions to an opioid treatment (methadone) program found that 34.8% had personality disorders, with higher rates among men than women (40.5% and 28.4%, respectively). Antisocial (25.1%) and borderline (5.2%) personality disorders accounted for much of this segment, with higher rates of antisocial personality among men, and higher rates of borderline personality disorder among women.[80] Other studies found even higher prevalence of personality disorders; one study of admissions to an inpatient substance abuse program demonstrated that 57 of 100 patients had a personality disorder.[81]

Substance use can worsen symptoms of personality disorder and, not surprisingly, substance users with personality disorders are at increased risk for other complications. For example, in a study of 615 heroin users, borderline and antisocial personality disorders were associated with overdoses, suicide attempts, and needle sharing.[82] As would be expected, injection drug users with personality disorders are at increased risk for acquiring HIV infection.[80] Although individuals with personality disorder benefit from addiction treatment, personality disorders appear to have a deleterious effect on treatment outcomes.[18,83] In one study of 266 individuals with alcoholism, APD was associated with poorer treatment outcomes at 1 year.[84] Similarly, in a prospective cohort study of 2,616 patients with substance use disorders, personality disorder was associated with deterioration after 1 year, more so than any other psychiatric disorder.[85] On the other hand, a study of a therapeutic community treatment approach reported that participants with APD did as well as those without it.[86] Interestingly, a study of patients on methadone maintenance found that although those with APD did not respond to treatment as well as those without the disorder, those with APD plus an additional psychiatric disorder performed as well as the non-APD patients.[87] This may indicate that patients with APD may be more responsive to treatment when under certain circumstances, such as psychiatric distress.

There are few conclusive data on the optimal treatment of individuals with co-occurring substance use and personality disorders. In general, it is thought that long-term, evidence-based treatments of both substance use and personality vulnerabilities should be applied concurrently, and ideally in an integrated and highly structured setting. Staff within and across settings should maintain a strong team mentality, communicate freely and often, and receive specific training in the management of patients with personality disorder. Other co-occurring psychiatric disorders should be treated aggressively, and case management services should be employed for patients with significant and complex life circumstances. One proven method of structuring treatment is contingency management, an approach that compared favorably to CBT in a study of 120 opioid- and cocaine-dependent persons with antisocial personality disorder on methadone maintenance.[88] In another behavioral study of two different, highly structured, behaviorally contingent approaches for patients with APD, patients improved significantly in both conditions, with no significant difference between groups.[19] For borderline personality disorder, a cognitive-behavioral approach that is often used with this population is called "dialectical behavior therapy." It combines directive, problem-oriented, and supportive techniques, balancing acceptance with change. The limited studies of patients with co-occurring borderline personality and substance use disorders failed to demonstrate advantages of this approach over standard addiction treatment.[89,90]

Regarding pharmacological treatments, there is a paucity of research on the use of medications as an adjunct to psychosocial treatments for personality disorders. Evaluations of medication trials among general populations of personality-disordered persons have generally revealed utility limited to particular features of limited disorders. For example, there is some evidence that antipsychotic medications can reduce some cognitive and affective symptoms in persons with schizotypal personality disorder, while SSRIs may help decrease symptoms of anger, aggression, and self-harm among persons with borderline personality disorder.[91,92,93]

Attention Deficit/Hyperactivity Disorder (ADHD)

Although not considered to be a cause of the acute morbidity of the psychiatric conditions just reviewed, ADHD, when persisting into adulthood, is associated with significant functional impairment, resulting in challenges to the addiction treatment patient and professional. The primary features of ADHD include a persistent pattern of inattention and/or hyperactivity-impulsivity that is inconsistent with developmental level and negatively impacts life functioning.[40] To meet diagnostic criteria, symptoms must have been present prior to the age of 12. Even when full criteria do not persist into adulthood, some impairing symptoms of the childhood disorder can persist into adulthood. ADHD affects 9.5% of children ages 3–17 in the United States, according to the National Health Interview Survey,[94] with boys being twice as likely to have current disorder as girls. Studies demonstrate that up to 60% of these individuals continue to have symptoms into adulthood. According to the National Comorbidity Survey Replication, the 12-month prevalence of ADHD persisting into adulthood is 4.1%, with 41.3% of cases (1.7% of the U.S. population) having severe disorder.[95] In studies of various substance abuse samples, ADHD is overrepresented compared to the general population, with prevalence rates of 5–25%[3], but those studies using more strict diagnostic criteria demonstrate rates between two and three times the general national averages. Among individuals with ADHD, substance use disorders are more common; in the National Comorbidity Survey

Replication, the prevalence of substance use disorder in individuals with ADHD was 15.2%, nearly three times the rate of those without ADHD (5.6%).[95] There is also a strong association between adult ADHD and nicotine dependence, with higher rates, earlier onset, and more frequent use of tobacco products.[96,97] The ability to detect ADHD in substance-using individuals can lie in the recognition of functional impairment inherent to this population, and especially the resultant inability to develop of a strong recovery foundation. This often results in a delay to remission of substance use.[98] ADHD features can impair these patients' ability to process content during counseling sessions; structure their time with work or educational pursuits; avoid impulsive decision-making, which often results in criminal behaviors; and develop healthy relationships and a positive social support network.

Although an assessment for ADHD is often absent from routine medical or substance abuse evaluations, patients with substance use disorder sometimes self-diagnose ADHD. While potentially valid, patients' identification with with the criteria list for ADHD may be a way to explain behaviors secondary to substance use or to another untreated psychiatric disorder. Some may report current ADHD as a means to gain access to stimulant medications that may be misused or sold. Therefore, when evaluating the patient for possible ADHD, especially the adult, it is important to seek out corroborating information. Useful evidence may be gleaned from parents or other past caregivers, as well as from academic records or medical and psychiatric documentation. A formal ADHD diagnosis need not have been made during childhood, as the diagnosis may have been missed—especially in the context of personal or parental substance use and related family dysfunction. That said, in the absence of clear documentation of childhood ADHD, diagnosis of the disorder in the individual with substance use disorder can be a challenge. Many of the features of ADHD overlap with those of substance intoxication, withdrawal, and related functional impairment. For this reason, there is no substitute for a drug-free time period during which to evaluate for symptoms and functionality. During this time, other psychiatric disorders can be ruled out as causing symptoms, such as poor attention and distractibility, which can occur with dysthymia or generalized anxiety; likewise, impulsivity and hyperactivity is a common feature of hypomania or mania in persons with bipolar disorder.

Staff managing the substance-using patient with ADHD can become particularly frustrated given the tendency of these individuals to act impulsively, not tolerate the typical 30- to 60-minute counseling session, and have problems with information processing. SAMHSA TIP 42[3] suggests the following general approach to the patient with co-occurring substance use disorder and ADHD:

- Educate the patient regarding ADHD and its interaction with substance use disorder.
- Provide ongoing feedback regarding elements of questions that the patient has and has not yet answered.
- Minimize distracting environmental stimuli.
- Use visual cues to convey information.
- Limit the duration of clinical contacts.
- Encourage the use of organizational tools (e.g., to-do lists and activity schedules).
- Evaluate the need for pharmacotherapy.

In addition, CBT, an integral component of most addiction treatment programs, has been shown to be effective for persons with co-occurring ADHD and substance use disorder.[99,100]

The pharmacological treatment of ADHD in substance-addicted populations presents a particular challenge because of the potential for misuse or diversion of the medications typically used for this disorder. Stimulants (amphetamine analogs and methylphenidate) are the most commonly used medications in the treatment of ADHD in children, adolescents, and adults. Nonstimulant medications are also used, including atomoxetine (a norepinephrine reuptake inhibitor), bupropion (an atypical antidepressant), tricyclic antidepressants, and venlafaxine (a serotonin-norepinephrine reuptake inhibitor). Some experts recommend that in this population of patients with substance use disorders, the treatment of ADHD should always start with a nonstimulant medication. However, a meta-analysis found that they tend to be less effective than stimulant medications in treating symptoms of ADHD.[101] Consistent with the general principle that shorter-acting, more rapidly available preparations of reinforcing medications carry a higher abuse potential, there is evidence that the longer-acting prescription stimulants may have lower abuse potential.[102] The other advantage of time-release preparations is that they tend to be more difficult to misuse via inhaled or injected routes. In choosing a pharmacotherapy, the risks of continued symptoms must be weighed against the risks associated with the medication. Levin and Mariani propose a rational approach for accomplishing this.[103] They devised a strategy that stratifies patients into three levels based on how temporally remote or active their substance use has been. Those with no current drug use (low risk) are prescribed delayed-release stimulants with general prescribing precautions. Those with some use but no current substance use disorder (moderate-risk) may be treated with long-acting stimulants with additional controls in place, or with nonstimulant medications. Those with current substance use disorder (high risk) are offered nonstimulants and more intensive nonpharmacological interventions.

Notes

1. Sadock BJ, Sadock VA, Ruiz, P (eds). *Kaplan & Sadock's Comprehensive Textbook of Psychiatry, 9th ed.* Philadelphia: Wolters Kluwer Health/Lippincott Williams & Wilkins; 2009.

2. Hales RE, Yudofsky SC, Gabbard GO (eds). *The American Psychiatric Publishing Textbook of Psychiatry, 5th ed.* Washington, DC: American Psychiatric Publishing; 2008.

3. Center for Substance Abuse Treatment. *Substance Abuse Treatment for Persons with Co-Occurring Disorders. Treatment Improvement Protocol (TIP) Series 42.* DHHS Publication No. (SMA) 05-3992. Rockville, MD: Substance Abuse and Mental Health Services Administration; 2005.

4. Regier DA, Farmer ME, Rae DS, et al. Comorbidity of mental disorders with alcohol and other drug abuse. Results from the Epidemiologic Catchment Area (ECA) Study. JAMA 1990;264:2511–8.

5. Substance Abuse and Mental Health Services Administration. *Results from the 2013 National Survey on Drug Use and Health: National Findings.* NSDUH Series H-48, HHS Publication No. (SMA) 14-4863. Rockville, MD: Substance Abuse and Mental Health Services Administration; 2014.

6. Merikangas KR, Mehta RL, Molnar BE, et al. Comorbidity of substance use disorders with mood and anxiety disorders: results of the International Consortium in Psychiatric Epidemiology. Addict Behav 1998;23:893–907.

7. Grant BF, Hasin DS, Chou SP, et al. Nicotine dependence and psychiatric disorders in the United States: results from the national epidemiologic survey on alcohol and related conditions. Arch Gen Psychiatry 2004;61:1107–15.

8. Derogatis LR. *SCL-90R; Administration, Soring, and Procedures Manual II,* 2nd ed. Baltimore: Clinical Psychometric Research; 1983.

9. Kroenke K, Spitzer RL, Williams JB. The PHQ-9: validity of a brief depression severity measure. J Gen Intern Med 2001;16:606–13.

10. Beck AT, Ward CH, Mendelson M, et al. An inventory for measuring depression. Arch Gen Psychiatry 1961;4:561–71.

11. First MB, Spitzer RL, Gibbon M, et al. *Structured Clinical Interview for DSM-IV Axis II Personality Disorders (SCID II).* Washington, DC: American Psychiatric Press; 1996.

12. First MB, Spitzer RL, Gibbon M, et al. *Structured Clinical Interview for DSM-IV-TR Axis I Disorders (SCID-I/P).* New York: Biometrics Research, New York State Psychiatric Institute; 2001.

13. Robbins LN, Cottler LB, Bucholz K, et al. *Diagnostic Interview Schedule (DIS) for DSM-IV.* St. Louis, MO: Washington University; 1995.

14. Brooner RK, King VL, Kidorf M, et al. Psychiatric and substance use comorbidity among treatment-seeking opioid abusers. Arch Gen Psychiatry 1997;54:71–80.

15. Miller NS. Comorbidity of psychiatric and alcohol/drug disorders: interactions and independent status. J Addict Dis 1993;12:5–16.

16. Kosten TR, Rounsaville BJ, Kleber HD. A 2.5-year follow-up of depression, life crises, and treatment effects on abstinence among opioid addicts. Arch Gen Psychiatry 1986;43:733–8.

17. Rounsaville BJ, Kosten TR, Weissman MM, et al. Prognostic significance of psychopathology in treated opiate addicts. A 2.5-year follow-up study. Arch Gen Psychiatry 1986;43:739–45.

18. Reich JH, Green AI. Effect of personality disorders on outcome of treatment. J Nerv Ment Dis 1991;179:74–82.

19. Brooner RK, Kidorf M, King VL, et al. Preliminary evidence of good treatment response in antisocial drug abusers. Drug Alcohol Depend. 1998;49:249–60.

20. Nunes EV, Levin FR. Treatment of depression in patients with alcohol or other drug dependence: a meta-analysis. JAMA 2004;21;291:1887–96.

21. McLellan AT, Arndt IO, Metzger DS, et al. The effects of psychosocial services in substance abuse treatment. JAMA 1993;269:1953–9.

22. Woody GE, McLellan AT, Luborsky L, et al. Psychotherapy in community methadone programs: a validation study. Am J Psychiatry 1995;152:1302–8.

23. Kidorf M, Brooner RK, Gandotra N, et al. Reinforcing integrated psychiatric service attendance in an opioid-agonist program: a randomized and controlled trial. Drug Alcohol Depend 2013;133:30–6.

24. King VL, Brooner RK, Peirce J, et al. Challenges and outcomes of parallel care for patients with co-occurring psychiatric disorder in methadone maintenance treatment. J Dual Diagn 2014;10:60–7.

25. Brooner RK, Kidorf MS, King VL, et al. Behavioral contingencies improve counseling attendance in an adaptive treatment model. J Subst Abuse Treat 2004;27:223–32.

26. Murphy SA, Lynch KG, Oslin D, et al. Developing adaptive treatment strategies in substance abuse research. Drug Alcohol Depend 2007;88(Suppl 2):S24–30.

27. Mee-Lee D (Ed.). *The ASAM Criteria: Treatment Criteria for Addictive, Substance-Related, and Co-Occurring Conditions*, Third Edition. Carson City, NV: The Change Companies; 2013.

28. Zimmerman M, Chelminski I, McDermut W. Major depressive disorder and axis I diagnostic comorbidity. J Clin Psychiatry 2002;63:187–93.

29. Mertens JR, Lu YW, Parthasarathy S, et al. Medical and psychiatric conditions of alcohol and drug treatment patients in an HMO: comparison with matched controls. Arch Intern Med 2003;163:2511–7.

30. King VL, Peirce J, Brooner RK. Comorbid psychiatric disorders. In Strain EC, Stitzer ML, Eds. *The Treatment of Opioid Dependence.* Baltimore: Johns Hopkins University Press; 2006:421–51.

31. Greenfield SF, Weiss RD, Muenz LR, et al. The effect of depression on return to drinking: a prospective study. Arch Gen Psychiatry 1998;55:259–65.

32. Hasin D, Liu X, Nunes E, et al. Effects of major depression on remission and relapse of substance dependence. Arch Gen Psychiatry 2002;59:375–80.

33. Samet S, Fenton MC, Nunes E, et al. Effects of independent and substance-induced major depressive disorder on remission and relapse of alcohol, cocaine and heroin dependence. Addiction 2013;108:115–23.

34. Schuckit MA, Monteiro MG. Alcoholism, anxiety and depression. Br J Addict 1988;83:1373–80.

35. Kosten TR, Morgan C, Kosten TA. Depressive symptoms during buprenorphine treatment of opioid abusers. J Subst Abuse Treat 1990;7:51–4.

36. Strain EC, Stitzer ML, Bigelow GE. Early treatment time course of depressive symptoms in opiate addicts. J Nerv Ment Dis 1991;179:215–21.

37. Landabaso-Vazquez MA, Iraurgi-Castillo I, Jiménez-Lerma JM, et al. Depressive symptomatology and response to treatment with antidepressants in patients with a dual diagnosis. Addict Disord Their Treat 2014;13:125–32.

38. Torrens M, Fonseca F, Mateu G, et al. Efficacy of antidepressants in substance use disorders with and without comorbid depression. A systematic review and meta-analysis. Drug Alcohol Depend 2005;4;78:1–22.

39. Hollon SD, DeRubeis RJ, Fawcett J, et al. Effect of cognitive therapy with antidepressant medications vs. antidepressants alone on the rate of recovery in major depressive disorder: a randomized clinical trial. JAMA Psychiatry 2014;711157–64.

40. American Psychiatric Association. *Diagnostic and Statistical Manual of Mental Disorders,* Fifth Edition. Arlington, VA: American Psychiatric publishing; 2013.

41. Salloum IM, Cornelius JR, Mezzich JE, et al. Impact of concurrent alcohol misuse on symptom presentation of acute mania at initial evaluation. Bipolar Disord 2002;4:418–21.

42. Goldberg JF, Garno JL, Leon AC, et al. A history of substance abuse complicates remission from acute mania in bipolar disorder. J Clin Psychiatry 1999;60:733–40.

43. Cassidy F, Ahearn EP, Carroll BJ. Substance abuse in bipolar disorder. Bipolar Disord 2001;3:181–8.

44. Dalton EJ, Cate-Carter TD, Mundo E, et al. Suicide risk in bipolar patients: the role of co-morbid substance use disorders. Bipolar Disord 2003;5:58–61.

45. McElroy SL, Altshuler LL, Suppes T, et al. Axis I psychiatric comorbidity and its relationship to historical illness variables in 288 patients with bipolar disorder. Am J Psychiatry 2001;158:420–6.

46. Weiss RD, Griffin ML, Greenfield SF, et al. Group therapy for patients with bipolar disorder and substance dependence: results of a pilot study. J Clin Psychiatry 2000;61:361–7.

47. Weiss RD & Connery HS. *Integrated Group Therapy for Bipolar Disorder and Substance Abuse*. New York: Guilford Press; 2012.

48. Grant BF, Hasin DS, Stinson FS, et al. Prevalence, correlates, and disability of personality disorders in the United States: results from the national epidemiologic survey on alcohol and related conditions. J Clin Psychiatry 2004;65:948–58.

49. Rounsaville BJ, Weissman MM, Kleber H, et al. Heterogeneity of psychiatric diagnosis in treated opiate addicts. Arch Gen Psychiatry 1982;39:161–8.

50. Muncie HL, Yasinian Y, Oge' L. Outpatient management of alcohol withdrawal syndrome. Am Fam Physician 2013;88:589–95.

51. Howland RH. Gabapentin for substance use disorders: is it safe and appropriate? J Psychosoc Nurs Ment Health Serv 2014;52(1):12–5.

52. Kessler RC, Sonnega A, Bromet E, et al. Posttraumatic stress disorder in the National Comorbidity Survey. Arch Gen Psychiatry 1995;52:1048–60.

53. Dansky BS, Saladin ME, Coffey SF, et al. Use of self-report measures of crime-related posttraumatic stress disorder with substance use disordered patients. J Subst Abuse Treat 1997;14:431–7.

54. Najavits LM, Gastfriend DR, Barber JP, et al. Cocaine dependence with and without PTSD among subjects in the National Institute on Drug Abuse Collaborative Cocaine Treatment Study. Am J Psychiatry 1998;155:214–9.

55. Cottler LB, Nishith P, Compton WM. Gender differences in risk factors for trauma exposure and post-traumatic stress disorder among inner-city drug abusers in and out of treatment. Compr Psychiatry 2001;42:111–7.

56. Peirce JM, Waesche MC, Kendrick A, et al. Association between PTSD and drug use and psychosocial problems in drug abusers. The Annual Scientific Conference of the College on Problems of Drug Dependence, Quebec City, Canada, 2002.

57. Hien DA, Nunes E, Levin FR, et al. Posttraumatic stress disorder and short-term outcome in early methadone treatment. J Subst Abuse Treat 2000;19:31–7.

58. Clark HW, Masson CL, Delucchi KL, et al. Violent traumatic events and drug abuse severity. J Subst Abuse Treat 2001;20:121–7.

59. Center for Substance Abuse Treatment. *Trauma-Informed Care in Behavioral Health Services. Treatment Improvement Protocol (TIP) Series 57.* DHHS Publication No. (SMA) 14-4816. Rockville, MD: Substance Abuse and Mental Health Services Administration; 2014.

60. Zatzick D, Roy-Byrne P, Russo J, et al. A randomized effectiveness trial of stepped collaborative care for acutely injured trauma survivors. Arch Gen Psychiatry 2004;61:498–506.

61. Zlotnick C, Najavits LM, Rohsenow DJ, et al. A cognitive-behavioral treatment for incarcerated women with substance abuse disorder and posttraumatic stress disorder: findings from a pilot study. J Subst Abuse Treat 2003;25:99–105.

62. Hien DA, Cohen LR, Miele GM, et al. Promising treatments for women with comorbid PTSD and substance use disorders. Am J Psychiatry 2004;161:1426–32.

63. Schoenfeld FB, Marmar CR, Neylan TC. Current concepts in pharmacotherapy for posttraumatic stress disorder. Psychiatr Serv 2004;55:519–31.

64. Watts BV, Schnurr PP, Mayo L, et al. Meta-analysis of the efficacy of treatments for posttraumatic stress disorder. J Clin Psychiatry 2013;74:e541–50.

65. Kung S, Espinel Z, Lapid MI. Treatment of nightmares with prazosin: a systematic review. Mayo Clin Proc 2012;87:890–900.

66. Green B. Prazosin in the treatment of PTSD. J Psychiatr Pract 2014;20:253–9.

67. Burns JK. Pathways from cannabis to psychosis: a review of the evidence. Front Psychiatry 2013;4:128.

68. Manrique-Garcia E, Zammit S, Dalman C, et al. Prognosis of schizophrenia in persons with and without a history of cannabis use. Psychol Med 2014;44:2513–21.

69. Fowler IL, Carr VJ, Carter NT, et al. Patterns of current and lifetime substance use in schizophrenia. Schizophr Bull 1998;24:443–55.

70. Dixon L, Haas G, Weiden PJ, et al. Drug abuse in schizophrenic patients: clinical correlates and reasons for use. Am J Psychiatry 1991;148:224–30.

71. Barrowclough C, Haddock G, Tarrier N, et al. Randomized controlled trial of motivational interviewing, cognitive behavior therapy, and family intervention for patients with comorbid schizophrenia and substance use disorders. Am J Psychiatry 2001;158:1706–13.

72. Hughes JR. Clinical implications of the association between smoking and alcoholism. In Fertig J, Fuller R, Eds. *Alcohol and Tobacco: From Basic Science to Policy*. NIAAA Research Monograph, Vol. 30 (pp. 171–181). Washington, DC: US Government Printing Office; 1995.

73. Hughes JR. Combining behavioral therapy and pharmacotherapy for smoking cessation: An update. *NIDA Research Monograph*, 1995;150:92–109.

74. Sagud M, Mihaljević-Peles A, Mück-Seler D, et al. Smoking and schizophrenia. Psychiatr Danub 2009;21:371–5.

75. Brizer DA, Hartman N, Sweeney J, et al. Effect of methadone plus neuroleptics on treatment-resistant chronic paranoid schizophrenia. Am J Psychiatry 1985;142:1106–7.

76. Schmauss C, Yassouridis A, Emrich HM. Antipsychotic effect of buprenorphine in schizophrenia. Am J Psychiatry 1987;144:1340–2.

77. Miotto P, Preti A, Frezza M. Heroin and schizophrenia: subjective responses to abused drugs in dually diagnosed patients. J Clin Psychopharmacol 2001;21:111–3.

78. Chou R, Cruciani RA, Fiellin DA, et al. Methadone safety: a clinical practice guideline from the American Pain Society and College on Problems of Drug Dependence, in collaboration with the Heart Rhythm Society. J Pain 2014;15:321–37.

79. Arboleda-Florez J, Holley HL. Antisocial burnout: an exploratory study. Bull Am Acad Psychiatry Law 1991;19:173–83.

80. Brooner RK, Greenfield L, Schmidt CW, et al. Antisocial personality disorder and HIV infection among intravenous drug abusers. Am J Psychiatry 1993;150:53–8.

81. Nace EP, Davis CW, Gaspari JP. Axis II comorbidity in substance abusers. Am J Psychiatry 1991;148:118–20.

82. Darke S, Williamson A, Ross J, et al. Borderline personality disorder, antisocial personality disorder and risk-taking among heroin users: findings from the Australian Treatment Outcome Study (ATOS). Drug Alcohol Depend 2004;9;74:77–83.

83. King VL, Kidorf MS, Stoller KB, et al. Influence of antisocial personality subtypes on drug abuse treatment response. J Nerv Ment Dis 2001;189:593–601.

84. Rounsaville BJ, Dolinsky ZS, Babor TF, et al. Psychopathology as a predictor of treatment outcome in alcoholics. Arch Gen Psychiatry 1987;44:505–13.

85. Moos RH, Moos BS, Finney JW. Predictors of deterioration among patients with substance-use disorders. J Clin Psychol 2001;57:1403–19.

86. Messina NP, Wish ED, Hoffman JA, et al. Antisocial personality disorder and TC treatment outcomes. Am J Drug Alcohol Abuse 2002;28:197–212.

87. Woody GE, McLellan AT, Luborsky L, et al. Sociopathy and psychotherapy outcome. Arch Gen Psychiatry 1985;42:1081–6.

88. Messina N, Farabee D, Rawson R. Treatment responsivity of cocaine-dependent patients with antisocial personality disorder to cognitive-behavioral and contingency management interventions. J Consult Clin Psychol 2003;71:320–9.

89. Linehan MM, Schmidt H, Dimeff LA, et al. Dialectical behavior therapy for patients with borderline personality disorder and drug-dependence. Am J Addict 1999;8:279–92.

90. Linehan MM, Dimeff LA, Reynolds SK, et al. Dialectical behavior therapy versus comprehensive validation therapy plus 12-step for the treatment of opioid dependent women meeting criteria for borderline personality disorder. Drug Alcohol Depend 2002;67:13–26.

91. Zanarini MC, Frankenburg FR, Parachini EA. A preliminary, randomized trial of fluoxetine, olanzapine, and the olanzapine-fluoxetine combination in women with borderline personality disorder. J Clin Psychiatry 2004;65:903–7.

92. Mercer D, Douglass AB, Links PS. Meta-analyses of mood stabilizers, antidepressants and antipsychotics in the treatment of borderline

personality disorder: effectiveness for depression and anger symptoms. J Pers Disord 2009;23:156–74.

93. Ingenhoven T, Lafay P, Rinne T, et al. Effectiveness of pharmacotherapy for severe personality disorders: meta-analyses of randomized controlled trials. J Clin Psychiatry 2010;71:14–25.

94. Center for Disease Control (2013). Summary Health Statistics for U.S. Children: National Health Interview Survey, 2012, Table VI. www.cdc.gov/nchs/data/series/sr_10/sr10_258.pdf. Accessed September 24, 2014.

95. Kessler RC, Chiu WT, Demler O, et al. Prevalence, severity, and comorbidity of 12-month DSM-IV disorders in the National Comorbidity Survey Replication. Arch Gen Psychiatry 2005;62:617–27.

96. Pomerleau OF, Downey KK, Stelson FW, et al. Cigarette smoking in adult patients diagnosed with attention deficit hyperactivity disorder. J Subst Abuse 1995;7:373–8.

97. Kollins SH, McClernon FJ, Fuemmeler BF. Association between smoking and attention-deficit/hyperactivity disorder symptoms in a population-based sample of young adults. Arch Gen Psychiatry 2005;62:1142–7.

98. Wilens TE, Biederman J, Mick E. Does ADHD affect the course of substance abuse? Findings from a sample of adults with and without ADHD. Am J Addict 1998;7:156–63.

99. Safren SA, Otto MW, Sprich S, et al. Cognitive-behavioral therapy for ADHD in medication-treated adults with continued symptoms. Behav Res Ther 2005;43:831–42.

100. Vidal-Estrada R, Bosch-Munso R, Nogueira-Morais M, et al. Psychological treatment of attention deficit hyperactivity disorder in adults: a systematic review. Actas Esp Psiquiatr 2012;40:147–54.

101. Faraone SV, Glatt SJ. A comparison of the efficacy of medications for adult attention-deficit/hyperactivity disorder using meta-analysis of effect sizes. J Clin Psychiatry 2010;71:754–63.

102. Mao AR, Babcock T, Brams M. ADHD in adults: current treatment trends with consideration of abuse potential of medications. J Psychiatr Pract 2011;17:241–50.

103. Levin FR & Mariani JJ. Co-occurring addictive disorder and attention deficit hyperactivity disorder. In Ries RK, Ed. *The ASAM Principles of Addiction Medicine*, 5th ed. Philadelphia: Wolters Kluwer Health; 2014:1365–1384.

16

Special Populations

Health Professionals   500

The prevalence of alcohol use disorders among health professionals is similar to that for the general population, although the use of illicit drugs is less common. Professional organizations have implemented programs to address impairment in the health professions.

Adolescents

Adolescent substance use poses serious public health problems. Adolescents tend to not perceive harm from drug use and often lack insight into the problems that result from use. However, educational efforts may have a beneficial effect, and a National Institute of Drug Abuse 2011 survey of adolescents revealed an increased perception of risk related to binge drinking.[1] Factors often associated with adolescent substance use include the following:

- Having a parent with a substance use disorder
- Mood disorder
- Learning disorder or poor school performance
- Low self-esteem
- Early sexual activity
- Dysfunctional family and parenting
- Drug- and alcohol-using peers
- Easy availability of drugs and alcohol in community

In caring for adolescents, clinicians must sensitively develop rapport and trust, in order to effectively screen, diagnose, and treat substance abuse disorders.

Epidemiology

According to the 2013 National Survey on Drug Use and Health, 11% of 12- to 17-year-olds reported current use of illicit drugs.[2] Approximately 31% of youth reported using an illicit drug at least once during their lifetime and 22% reported using an illicit drug within the past year. Overall, marijuana was the most used drug, with 40% of high school students reporting having used marijuana in their lifetime and 7.9% of youth reporting current marijuana use. Adolescents' use of heroin was low and primarily by non-injection routes—smoking or sniffing. Compared to previous surveys, use of most other drugs by adolescents was similar or less, with the exception of an increase in the use of MDMA (ecstasy) by older teens. Inhalant use is primarily seen among younger teens. Initiating inhalant use prior to the age of 13 is associated with increased risk of involvement in violence, criminal activity, developing dependence on another drug, and school dropout.[3]

Among college students, depressive symptoms and suicidality are significantly associated with greater odds of any nonmedical prescription drug use (especially for females).[4] These results suggest that students may be inappropriately self-medicating psychological distress with prescription medications. An analysis of trends in nonmedical use of prescription medications among college students showed that about one in five students reported nonmedical use of at least one prescription medication class in their lifetime.[5] Stimulant use appears to be on the rise, while opioid use is decreasing. The odds of past-year nonmedical use of each prescription medication class were generally greater among males, members of social fraternities and sororities, and those with a lifetime history of medical use of prescription medications or a past-year history of being approached to divert their prescription medications.

Screening and Assessment

The American Academy of Pediatrics Committee on Substance Abuse recommends that all pediatricians evaluate the nature and extent of tobacco, alcohol, and other drug use among their patients; offer appropriate counseling about the risks of substance abuse; and make an assessment as to whether additional counseling and referral may be needed.[6] The medical interview of adolescents related to substance use should be done in private, without the presence of parents. Tools for assessing substance use in adolescents are

limited, as it is often difficult to distinguish limited experimenta-
tion from problem use. The drug and alcohol screening tools used
in adults are described in Chapters 2 and 4. Studies vary as to the
effectiveness of these screening tools in adolescents, and they are
specifically validated for alcohol. The CRAFFT (Box 16.1) is a reliable, easy-to-administer screening tool for assessing substance
abuse (not just alcohol) in adolescents.[7,8,9] The CRAFFT can enable
providers to identify adolescents with problem use who would not
have otherwise been identified.[10]

The diagnostic criteria for substance use disorders in adolescents are generally the same as in adults. Obviously, for adolescents,
any use of alcohol may be judged problematic, as use of alcohol by
adolescents is illegal. Unlike adults, whose drug use may impact job
performance, adolescent use may impact school performance. For
adolescents, experimental use of drugs that transitions into social
use may, in some instances, result in an adverse consequence that

---

**BOX 16.1 CRAFFT: A Brief Screening Test for Adolescent
Substance Abuse***

C—Have you ever ridden in a CAR driven by someone (including yourself) who was high or had been using alcohol or drugs?
R—Do you ever use alcohol or drugs to RELAX, feel better
about yourself, or fit in?
A—Do you ever use alcohol or drugs while you are by
yourself, ALONE?
F—Do your family or FRIENDS ever tell you that you should
cut down on your drinking or drug use?
F—Do you ever FORGET things you did while using alcohol
or drugs?
T—Have you gotten into TROUBLE while you were using
alcohol or drugs?

---

*2 or more yes answers suggests a significant problem.

motivates abstinence without the need for formal treatment. Most adolescent drug use fits into the DSM-5 diagnoses of a mild substance use disorder. For example, it is unusual for an adolescent to develop alcohol dependence such that abstinence results in significant alcohol withdrawal.[11] Signs and symptoms related to substance use in adolescents may include weight loss, sleep disorder, memory and focusing problems, hoarse voice, unexplained injuries, nasal erythema (from sniffing), teary red eyes (from inhalants), and needle marks.

Effects of Substance Use

The common complications of substance use disorder in adolescents are poor school performance, poor peer relations, family problems, and involvement with the juvenile justice system. According to the Federal Bureau of Investigation, there were approximately 1.6 million juveniles (under the age of 18) arrested by state and local law enforcement agencies for drug violations during 2010.[12] Binge drinking among adolescents is associated with road accidents and violence, and increases the risk of contracting a sexually transmitted disease as well as becoming pregnant.[13] Binge drinking can result in blackouts and amnesia for events, and deaths may occur in adolescents who drink large amounts of high-proof alcohol quickly, resulting in respiratory depression.

In 2011, emergency department treatment of adolescents related to pharmaceuticals was most common for opioids (38 per 100,000 age 12–17) and antianxiety medications (73 per 100,000 age 12–17).[14] Psychiatric illness, including behavioral disorders, learning disabilities, depression, and anxiety, generally precede the onset of substance abuse disorders.[15,16] Suicide, a leading cause of mortality in adolescents, has been shown in several studies to be more common in adolescents with substance use disorders than in nonusers.[17]

Most medical complications of substance use seen in adults are less common in adolescents. For example, liver abnormalities related to alcohol are rarely seen in adolescents.[18] Medical complications of specific drugs are discussed in Chapters 4–12, on specific substances.

Treatment

The types of treatment available for adolescents are similar to those used for adults, but there tends to be less evidence to support them. Adolescents' right to consent to treatment for substance use disorders varies by state, and the age at which consent is allowed also varies.[19] Most treatments for adolescent substance use disorders have been limited to psychosocial interventions, often involving individual and family therapy. Treatment approaches vary, and there is a need for studies comparing treatment outcomes.[20]

Brief Interventions

As for adults, the evidence supporting the efficacy of brief interventions in adolescents is mixed. A 2012 meta-analysis of 39 studies of motivational interviewing for substance use among adolescents found that 67% of studies reported statistically significant improvement in substance use outcomes.[21] These interventions occurred in a variety of settings, most not in the primary care setting. Among adolescents identified in an emergency room with alcohol use and aggression, brief intervention has been reported to decrease future consequences related to alcohol use.[22] A 2014 systematic review for the U.S. Preventive Services Task Force, however, found inadequate evidence for the benefit of primary care behavioral interventions in reducing self-reported illicit and pharmaceutical use among adolescents.[23] Furthermore, in a study of college students, a Web-based alcohol screening and brief intervention did not reduce the frequency or volume of drinking or number of academic problems.[24] Brief interventions and motivational interviewing are covered further in Chapter 2.

Medically Supervised Withdrawal

Most adolescents do not require acute treatment of alcohol or other drug withdrawal. The treatment of alcohol and opioid withdrawal is discussed in Chapters 4 and 6. Treatment after cessation of use generally consists of supportive care and should start with motivational interviewing as outlined in Chapter 2. The mechanisms for change in adolescents with substance use disorders are not well understood, and there are few data on neurochemical changes associated with addiction or recovery.[25]

Self-Help Groups

There are insufficient data to evaluate the effectiveness of self-help groups or 12-step meetings for the treatment of substance use disorders in adolescents, and perceptions of value are mixed.[26] Currently, most adolescents identified with substance use problems are referred for treatment, and part of the treatment consists of group therapy that follows much the same philosophy as Alcoholics Anonymous or Narcotics Anonymous. The impact of comorbid depression on treatment outcomes is mixed, with studies showing negative, positive, or nonsignificant impact.[27]

Drug Courts

For adolescents with legal problems, drug treatment often involves a juvenile drug court.[28] The juvenile drug court is a recently introduced model developed in response to a need to intervene more effectively in the substance abuse–delinquency cycle. Reports of positive experiences with adult drug courts helped trigger interest in adapting the drug court model for juveniles. Currently, little is known about the impact of juvenile drug courts.

Pharmacotherapy

There are few studies of pharmacotherapy in the treatment of substance use disorders in adolescents. None of the medications used for alcohol use disorders in adults (disulfiram, acamprosate, and naltrexone) have been sufficiently studied for treatment of adolescents.

There are limited data on long-term medication treatment for opioid-dependent adolescents, with a need for randomized controlled trials.[29] The use of naltrexone for opiate use disorder in adolescents is limited to a case series.[30] A 1979 study of heroin-dependent adolescents showed methadone maintenance to be more effective than other drug-free modalities.[31] However, currently, most methadone maintenance treatment programs exclude adolescents. Buprenorphine is approved for treatment of adolescents ages 16 and higher; 12 weeks of buprenorphine treatment has been shown to be superior to a taper alone.[32]

Women

According to the 2013 National Survey of Drug Use and Health, 7.3% of women over the age of 12 reported using an illicit drug in the past year, and 5.8% met criteria for substance abuse or dependence.[2] In 2011, there were 442,000 emergency room visits related to drug use in women, the greatest number being related to alcohol, followed by cocaine.[14] In 2012, 583,000 women were admitted to drug treatment facilities in the United States, representing 33% of admissions.[33] Sedatives were the only drug category for which more women than men were admitted into treatment.

In 2013, 48% of females (compared to 57% of males) aged 12 or older in the United States were current drinkers.[2] Women tend to drink more covertly and women with alcohol use disorder are more likely to have alcoholic spouses.[34] The CAGE questionnaire (see Chapter 4), although originally validated on a group of men, has also been validated for women.[35,36] An additional tool similar to the CAGE, the TWEAK (see Box 16.2), was developed and validated for assessing alcohol misuse in pregnant women and may perform better than the CAGE in assessing alcohol misuse among women in general.[37]

Women are more likely to develop alcohol dependence after a shorter duration of drinking, and suicide, trauma, and liver disease are more common in female than male alcoholics.[38] Complications

BOX 16.2 The TWEAK Questionnaire

Prior to administering TWEAK, drinkers are identified by a positive response to the question, "Do you or have you ever consumed beer, wine, wine coolers, or drinks containing liquor (i.e., whiskey, rum, or vodka)?"

Points

(1–2) Tolerance—How many drinks can you hold? **OR** How many drinks do you need to feel high?

(1–2) Worried—Have close friends or relatives worried or complained about your drinking in the past year?

(1) Eye-openers—Do you sometimes take a drink in the morning when you first get up?

(1) Amnesia (blackouts)—Has a friend or family member ever told you about things you said or did while you were drinking that you could not remember?

(1) K (C) Cut Down—Do you sometimes feel the need to cut down on your drinking?

- To score the test, a 7-point scale is used
- The Tolerance-hold question scores 2 points if the respondent is able to hold six or more drinks
- The Tolerance-high question scores 2 points if three or more drinks are needed to feel high

A total score of 2 or more indicates that patients are likely to be risk drinkers. A score of 3 or greater identifies harmful drinking or alcoholism.

of alcoholism are discussed further in Chapter 4. Women who initiate heroin use are more likely than men to have been influenced by a partner who uses heroin.[39,40] Women tend to be less likely than men to inject heroin.[41] One study suggests that women who use heroin develop dependence more quickly than men.[42] Women heroin users report more chronic health problems and psychological stress compared with men.[43] There appears to be no gender differences in complications or mortality related to heroin addiction.

Compared to men, women who use cocaine at an earlier age develop a problem earlier, are more frequently living with an addicted partner, are of lower socioeconomic status, and are more likely to have comorbid depression.[44] Women are more likely than men to use cocaine by smoking and injection, rather than intranasally.[45] Women also trade sex for crack cocaine, putting themselves at high risk for sexually transmitted diseases.

There are few data on gender differences related to marijuana use. Cigarette smoking, however, appears to be particularly problematic for women, with a common belief that smoking can control weight and cessation will contribute to unacceptable weight gain.[46] Women are also more likely than men to identify smoking as a way to reduce stress.[47]

Treatment

There are potentially unique obstacles to addiction treatment for women. Historically, because of stigma, women have been more likely to be hidden users of alcohol and other drugs. Women are more likely to need provision of child care while they are in treatment, and alcoholic women tend to have less spousal support than alcoholic men do.

Women have been found to respond well to brief intervention for alcoholism, especially if they are pregnant.[48] Many treatment programs have been developed specifically for women, but there are no studies that have been specifically designed to show that gender-specific treatment is more effective.[49] However, gender-specific programs may help address issues specific to women; for example, some provide child care.[50] Women attending 12-step groups should seek other women to be their sponsors. An additional goal of treatment specific to women with addiction is reunification of mothers with their children. Women competing 90 days in treatment double the likelihood of reunification.[51]

Pregnancy

Among pregnant women aged 15–44, 5.4% were current illicit drug users, based on data from 2012 and 2013.[2] Many reported effects of drugs of abuse on fetal development are based on animal studies (in which massive doses of drugs are administered) or case reports. For most substances, the major risk to the fetus appears to be possible growth retardation. A summary of reported effects of alcohol and other drugs on the fetus is given in Table 16.1.

Of the drugs of abuse, alcohol is the most harmful to the fetus. Fetal alcohol syndrome (FAS), the most preventable cause of mental retardation,[52] was first described as a well-defined syndrome in 1973.[53] FAS is defined by (1) maternal drinking during pregnancy; (2) characteristic pattern of facial anomalies: short palpebral fissures and abnormalities of the premaxillary area—flat upper lip, flattened philtrum, flat midface; (3) growth retardation and neurodevelopmental abnormalities; and (4) structural brain abnormalities. The amount of alcohol intake needed to cause FAS is unknown, so all pregnant women should be advised to abstain from alcohol.

Cocaine use during pregnancy has been associated with increased risk of placenta previa, placental abruption, and premature labor.[54,55] Much political clamor on the detrimental long-term developmental effects of prenatal cocaine exposure led some states to attempt to criminalize cocaine use during pregnancy. However, subjects abusing other drugs, including alcohol and opioids, have confounded most studies of cocaine risk during pregnancy. Studies differ as to whether infants born to cocaine-using women have lower birth weight.[56,57] Environmental factors appear to play a role in reports of neurobehavioral effects of prenatal exposure to cocaine.[58,59] A 2001 systematic review of the literature, which included 36 papers, failed to find evidence that prenatal cocaine exposure was associated with developmental toxic effects in children.[60]

For opioid-dependent pregnant women, the infant may be born opioid-dependent and require treatment for withdrawal at birth.[61,62] Signs of opioid withdrawal in a neonate include tremor, high-pitched cry, increased muscle tone, hyperactivity, poor feeding, diarrhea,

TABLE 16.1 Reported Abnormalities of the Fetus or Neonate by Substance of Exposure

Substance	Impact
Alcohol	Spontaneous abortion, microcephaly; intrauterine growth restriction' central nervous system dysfunction, including mental retardation and behavioral abnormalities; craniofacial abnormalities; behavioral abnormalities
Sedatives—benzodiazepines	Mild reduction in head circumference at birth, hypotonia and decreased sucking at birth, mild impairment in gross motor development
Opioids	No anomalies; intrauterine growth restriction; depressed breathing movements, preterm rupture of the membranes, preterm labor, meconium-stained amniotic fluid
Marijuana	No anomalies; possible mild behavioral alterations
Stimulants: methamphetamines, cocaine, methylphenidate,	Urinary tract defects; intrauterine growth restriction, hyperactivity in utero, placental abruption, neonatal necrotizing enterocolitis
Hallucinogens	No anomalies; increased spontaneous abortions, dysmorphic face, behavioral problems
Inhalants	Similar to alcohol; increases risk of childhood leukemia
Nicotine	No anomalies; spontaneous abortion, mild intrauterine growth restriction, preterm birth, placenta previa, placental abruption

and sweating. Prenatal marijuana exposure has been reported to cause placental abruption,[63] low birth weight,[64] increased risk of prematurity,[65] and neurological disturbances.[66]

Treatment of Pregnant Women

Treatment of addiction in pregnant women is mostly similar to that for other individuals; however, there are special considerations, such as education related to pregnancy and parenting, as well as the safety of some medications during pregnancy. Most clinical trials of pharmacotherapy for addiction, including treatment of withdrawal, have excluded pregnant women. As a result, recommendations for treatment of addiction in pregnant women have been based on expert opinion, with avoidance of medications that clearly put the fetus at risk for developing abnormalities. Additional consideration must be given after delivery, as most medications pass into breast milk. The World Health Organization (WHO) issued guidelines in 2014 for the identification and treatment of substance use disorders; these guidelines are available online.[67]

For treatment of alcohol withdrawal in pregnant women, benzodiazepines should be prescribed as described in Chapter 4. Both prospective and retrospective clinical trials have not found an association between diazepam use and birth defects.[68,69] The anticonvulsant drugs, carbamazepine and valproic acid, sometimes prescribed for treatment of alcohol withdrawal, should not be used in pregnant women because of teratogenic risk.

For prevention of relapse to drinking, disulfiram should be avoided in pregnant women. Drinking after taking disulfiram could lead to high levels of acetaldehyde that may be dangerous to the mother and fetus. Additionally, fetal abnormalities have been reported with first-trimester exposure to disulfiram.[70,71] There are few data to support the use or safety of naltrexone or acamprosate in treating alcohol dependence in pregnant women.

Opioid dependence in pregnant women has traditionally been treated with a methadone taper or maintenance. The advantage of maintenance is the continued engagement of pregnant women in addiction treatment. There are no reports of birth defects associated with methadone; however, there are reports of lower birth weight and smaller head circumference.[72] Babies born to women receiving methadone generally require treatment for withdrawal. There is no evidence that these babies will have long-term cognitive abnormalities.[73] Buprenorphine, discussed further in Chapter 6, has been used successfully in several clinical trials to treat opioid dependence in pregnant women.[74] Babies born to women receiving buprenorphine maintenance have less opioid withdrawal, not always requiring treatment.[75,76] A 2013 Cochrane review of maintenance agonist treatments for opiate-dependent pregnant women deemed both methadone and buprenorphine to be effective, with methadone superior for retaining patients in treatment and buprenorphine leading to less severe neonatal abstinence syndrome.[77] Reports on the use of naltrexone for opiate dependence in pregnant women are limited to a study of seven women who received oral naltrexone[78] and a study of eight women who received subcutaneous pellet implants of naltrexone;[79] both study groups reported no adverse outcomes.

All pregnant women should be encouraged to quit smoking. Nicotine replacement therapies in pregnant women result in serum nicotine levels similar to those obtained from cigarettes.[80] Tapered use of nicotine replacement is preferable to maintenance, as nicotine may reduce uterine blood flow.[81] The safety of the use of bupropion or varenicline for smoking cessation during pregnancy is unclear, with both agents being pregnancy class C.

Intimate Partner Violence

Intimate partner violence (IPV) or abuse (also referred to as domestic violence or victimization) can be defined as the debilitating experience of physical, psychological, or sexual abuse, often associated with increased isolation from the outside world and limited personal freedom and accessibility to resources. This occurs in all demographic and socioeconomic strata[82] but is especially prevalent among women whose partners have a substance use disorder or who themselves have a substance use disorder.[83,84] A study of female college students found a direct relationship between amount of weekly drinking and the risk sexual victimization.[85] Similarly, female high school students who drink alcohol are more likely to be victims of date violence.[86] In a survey of women in a residential drug treatment center, 73% of women had been raped at least once during their lifetime,[87] and in a similar study of women in a methadone treatment program, 60% reported physical or sexual abuse by an intimate partner.[88] A history of sexual abuse is also associated with poorer global functioning in women otherwise in recovery from alcohol use disorder.[89]

An estimated 1 in 17 women experiences rape, physical violence, or stalking by an intimate partner in the past year.[90] Most of these women never seek help from healthcare practitioners for the consequences of domestic violence. Brief screening for IPV should be incorporated into the medical interview of all women, particularly those of childbearing age; this is endorsed by the U.S. Preventive Services Task Force.[91] Because some women may not initially recognize themselves as victims of IPV, questioning should be specific (Box 16.3). The issue should be dealt with sensitively, validating the difficulty most women have in discussing the issue. There may be reluctance to disclose information because of shame, humiliation, low self-esteem, or fear of retaliation by the perpetrator. Some women may also believe that they deserve the abuse and do not deserve help or that they need to protect their partner, who is often their only source of affection and support. There may also be a belief on the part of the victim that the clinician will not understand the problem or believe her.

In addition to screening, certain patient problems should alert the practitioner to the possibility of IPV (Box 16.4). Women with a history of IPV report 60% higher rates of all health problems than those of women with no history of abuse.[92] Problems may range from direct evidence of physical trauma (contusions, abrasions, broken bones) to nonspecific complaints of fatigue and difficulty concentrating. The screening information and medical history related

---

BOX 16.3 Screening Patients for Intimate Partner Violence

Integrating intimate partner violence inquiry into interview as part of social history:

"Because abuse and violence have unfortunately become a common part of a woman's life, I ask all my patients about it routinely."

> We all occasionally fight at home. What happens when you and your partner disagree?
>
> Have you ever been treated badly or threatened by your partner?
>
> Has your partner ever prevented you from leaving the house, seeing friends, getting a job, or continuing your education?
>
> Does your partner ever force you to have sex or force you to engage in sex that is uncomfortable to you?

(if appropriate) You mentioned your partner drinks (uses drugs). How does he (or she) act when he is drinking (using drugs)?

---

to IPV must be well documented in the medical record, because they can provide evidence that may be used in a legal case. The record should include detailed descriptions of any injuries and, if possible, photographs of injuries sustained.

Once evidence of IPV is obtained, one must assess the seriousness of the situation and the safety of the woman. This must occur even if she is not yet ready to leave the abusive partner. Unfortunately, the level of severity of past violence may not be a predictor of the future severity. If safety is in question, the woman (and her children) should be advised to stay with family or friends, or at a shelter that specializes in caring for abused women and their

---

**BOX 16.4 Clinical Signs and Symptoms Suggestive
of Intimate Partner Violence**

Alcohol or drug abuse

Anxiety

Atypical chest pain

Change in appetite

Chronic headaches

Chronic pain of unclear etiology

Depressed mood

Difficulty concentrating

Dizziness

Fatigue

Frequent minor trauma

Frequent requests for pain medications or tranquilizers

Frequent vague somatic complaints

Gastrointestinal upset, diarrhea, or dyspepsia

Insomnia

Palpitations

Panic attacks

Paresthesias

Pelvic pain

Suicide attempts or gestures

---

families. Medical attention may also be needed for abused children in the household. When women resist taking action, the clinician should continue to show concern and work to motivate the patient toward taking action. The National Domestic Violence Hotline (1-800-799-7233) is a 24-hour service that helps women with crisis intervention. Unfortunately, women with active substance use disorders are sometimes denied shelter by organizations that assist victims of IPV. As an alternative, women's recovery houses that are sensitive and able to meet the needs of women in crisis should be sought. For women with addiction and victimization, recovery from addiction is closely tied to recovery from victimization.[93]

Older Adults

Most substance use problems in the elderly are related to alcohol. However, many older adults take prescribed scheduled drugs for insomnia, chronic pain, and anxiety. It is estimated that up to 11% of older women misuse prescription drugs and that nonmedical use of prescription drugs among all adults over age 50 will increase to 5.7 million by the year 2020.[94]

Literature related to screening, brief intervention, and referral to treatment (SBIRT) in older adults is just emerging.[95] The probability of an alcohol-related discussion between physician and patient declines with patient age.[96] There are no validated screening or assessment instruments available for specifically identifying or diagnosing substance use disorders in the older population.

Alcohol

Longitudinally, drinking amounts typically decrease with advancing age.[97] However, even with the decrease, many drink amounts that are considered unhealthy; the National Institute on Alcohol Abuse and Alcoholism (NIAAA)'s healthy limits for men over 65 are the same as for women (1 drink/day, 7 drinks/week). The 2008 National Health and Nutrition Examination Survey of adults aged 65 and over found that 15% of older drinkers consume alcohol above the NIAAA's recommended limits.[98] However, when health status was taken into account, 53% had potentially harmful consumption. Male drinkers had significantly greater odds of hazardous or harmful consumption than female drinkers. This study did not take into account the additional risk of interaction between alcohol and prescribed drugs, as older adults have been found to lack knowledge of prescription drug risks related to interactions with alcohol.[99,100]

In older adults, the diagnosis of alcohol use disorder may be more difficult, as older adults are less likely to experience loss of a job or legal problems, and more likely to be unemployed and isolated. A change in functional status related to drinking may help define a problem related to alcohol use. Self-report of alcohol use in the elderly may be unreliable, with recall amounts less than diary-recorded amounts.[101]

The performance of the CAGE questionnaire in elderly populations has been assessed in several studies. In a study of 323 general medical outpatients over the age of 60, a CAGE score ≥1 had a sensitivity of 86% and a specificity of 78%.[102] Another study of 154 medical outpatients over the age of 64 found a CAGE score >1 had a sensitivity and specificity of 88%.[103] A study of 103 frail homebound elderly found the CAGE questionnaire had a sensitivity of 60% and a specificity of 100%.[104] Use of the CAGE may not effectively discriminate elderly patients currently drinking from those with a prior history of a drinking problem. Further questioning should distinguish the current pattern of use from past use. The CAGE performs poorly in detecting elderly binge drinkers.[105] To aid further in the diagnosis of alcoholism among the elderly, a geriatric version of the Michigan Alcoholism Screening Test (MAST) can be used.[106] Greater than five "yes" answers indicates an alcohol use disorder, with a sensitivity of 91–93% and a specificity of 65–84%.[107,108]

Elderly individuals with alcoholism tend to fall into two groups: early onset and late onset, and two-thirds fall into the early-onset group.[109,110,111] Those in the early-onset group have had ongoing alcoholism for most of their lives but have often avoided some of the usual morbidities. The late-onset individual may have had a recent stressful life event: loss of spouse, retirement, or a new impairment in activities of daily life. There are no significant differences in age, marital status, employment, or education between individuals in the early- and late-onset alcoholism groups. Women represent a greater proportion of the late-onset group than the early-onset group, but this may be related to the overall higher life expectancy of females. The early-onset group is more likely to drink to intoxication; more likely to have been in alcohol treatment in the past; more likely to have legal, financial, or job problems; and less likely to have social support. The late-onset group is more likely to enter treatment as a result of a crisis, have symptoms of depression or loneliness, and be in denial.

In older adults, alcohol tends to cause dysphoria, rather than euphoria. Tolerance may decrease with aging due to changes in absorption and change in distribution of alcohol in the body.[112,113] Age-related decrease in gastric alcohol dehydrogenase increases the amount of alcohol that enters the bloodstream.[114] This effect may be increased by the use of H2 blockers and proton pump inhibitors commonly prescribed among the elderly. There is no evidence that liver metabolism of alcohol is significantly changed with aging.

The complications of alcohol use in the elderly are mostly the same as those discussed in Chapter 4. Sensitivity to the acute effects of alcohol is heightened in the elderly, with increased risk of harm related to falls.[115] Alcohol-related liver disease as defined by fatty liver on liver biopsy is present in 90–100% of elderly individuals with alcoholism.[116] The probability of cirrhosis increases with the duration of drinking. In the first year after diagnosis of cirrhosis, the mortality rate is 50% in individuals over age 60, compared to 7% in those under age 60.[117] Psychiatric complications of alcoholism in the elderly are similar to those seen in younger individuals.

In the elderly, the onset of withdrawal may not occur until several days after cessation. Confusion rather than tremor is often the predominant clinical sign, and the severity and duration of withdrawal tend to increase with age.[118] Delirium tremens should be part of the differential in any confused older patient, and the diagnosis may depend on interviewing family members.

Elderly alcoholics without a history of severe withdrawal and without comorbid medical conditions can be managed with supportive care at home. The older alcoholic with a history of severe withdrawal is best monitored in the inpatient setting. Additionally, the elderly are at increased risk of adverse effects from the pharmacological treatment of withdrawal, warranting close monitoring. Benzodiazepines, prescribed for treatment of withdrawal, may cause gait disturbance, cognitive impairment, and incontinence.

As with others, treatment of alcohol withdrawal with benzodiazepines should be symptom triggered, and it may be preferable to give shorter-acting agents such as lorazepam.[119]

Over a decade ago, it was reported that only 15% of alcoholics over the age of 60 were receiving adequate treatment.[120] No report has been issued since that time, but it is likely the percentage is now even lower. Few treatment studies include older patients or reported outcomes specific to older age. Evidence suggests alcohol treatment outcome success is optimized when older patients receive age-specific treatment.[121,122] Treatment plans for older patients should focus on overcoming isolation and on establishing social supports.[123] Abstinence may not be required. Older unhealthy drinkers may diminish alcohol consumption if they perceive benefit.[124,125] Senior center involvement is often a way for the elderly alcoholic to find new interests, socialize, and spend time. A telephone intervention to reduce at-risk drinking in older adults in primary care showed moderate impact at 3 months, but no impact at 1 year.[126] Treatment outcomes in elderly alcoholics are comparable to those found in younger alcoholics, with individuals with late-onset alcoholism having a greater likelihood of maintaining abstinence.[127] The pharmacological agents available for use in the treatment of alcoholism (disulfiram, acamprosate, and naltrexone) have not been studied adequately in the elderly.[128] Drug interactions and comorbid medical conditions often limit the use of disulfiram in the elderly.

Illicit Drugs

There are few studies examining the prevalence of illicit drug use among the elderly. Older adults are less likely to be involved in the drug culture. Most elderly heroin users began when they were younger and have survived and avoided serious medical complications. Additionally, the need for treatment may diminish, as in some individuals, addiction wanes with age. There are no data on medication-assisted treatment with buprenorphine or methadone in older adults.

Sedatives

Depression in the elderly often presents with features of anxiety and may be inappropriately treated with sedatives rather than an anti-depressant. Benzodiazepine use increases with age (8.7% of those age 65–80), and the elderly tend to be on high doses of long-acting agents.[129] Use is greater among elderly women than among elderly men. Older adults are also more likely to suffer from insomnia, resulting in prescribing of benzodiazepines. Morbidity related to benzodiazepine use and the treatment of benzodiazepine use disorder are discussed in Chapter 5.

Prescription Opioids

The elderly frequently suffer from chronic pain related to arthritis and other degenerative disorders. Nonpharmacological measures often fail, and the use of nonsteroidal anti-inflammatory drugs (NSAIDs) may be contraindicated by other medical disorders. In most circumstances, opioids can be safely prescribed for chronic pain with good pain relief and improvement in functional status. Many patients can be prescribed a stable, moderate dose of opioid for pain relief without the need for dose escalation. It has generally been thought that adverse consequences most often occur when a drug is used for the wrong purpose, excessive dosages are used, or mental illness is present. However, a 2010 analysis of Medicare claims data raised concerns about the safety of opioids in older adults; in this study, older adults who were prescribed opioids (in comparison to those prescribed NSAIDs), had significantly higher rates of cardio-vascular events, fractures, hospitalizations, and death. Moreover, their risk for gastrointestinal bleeding was not any lower.[130]

Medically supervised withdrawal, or detoxification, of elderly individuals from prescribed opioids follows the same principles as those used for younger individuals. Inpatient treatment is gener-ally reserved for individuals with high potential for morbidity with withdrawal, lack of social support, major medical illness, or fail-ure at attempted outpatient tapering. The long-term treatment of elderly who have misused prescription opioids should be individualized. An elderly person who has misused prescription opioids is unlikely to benefit from attendance at NA meetings dominated by young people who have been using heroin. Group therapy specific to the elderly should be sought. Primary care practitioner involvement is essential, both for counseling and for coordination of a treatment plan. For those with chronic pain, nonpharmacological treatment plays an essential role in long-term success.

Families and Codependence

Codependence is maladaptive or dysfunctional behavior that is associated with living with, working with, treating, or being close to a person with addiction.[131] Codependence affects families, friends, professionals, and communities. Signs and symptoms of codependence include behaviors aimed at protecting the individual with addiction (enabling), psychological symptoms (anxiety, depression, insomnia, aggressiveness, eating disorder, or suicidal gestures), psychosomatic illness, family violence, and drug addiction.[132] Health professionals may fail to diagnose addiction and incorrectly treat symptoms with sedatives, antidepressants, or opioids. Society often chooses not to confront relatives, friends, and colleagues who are obviously impaired by addiction.

When a patient has unexplained somatic or psychological symptoms, it is helpful to ask whether the patient is concerned about the drinking or drug use of someone close to him or her. For an affirmative response, the patient should be asked to describe the problem. One can also ask the patient with possible codependence to answer CAGE questions or the questions on other screening tools as though they were addressed to, and answered honestly by, the "someone." A positive score on one of these is a strong indication of codependence.

Initially, the psychological and behavioral expressions of individuals with codependence are normal responses to an abnormal situation. However, these adaptive responses eventually become dysfunctional. Codependence is chronic and progressive, characterized by denial, ill health, and/or maladaptive behavior and by a lack of knowledge about addiction.

The major strategies in treating a patient with codependence are similar to those for treating an individual with addiction—gaining acceptance of the diagnosis of codependence, motivating the patient to get help, and referring the patient to Al-Anon or Nar-Anon (as with AA or NA referrals, a good understanding of the Al-Anon or Nar-Anon process on the part of the referring clinician is critical to successful referral). Attendees of Al-Anon report better quality of life and decreased stress.[133] Al-Anon attendees referred to the program by their drinkers' healthcare practitioner are more likely to continue to attend Al-Anon meetings.[134] Clinicians should try especially to encourage men to attend Al-Anon, as there continues to be a significant gender difference in Al-Anon—only 16% of members are men.[135] Additionally, the clinician may refer the patient or the family for additional therapy, especially group therapy. If appropriate, assistance in getting the individual with addiction into treatment can be provided.

Codependence includes actions of healthcare practitioners that enable individuals with addiction to remain enmeshed in their disease. Enabling behavior often coexists with otherwise excellent clinical skills.[136] Societal norms, one's own beliefs related to the use of alcohol or other drugs, and a lack of awareness of approaches to diagnosis, motivation, and treatment of individuals with substance use disorders are the major reasons for codependence among clinicians. To overcome enabling behavior, clinicians should update their knowledge of addiction, attend some AA, NA, and Al-Anon meetings, and use the interviewing skills described in Chapter 2. Increased comfort in treating codependence occurs as the clinician helps increasing numbers of patients and their families through the recovery process.

Prisoners

Historically, society has approached the problem of substance use disorders by criminalizing all aspects of addiction. Drug users frequently commit crimes to obtain money for the drugs they use or are arrested in the midst of buying or selling illicit drugs. Drug laws in many states impose mandatory long sentences on those who are arrested for crack cocaine possession. Individuals with alcoholism may be arrested for vagrancy or disorderly conduct. Newly incarcerated individuals show high rates of recent drug use at the time of incarceration. There are calls to transform how the criminal justice system deals with arrested individuals with substance use disorder.[137] Many local jurisdictions have created drug courts with court-ordered drug treatment as an alternative to incarceration, but barriers to effective treatment include cost and court policy.[138] Data for effectiveness are still limited.

The majority of inmates perceive a need for drug treatment, this perception being greatest for individuals using opioids and cocaine.[139] Despite the obvious need for prison-based drug treatment, availability is severely limited, but the need for prison-based treatment has received increasing attention.[140] There has been an effort to increase the number of inmates receiving drug education while in prison; in 2012, 12,000 individuals were transitioned into drug treatment at release.[141] However, this number represents a small fraction of individuals who could benefit from drug treatment.

Arrestees dependent on opioids are often forced to undergo withdrawal without medications, and at most facilities, those who had been receiving methadone or buprenorphine prior to arrest have no possibility for continued maintenance while incarcerated. Clearly, the prison system must do more to provide drug treatment to inmates and facilitate ongoing treatment at release in order to prevent the revolving door of incarceration that many inmates with addiction go through.[142] A study has shown effectiveness of linking inmates to buprenorphine treatment following release from jail.[143] Additionally, another study has shown that initiating methadone treatment in the weeks prior to release from incarceration is an effective way to improve methadone access post-release and to decrease relapse to opioid use.[144]

Health Professionals

The prevalence of substance use disorders among health professionals is regarded to be similar to that of the general population. For example, among American surgeons, a survey found that 15% had a score on the AUDIT-C consistent with an alcohol use disorder.[145] Surgeons who reported being "burned out" were more likely to have alcohol use disorder. Surgeons are also more likely than non-surgeons to enroll in a physician health program (PHP) because of alcohol-related problems (and less likely to enroll because of opioid use).[146] Physicians referred to a PHP have significantly higher odds of substance use disorders for cannabinoids or cocaine compared with a matched general population sample that had ever sought treatment for substance use disorders, even though physicians are less likely to report use of these substances.[147]

Physicians may self-prescribe and self-medicate with controlled substances, and this must be viewed as problematic. Nurses with substance use disorders may have access to opioids intended for patients, and problematic use of opioids by anesthesiologists often occurs through diversion from the operating room.[148]

Many clinicians continue to practice despite being impaired. Professional organizations have implemented programs to address impairment in the health professions. Timely intervention with appropriate treatment as soon as a problem is recognized is imperative. In caring for a health professional with substance use disorder, the interviewing approach outlined in Chapter 2 should be used. It is especially important to show concern and address the often-dominant issues of shame and low self-esteem.

The manifestations of impairment from substance use disorders among health professionals are the same as those seen in other individuals. When one is concerned about impairment in a colleague, it is advisable to contact one or more close associates of that colleague to confirm this. Notably, only 64% of physicians agree with the professional commitment to report physicians who are significantly impaired.[149] When caring for physicians with substance use disorders, the treating physician should openly discuss the issue of physician-patients writing prescriptions for themselves—both in terms of misuse and attempts at self-medicating symptoms.

Persuasion of an impaired professional to accept the existence of a problem and agree to treatment can be attempted by a concerned colleague. Such efforts are often initially met with anger and denial. Most physicians participating in state monitoring programs are not self-referred,[150] and in fact, physicians who are in treatment have had a problem for a mean of 6 years prior to entering treatment.[151] The involvement of a state's physician or nurse rehabilitation committee is generally required. A directory of these programs is available through the website www.fsphp.org. State boards will directly confront the impaired health provider using a formal intervention. The goal of this process is provide help, usually in the form of treatment, with the requirement to complete treatment in order to maintain a professional license. All PHPs require random drug testing and are generally 5 years in duration.[152] In a survey of physicians who completed a PHP, 93% would recommend it to others, and 85% continued participation in 12-step meetings after the 5-year mandate.[153]

There are few clinical trials on the optimal type or length of addiction treatment for health professionals. After rehabilitation, individuals may seek 12-step group meetings specifically aimed at professionals that are available in most communities. In surveys, health professionals' acceptance of 12-step groups tends to be high;[154,155] indeed, one of the founders of AA was a physician.

Some states have created treatment requirements specific to specialty, such as in Florida, where anesthesiologists referred to the PHP for an opioid use disorder must take naltrexone for 2 years, with one study showing efficacy for this requirement.[156] Buprenorphine maintenance therapy for opioid-dependent physicians or nurses is permitted in some states and prohibited by others, and many states do not have an official policy.[157]

As in other individuals, relapse is not uncommon in healthcare professionals. Use of opioids with coexisting psychiatric illness and a family history of substance use disorders appear to be risk factors for relapse among healthcare professionals.[158] Overall success rates for physicians are quite high, with a cohort of 904 physicians in 16 state PHPs showing 78% of physicians never having a positive test for alcohol or drugs over a 5-year period.[159] In other reports on this cohort, psychiatrists, anesthesiologists, and emergency physicians with a substance use disorder fared as well as physicians in other specialties.[160,161,162]

Notes

1. Johnston LD, O'Malley PM, Bachman JG, Schulenberg, JE. Monitoring the future. National results on adolescent drug use: overview of key findings, 2011. Ann Arbor: Institute for Social Research, University of Michigan.

2. Substance Abuse and Mental Health Services Administration. *Results from the 2013 National Survey on Drug Use and Health: Summary of National Findings*. NSDUH Series H-48, HHS Publication No. (SMA) 14-4863. Rockville, MD: Substance Abuse and Mental Health Services Administration; 2014.

3. Howard MO, Bowen SE, Garland EL, et al. Inhalant use and inhalant use disorders in the United States. Addict Sci Clin Pract 2011;6:18–31.

4. Zullig KJ, Divin AL. The association between non-medical prescription drug use, depressive symptoms, and suicidality among college students. Addict Behav 2012;37:890–9.

5. McCabe SE, West BT, Teter CJ, Boyd CJ. Trends in medical use, diversion, and nonmedical use of prescription medications among college students from 2003 to 2013: connecting the dots. Addict Behav 2014;39:1176–82.

6. Committee on Substance Abuse. American Academy of Pediatrics. Substance use screening, brief intervention, and referral to treatment for pediatricians. Pediatrics 2011;128:e1330–40.

7. Knight JR, Shrier LA, Bravender TD, et al. A new brief screen for adolescent substance abuse. Arch Pediatr Adolesc Med 1999;153:591–6.

8. **Knight JR, Sherritt L, Shrier LA, et al. Validity of the CRAFFT substance abuse screening test among general adolescent clinic patients. Arch Pediatr Adolesc Med 2002;156:607–14**. *In this cohort of 538 patients ages 14–18 (68% female and 76% racial/ethnic minorities),*

50% had practiced no substance use in the past 12 months; 24%, occasional use; 11%, problem use; 9.5% had experienced abuse; and 6.7%, dependence. A CRAFFT score of 2 or higher was optimal for identifying any problem (sensitivity, 0.76; specificity, 0.94; positive predictive value [PPV], 0.83; negative predictive value [NPV], 0.91) and dependence (sensitivity, 0.92; specificity, 0.80; PPV, 0.25; NPV, 0.99). Validity was not significantly affected by age, sex, or race.

9. Mitchell SG, Kelly SM, Gryczynski J, et al. The CRAFFT cut-points and DSM-5 criteria for alcohol and other drugs: a reevaluation and reexamination. Subst Abuse 2014;35:376–80.

10. **Wilson CR, Sherritt L, Gates E, Knight JR. Are clinical impressions of adolescent substance use accurate? Pediatrics 2004;114:536–40.** *This study involved secondary analysis of data from a validation study of the CRAFFT in 14- to 18-year-old medical clinic patients (n = 533) and their corresponding clinicians (n = 109). Of 100 patients with problem substance use, clinicians correctly identified 18; of 50 patients with a diagnosis of alcohol or drug abuse, clinicians correctly identified 10; and of 36 patients with a diagnosis of alcohol or drug dependence, clinicians correctly identified none.*

11. Cornelius JR, Maisto SA, Pollock NK, et al. Withdrawal and dependency symptoms among adolescent alcohol and drug abusers. Addiction 1995;90:627–35.

12. Federal Bureau of Investigation. Crime in the United States, 2010. http://www.fbi.gov/about-us/cjis/ucr/crime-in-the-u.s/2010/crime-in-the-u.s.-2010/persons-arrested

13. Kann L, PhD, Kinchen S, Shanklin SL, et al. Youth risk behavior surveillance—United States. MMWR Morbid Mortal Wkly Rep 2014;63:1–47.

14. Substance Abuse and Mental Health Services Administration, *Drug Abuse Warning Network, 2011: National Estimates of Drug-Related Emergency Department Visits.* HHS Publication No. (SMA) 13-4760, DAWN Series D-39. Rockville, MD: Substance Abuse and Mental Health Services Administration; 2013.

15. Biederman J, Wilens T, Mick E, et al. Is ADHD a risk factor for psychoactive substance use disorders? Findings from a four-year prospective follow-up study. J Am Acad Child Adolesc Psychiatry 1997;36:21–9.

16. Molina BS, Pelham WE. Childhood predictors of adolescent substance use in a longitudinal study of children with ADHD. J Abnormal Psychol 2003;112:497–507.

17. Esposito-Smythers C, Spirito A. Adolescent substance use and suicidal behavior: a review with implications for treatment research. Alcohol Clin Exp Res 2004;28:77S–88S.

18. Clark DB, Lynch KG, Donovan JD, et al. Health problems in adolescents with alcohol use disorders: self-report, liver injury and physical examination findings. Alcohol Clin Exp Res 2001;25:1350–9.

19. Weddle M, Kokotailo P. Adolescent substance abuse. Confidentiality and consent. Pediatr Clin North Am 2002;49:301–15.

20. Winters KC, Botzet A, Fahnhorst T. Advances in adolescent substance abuse treatment. Curr Psychiatry Rep 2011;13:416–21.

21. Barnett E, Sussman S, Smith C, et al. Motivational interviewing for adolescent substance use: a review of the literature. Addict Behav 2012;37:1325–34.

22. Walton MA, CHermack ST, Shope JT. Effects of a brief intervention for reducing violence and alcohol misuse among adolescents: a randomized controlled trial. JAMA 2010;304:527–35.

23. Patnode CD, O'Connor E, Rowland M, et al. Primary care behavioral interventions to prevent or reduce illicit drug use and nonmedical pharmaceutical use in children and adolescents: a systematic evidence review for the U.S. Preventive Services Task Force. Ann Intern Med 2014;160:612–20.

24. Kypri K, Vater T, Bowe SJ, et al. Web-based alcohol screening and brief intervention for university students: a randomized trial. JAMA 2014;311:1218–24.

25. Black JJ, Chung T. Mechanisms of change in adolescent substance abuse treatment: how does treatment work? Subst Abuse 2014;35:344–51.

26. Labbe AK, Slaymaker V, Kelly JF. Toward enhancing 12-step facilitation among young people: a systematic qualitative investigation of young adults' 12-step experiences. Subst Abuse 2014;35:399–407.

27. Hersh J, John F. Curry JF, Kaminer Y. What is the impact of comorbid depression on adolescent substance abuse treatment? Subst Abuse 2014;35:364–75.

28. Hiller ML, Malluche D, Bryan V. A multisite description of juvenile drug courts: program models and during-program outcomes. Int J Offender Ther Comp Criminol 2010;54:213–35.

29. Minozzi S, Amato L, Bellisario C, Davoli M. Maintenance treatments for opiate-dependent adolescents. Cochrane Database Syst Rev 2014;6:CD007210.

30. Fishman MJ, Winstanley EL, Curran E, et al. Treatment of opioid dependence in adolescents and young adults with extended release naltrexone: preliminary case-series and feasibility. Addiction 2010;105:1669–76.

31. Sells SB, Simpson DD. The case for drug abuse treatment effectiveness, based on the DARP research program. Br J Addict 1980;75:117–31.

32. **Woody GE, Poole SA, Subramaniam G. Extended vs. short-term buprenorphine-naloxone for treatment of opioid-addicted youth: a randomized trial. JAMA 2008;300:2003–11.** *In this 12-week trial of 152 patients aged 15–21 years, 21% of those who received a 4-week taper remained in treatment compared to 70% of those who received 12 weeks of buprenorphine (p < 0.001).*

33. Substance Abuse and Mental Health Services Administration, Center for Behavioral Health Statistics and Quality. *Treatment Episode Data Set (TEDS): 2002–2012. National Admissions to Substance Abuse Treatment Services.* BHSIS Series S-71, HHS Publication No. (SMA) 14-4850. Rockville, MD: Substance Abuse and Mental Health Services Administration; 2014.

34. Redgrave GW, Swartz KL, Romanoski AJ. Alcohol misuse by women. Int Rev Psychiatry 2003;15:256–68.

35. Bradley KA, Boyd-Wickizer J, Powell SH, Burman ML. Alcohol screening questionnaires in women: a critical review. JAMA 1998;280:166–71.

36. Cherpital CJ. Screening for alcohol problems in the US general population: a comparison of the CAGE and TWEAK by gender, ethnicity, and services utilization. J Stud Alcohol 1999;60:705–11.

37. Russell M, Martier SS, Sokol RJ, et al. Screening for pregnancy risk-drinking. Alcohol Clin Exp Res 1994;18:1156–61.

38. Wilsnack SC, Wilsnack RW. Epidemiology of women's drinking. J Subst Abuse Treat 1991;3:133–57.

39. Hser Y, Anglin M, McGlothin W. Sex differences in addict careers, I: initiation of use. Am J Drug Alcohol Abuse 1987;13:33–57.

40. Gossop M, Griffiths P, Strang J. Sex differences in patterns of drug taking behavior: a study at a London community drug team. Br J Psychiatry 1994;164:101–4.

41. Powis B, Griffiths P, Gossop M, Strang M. The differences between male and female drug users: community samples of heroin and cocaine users compared. Subst Use Misuse 1996;31:529–43.

42. Ellinwood E, Smith W, Vaillant G. Narcotic addictions in males and females: a comparison. Int J Addict 1966;1:33–45.

43. Grella CE, Loviger K. Gender differences in physical and mental health outcomes among an aging cohort of individuals with a history of heroin dependence. Addictive Behav 2012;37:306–12.

44. Griffin ML, Weiss RD, Mirin SM, Lange U. A comparison of male and female cocaine abusers. Arch Gen Psychiatry 1989;46:122–6.

45. McCance-Katz E, Carroll K, Rounsaville B. Gender differences in treatment-seeking cocaine abusers-implications for treatment and prognosis. Am J Addict 1999;8:300–11.

46. Rigotti N. Cigarette smoking and body weight. N Engl J Med 1989;320:931–3.

47. Gritz E, Nielsen I, Brooks L. Smoking cessation and gender: the influence of physiological, psychological, and behavioral factors. J Am Med Womens Assoc 1996;51:35–42.

48. **Manwell LB, Fleming MF, Mundt MP, et al. Treatment of problem alcohol use in women of childbearing age: results of a brief intervention trial. Alcohol Clin Exp Res 2000;24:1517–24.** *In this study, 205 female patients ages 18–40 were randomized to control or brief intervention (BI)—two 15-minute, physician-delivered counseling visits. BI significantly reduced both 7-day alcohol use (p = 0.004) and binge drinking episodes (p = 0.002) over the 48-month follow-up. A logistic regression model found an odds ratio of 1.9 of a 20% or greater reduction in drinking in the sample exposed to BI.*

49. Greenfield SF, Brooks AJ, Gordon SM, et al. Substance abuse treatment entry, retention, and outcome in women: a review of the literature. Drug Alcohol Depend 2007;86:1–21.

50. Niv N, Hser YH. Women-only and mixed-gender drug abuse treatment programs: service needs, utilization and outcomes. Drug Alcohol Depend 2007;87:194–201.

51. Grella CE, Needell B, Shi Y, Hser YI. Do drug treatment services predict reunification outcomes of mothers and their children in child welfare? J Subst Abuse Treat 2009;36:278–93.

52. Warren K, Foudin L. Alcohol-related birth defects, the past, present and future. Alcohol Res Health 2001;25:153–8.

53. Jones K, Smith D, Ulleland C, Streissguth P. Pattern of malformation in offspring of chronic alcoholic mothers. Lancet 1973;1(7815):1267–71.

54. Macones G, Sehdev H, Parry S, et al. The association between maternal cocaine use and placenta previa. Am J Obstet Gynecol 1997;177:1097–100.

55. Acker D, Sachs BP, Tracey KJ, Wise WE. Abruptio placentae associated with cocaine use. Am J Obstet Gynecol 1983;146:220–1.

56. Miller J, Boudreaux M, Regan F. A case-control study of cocaine use in pregnancy. Am J Obstet Gynecol 1995;172:180–5.

57. **Hulse G, English D, Milne E, et al. Maternal cocaine use and low birth weight newborns: a meta-analysis. Addiction 1997;92:1561–70.** *A meta-analysis of five studies presenting data for "any" prenatal cocaine exposure, adjusted for tobacco smoking but unadjusted for gestational age, produced a pooled relative risk estimate of 2.15 (95% CI 1.75–2.64). However, other lifestyle factors not controlled for may account for the observed effects.*

58. **Chasnoff I, Anson A, Hatcher R, et al. Prenatal exposure to cocaine and other drugs. Outcome at four to six years. Ann N Y Acad Sci 1998;846:314–28.** *This longitudinal, prospective study compared 95 children born to mothers who used cocaine and other drugs during pregnancy and 75 matched, non-exposed children born to mothers who had no evidence of alcohol or illicit substance use during pregnancy. Prenatal exposure to cocaine and other drugs had no direct effect on the child's cognitive outcome (measured as IQ), but there was an effect mediated through the home environment.*

59. Koren G, Nulman I, Rovet J, et al. Long-term neurodevelopmental risks in children exposed in utero to cocaine. The Toronto Adoption Study. Ann N Y Acad Sci 1998;846:306–13.

60. Frank DA, Augustyn M, Knight WG, et al. Growth, development, and behavior in early childhood following prenatal cocaine exposure: a systematic review. JAMA 2001;285:1613–25.

61. Werler MM, Pober BR, Holmes LB, Smoking and pregnancy. Teratology 1985;32:473–81.

62. Himmelberger D, Brown B, Cohen E. Cigarette smoking during pregnancy and the occurrence of spontaneous abortion and congenital abnormality. Am J Epidemiol 1978;108:470–9.

63. Williams MA, Lieberman E, Mittendorf R, et al. Risk factors for abruptio placentae. Am J Epidemiol 1991;134:965–72.

64. Zuckerman B, Frank DA, Hingson R, et al. Effects of maternal marijuana and cocaine use on fetal growth. N Engl J Med 1989;320:762–8.

65. Gibson GT, Baghurst PA, Colley DP. Maternal alcohol, tobacco and cannabis consumption and the outcome of pregnancy. Aust N Z J Obstet Gynaecol 1983;23:15–19.

66. Fried PA. Marihuana use by pregnant women and effects on offspring: an update. Neurobehav Toxicol Teratol 1982;4:451–4.

67. World Health Organization. *Guidelines for the Identification and Management of Substance Use Disorders in Pregnancy.* Geneva: WHO Press; 2014. http://apps.who.int/iris/bitstream/10665/107130/1/9789241548731_eng.pdf

68. Rosenberg L, Mitchell AA, Parsells JL, et al. Lack of relation of oral clefts to diazepam use during pregnancy. N Engl J Med 1983;309:1282–5.

69. **Ornoy A, Arnon J, Shechtman S, et al. Is benzodiazepine use during pregnancy really teratogenic? Reprod Toxicol 1998;12:511–5.** *This follow-up study of 460 pregnancies in which women reported using benzodiazepines found that the incidence of congenital anomalies (3.1%) in the exposure group was not significantly different from that found in 424 control pregnancies (2.6%).*

70. Helmbrecht GD, Hoskins IA. First trimester disulfiram exposure: report of two cases. Am J Perinatal 1993;10:5–7.

71. Reitnauer J, Callanan NP, Farber RA, Aylsworth AS, Prenatal exposure to disulfiram implicated in the cause of malformations in discordant monozygotic twins. Teratology 1997;56:358–62.

72. Blinick GE, Jerez E, Wallach RC. Methadone maintenance, pregnancy and progeny. JAMA 1973;225:477–9.

73. Kaltenbach KA, Finnegan LP, Prenatal narcotic exposure: perinatal and developmental effects, Neurotoxicology 1989;10:597–604.

74. **Fischer G, Johnson RE, Eder H, et al. Treatment of opioid-dependent pregnant women with buprenorphine. Addiction 2000;95:239–44.** *This case series involved 15 opioid-dependent pregnant women who received sublingual buprenorphine for opioid withdrawal. Buprenorphine was well tolerated during induction and 91% of women remained opioid negative. All maternal, fetal, and neonatal safety laboratory measures were within normal limits or not of clinical significance. Opioid withdrawal was absent, mild (without treatment), and moderate (with treatment) in eight, four, and three neonates, respectively. The mean duration of withdrawal was 1.1 days.*

75. **Johnson RE, Jones HE, Fischer G. Use of buprenorphine in pregnancy: patient management and effects on the neonate. Drug**

Alcohol Depend 2003;70:S87–101. *This review consisted of 15 cohorts of infants exposed to buprenorphine in utero. Of approximately 309 infants exposed, a neonatal abstinence syndrome (NAS) occurred in 62% infants with 48% requiring treatment; 40% of these cases are confounded by illicit drug use.*

76. Jones HE, Kaltenbach K, Heil SH. Neonatal abstinence syndrome after methadone or buprenorphine exposure. N Engl J Med 2010;363:2320–31.

77. Minozzi S, Amato L, Bellisano C, et al. Maintenance agonist treatments for opiate dependent pregnant women. Cochrane Database Syst Rev 2013;12:CD006318.

78. Hulse GK, G. O'Neill G, Pereira C, Brewer C. Obstetric and neonatal outcomes associated with maternal naltrexone exposure. Aust N Z J Obstet Gynaecol 2001;41:424–8.

79. Hulse G, O'Neil G. Using naltrexone implants in the management of the pregnant heroin user. Aust N Z J Obstet Gynaecol 2002;42:569–73.

80. Ogburn PL, Hurt RD, Croghan IT, et al. Nicotine patch use in pregnancy: nicotine and cotinine levels and fetal effects, Am J Obstet Gynecol 1999;181:736–43.

81. Clark KE, Irion GL. Fetal hemodynamic response to maternal intravenous nicotine administration. Am J Obstet Gynecol 1992;167:1624–31.

82. Heise L, Garcia-Moreno C. Violence by Intimate Partners. World Report on Violence and Health. Geneva: World Health Organization; 2002.

83. **Weinsheimer RL, Schermer CR, Malcoe LH, et al. Severe intimate partner violence and alcohol use among female trauma patients. J Trauma 2005;58:22–9.** *In this survey of 95 consecutive adult female trauma patients, 46% reported a lifetime history of severe intimate partner violence (IPV), and 26% experienced severe IPV in the past year. Past-year IPV was identified in 59% of women screening positive for drinking problems, but in only 13% of those screening negative for drinking problems (p = 0.001). Past-year IPV prevalence was 55% when the partner was a problem drinker and was 8% when he was not (p = 0.001). Multivariate analysis showed that female problem drinking (odds ratio [OR] = 5.8) and partner problem drinking (OR = 8.9) were independent predictors of past-year severe IPV.*

84. Miller BA, Wilsnack SC, Cunradi CB. Family violence and victimization: treatment issues for women with alcohol problems. Alcohol Clin Exp Res 2000;24:1287–97.

85. Gross W, Billingham R. Alcohol consumption and sexual victimization among college women. Psychol Rep 1998;82:80–2.

86. Malik S, Sorenson S, Aneshensel C. Community and dating violence among adolescents: perpetration and victimization. J Adolesc Health 1997;21:291–302.

87. Teets JM. The incidence and experience of rape among chemically dependent women. J Psychoactive Drugs 1997;29:331–6.

88. Gilbert L, el-Bassel N, Schilling RF, Friedman E. Childhood abuse as a risk for partner abuse among women in methadone maintenance. Am J Drug Alcohol Abuse 1997;23:581–95.

89. Sugarman DE, Kaufman JS, Trucco EM, et al. Predictors of drinking and functional outcomes for men and women following inpatient alcohol treatment. Am J Addict 2014;23:226–33.

90. Black MC, Basile KC, Breiding MJ, et al. *The National Intimate Partner and Sexual Violence Survey (NISVS): 2010 Summary Report*. Atlanta, GA: National Center for Injury Prevention and Control, Centers for Disease Control and Prevention; 2011.

91. Nelson HD, Bougatsos C, Blazina I. Screening women for intimate partner violence: a systematic review to update the U.S. Preventive Services Task Force recommendation. Ann Intern Med 2012;156:796–808.

92. Campbell J, Jones AS, Dienemann J, et al. Intimate partner violence and physical health consequences. Arch Intern Med 2002;162:1157–63.

93. Liebschutz JM, Mulvey KP, Samet JH. Victimization among substance-abusing women. Worse health outcomes. Arch Intern Med. 1997;157:1093–7.

94. Han B, Gfroerer JC, Colliver JD, Penne MA. Substance use disorder among older adults in the United States in 2020. Addiction. 2009;104:88–96.

95. Schonfeld L, Hazlett RW, Hedgecock DK, et al. Screening, brief intervention, and referral to treatment for older adults with substance misuse. Am J Public Health 2015;105:205–11.

96. Duru OK, Xu H, Tseng CH, et al. Correlates of alcohol-related discussions between older adults and their physicians. J Am Geriatr Soc 2010;58:2369–74.

97. McEvoy LK, Kritz-Silverstein D, Barrett-Connor E, et al. Changes in alcohol intake and their relationship with health status over a 24-year

follow-up period in community-dwelling older adults. J Am Geriatr Soc 2013;61:1303–8.

98. Wilson SR, Knowles SB, Huang Q, Fink A. The prevalence of harmful and hazardous alcohol consumption in older U.S. adults: data from the 2005–2008 National Health and Nutrition Examination Survey (NHANES). J Gen Intern Med 2014;29:312–9.

99. Zanjani F, Hoogland AI, Downer BG. Alcohol and prescription drug safety in older adults. Drug Health Patient Saf 2013;5:13–27.

100. Cousins G, Galvin R, Flood M, et al. Potential for alcohol and drug interactions in older adults: evidence from the Irish longitudinal study on ageing. BMC Geriatr 2014;14:57.

101. Graham K. Identifying and measuring alcohol abuse among the elderly: serious problems with existing instrumentation. J Stud Alcohol 1986;47:322–6.

102. Buchsbaum DG, Buchanan RG, Welsh J, et al. Screening for drinking disorders in the elderly using the CAGE questionnaire. J Am Geriatr Soc 1992;40:662–5.

103. Jones TV, Lindsey BA, Yount P, et al. Alcoholism screening questionnaires: are they valid in elderly medical outpatients? J Gen Intern Med 1993;8:674–8.

104. Bercsi SJ, Brickner PW, Saha DC. Alcohol use and abuse in the frail, homebound elderly: a clinical analysis of 103 persons. Drug Alcohol Depend 1993;33:139–49.

105. **Adams WL, Barry KL, Fleming MF. Screening for problem drinking in older primary care patients. JAMA 1996;276:1964–7.** *A total of 5,065 consecutive patients over 60 years old were administered questions about the quantity and frequency of regular drinking in the last 3 months, the number of episodes of binge drinking (≥6 drinks per occasion), and the CAGE questionnaire—15% of men and 12% of women drank in excess of recommended limits (>7 drinks/week for women and >14 drinks/ week for men), while 9% of men and 3% of women screened positive on the CAGE (≥2 positive answers) for alcohol abuse within the past 3 months. The authors concluded that asking questions on the quantity and frequency of drinking, in addition to administering the CAGE, increases the number of problem drinkers detected.*

106. Blow FC, Brower KJ, Schulenberg JE, et al. The Michigan Alcoholism Screening Test-Geriatric version (MAST-G): a new elderly-specific screening instrument. Alcohol Clin Exp Res 1992;16:372–4.

107. Joseph CL, Ganzin L, Atkinson RM. Screening for alcohol use disorders in the nursing home. J Am Geriatr Soc 1995;43:368–73.

108. MacNeil, PD, Campbell JW, Vernon L. Screening for alcoholism in the elderly. J Am Geriatr Soc 1994;42:SA7.

109. Adams SL, Waskel SA. Late onset of alcoholism among older Midwestern men in treatment. Psychol Rep 1991;68:432–4.

110. Atkinson RM, Tolson RL, Turner JA. Late versus early onset drinking in older men. Alcohol Clin Exp Res 1990;14:574–9.

111. Brennan PL, Moos RH. Functioning, life context and help-seeking among late-onset problem drinkers: comparison with non-problem and early onset heavy drinkers on skid row. Br J Addict 1991;86:1139–50.

112. Pozzato G, Moretti M, Franzin F, et al. Ethanol metabolism and aging: the role of first-pass metabolism and gastric alcohol dehydrogenase activity. J Gerontol A Biol Sci Med Sci 1995;50:135–41.

113. Vestal RE, McGuire EA, Tobin JD, et al. Aging and ethanol metabolism. Clin Pharmacol Ther 1977; 21:343–54.

114. Seitz HK, Simanowski UA, Waldherr R, et al. Human gastric alcohol dehydrogenase activity: effect of age, sex and alcoholism. Gut 1993;34:1433–7.

115. Wadd S, Papadopoulos C. Drinking behaviour and alcohol-related harm amongst older adults: analysis of existing UK datasets. BMC Res Notes. 2014;7:741.

116. 38. Grant BF, Dufour MC, Hartford TC. Epidemiology of alcoholic liver disease. Semin Liver Dis 1988;8:12–25.

117. Potter JF, James OF. Clinical features and prognosis of alcoholic liver disease in respect to advancing age. Gerontology 1987;33:380–7.

118. Brower KJ, Mudd S, Blow FC, et al Severity and treatment of alcohol withdrawal in elderly versus younger patients. Alcohol Clin Exp Res 1994;18:196–201.

119. Taheri A, Dahri K, Chan P, et al. Evaluation of a symptom-triggered protocol approach to the management of alcohol withdrawal syndrome in older adults. J Am Geriatr Soc 2014;62:1551–5.

120. National Institute on Alcohol Abuse and Alcoholism. Alcohol and Health, Tenth Special Report to the U.S. Congress from the Secretary of Health and Human Services, 2000.

121. Amadeo M. Treating the late life alcoholic. Guidelines for working through denial—integrating individual, family and group approaches. J Geriatr Psychol 1990;23:91–105.

122. Kofoed LL, Tolson RL, Atkinson RM, et al. Treatment compliance of older alcoholics: an elder-specific approach is superior to mainstreaming. J Stud Alcohol 1987;48:47–51.

123. Schonfeld L, Dupree LW. Treatment approaches for older problem drinkers. Int J Addiction 1995;30:1819–42.

124. Borok J, Galier P, Dinolfo M, et al. Why do older unhealthy drinkers decide to make changes or not in their alcohol consumption? Data from the Healthy Living as You Age study. J Am Geriatr Soc 2013;61:1296–302.

125. Fink A, Elliott MN, Tsai M, Beck JC. An evaluation of an intervention to assist primary care physicians in screening and educating older patients who use alcohol. J Am Geriatr Soc 2005;53:1937–43.

126. Lin JC, Karno MP, Tang L, et al. Do health educator telephone calls reduce at-risk drinking among older adults in primary care? J Gen Intern Med 2010;25:334–9.

127. Atkinson RM, Tolson RL, Turner JA. Factors affecting outpatient treatment compliance of older male problem drinkers. J Stud Alcohol 1993;54:102–6.

128. Kuerbis A, Sacco P. A review of existing treatments for substance abuse among the elderly and recommendations for future directions. Subst Abuse 2013;7:13–37.

129. Olfson M, King M, Schoenbaum M. Benzodiazepine use in the United States. JAMA Psychiatry. 2015;72(2):136–42.

130. Solomon DH, Rassen JA, Glynn RJ, et al. The comparative safety of analgesics in older adults with arthritis. Arch Intern Med 2010;170:1968–76.

131. Young LB, Timko C. Benefits and costs of alcoholic relationships and recovery through Al-Anon. Subst Use Misuse 2015;50:62–71.

132. Hurcom C, Copello A, Orford J. The family and alcohol: effects of excessive drinking and conceptualizations of spouses over recent decades. Subst Use Misuse 2000;35:473–502.

133. Timko C, Cronkite R, Kaskutas LA, et al. Al-Anon family groups: newcomers and members. J Stud Alcohol Drugs 2013;74:965–76.

134. Timko C, Laudet A, Moos RH. Newcomers to Al-Anon: who stays and who drops out? Addictive Behav 2014;39:1042–9.

135. Short NA, Cronkite R, Moos R, Timko C. Men and women who attend Al-Anon: gender differences in reasons for attendance, health status and personal functioning, and drinker characteristics. Subst Use Misuse 2015;50:53–61.

136. Williams E, Bissell L, Sullivan E. The effects of co-dependence on physicians and nurses. Br J Addict 1991;86:37–42.

137. Office of National Drug Control Policy. National Drug Control Strategy. Washington, DC: Executive Office of the President, The White House; 2014.

138. Matusow H, Dickman SL, Rich JD. Medication-assisted treatment in US drug courts: results from a nationwide survey of availability, barriers and attitudes. J Subst Abuse Treat 2013;44:473–80.

139. Lo CC, Stephens RC. Drugs and prisoners: treatment needs on entering prison. Am J Drug Alcohol Abuse 2000;26:229–45.

140. Chandler RK, Fletcher BW, Volkow ND. Treating drug abuse and addiction in the criminal justice system: improving public health and safety. JAMA 2009;301:183–90.

141. Federal Bureau of Prisons. Annual Report on Substance Abuse Treatment Programs—Fiscal Year 2012. http://www.bop.gov/inmates/custody_and_care/docs/annual_report_fy_2012.pdf

142. Lee JD, Rich JD. Opioid pharmacotherapy in criminal justice settings: now is the time. Subst Abuse 2012;33:1–4.

143. Lee JD, Grossman E, Truncali A, et al. Buprenorphine-naloxone maintenance following release from jail. Subst Abuse 2012;33:40–47.

144. McKenzie A randomized trial of methadone initiation prior to release from incarceration. Subst Abuse 2012;33:19–29.

145. Oreskovich MR, Kaups KL, Balch CM, et al. Prevalence of alcohol use disorders among American surgeons. Arch Surg 2012;147:168–74.

146. Buhl A, Oreskovich, Meredith CW, et al. Prognosis for the recovery of surgeons from chemical dependency: a 5-year outcome study. Arch Surg 2011;146:1286–91.

147. Cottler LB, Ajinkya S, Merlo LJ. Lifetime psychiatric and substance use disorders among impaired physicians in a physicians health program: comparison to a general treatment population: psychopathology of impaired physicians. J Addict Med 2013;7:108–12.

148. Cummings SM, Merlo L, Cottler LB. Mechanisms of prescription drug diversion among impaired physicians. J Addict Dis 2011;30:195–202.

149. DesRoches CM, Rao SR, Fromson JA, et al. Physicians' perceptions, preparedness for reporting, and experiences related to impaired and incompetent colleagues. JAMA 2010;304:187–93.

150. **Knight JR, Sanchez LT, Sherritt L, et al. Monitoring physician drug problems: attitudes of participants. J Addict Dis 2002;21:27–36.** *Among 87 physicians in a treatment program, identified sources of referral were self (32%), a friend/colleague (31%), the state medical board (15%), hospital chief (12%), and family member (3%).*

151. **Brooke D, Edwards G, Taylor C. Addiction as an occupational hazard: 144 doctors with drug and alcohol problems. Br J Addict 1991;86:1011–16.** *In this retrospective study of 144 doctors (mean age 43) who had received treatment for alcohol and other drug use disorders, mean duration of problematic use prior to entering treatment was 6.7 years for alcohol users and 6.4 years for other drug users. Alcohol was the current problem for 42% and other drugs for 26%; 31% were using both alcohol and other drugs.*

152. Dupont RL, McLellan AT, Carr G, et al. How are addicted physicians treated? A national survey of physician health programs. J Subst Abuse Treat 2009;37:1–7.

153. Merlo LJ, Greene W. Physician views regarding substance use related participation in a state physician health program. Am J Addict 2010;19:529–33.

154. Carlson HB, Dilts SL, Radcliff S. Physicians with substance abuse problems and their recovery environment: a survey. J Subst Abuse Treat 1994;11:113–9.

155. Galanter M, Talbott D, Gallegos K, Rubenstone E. Combined Alcoholics Anonymous and professional care for addicted physicians. Am J Psychiatry 1990;147:64–8.

156. Merlo LH, Greene WM, Pomm R. Mandatory naltrexone treatment prevents relapse among opiate dependent anesthesiologists returning to practice. J Addict Med 2011;5:279–83.

157. Hamza H, Bryson EO. Buprenorphine maintenance therapy in opioid addicted health care professionals returning to clinical practice: a hidden controversy. Mayo Clin Proc 2012;87:260–7.

158. **Domino KB, Hornbein TF, Polissar NL, et al. Risk factors for relapse in health care professionals with substance use disorders.**

JAMA 2005;293:1453–60. *In this retrospective cohort study of 292 health care professionals, 25% had at least one relapse. The risk of relapse increased with family history of a substance use disorder (hazard ratio [HR], 2.3; 95% CI, 1.4–3.6), and use of an opioid increased the risk of relapse significantly in the presence of a coexisting psychiatric disorder (HR, 5.8; 95% CI, 2.9–11.4) but not in the absence of a coexisting psychiatric disorder (HR, 0.9; 95% CI, 0.3–2.2). The presence of all three factors (opioid use, psychiatric illness, and family history) markedly increased the risk of relapse (HR, 13.2; 95% CI, 5.2–33.6). The risk of subsequent relapses increased after the first relapse (HR, 1.7; 95% CI, 1.1–2.5).*

159. Dupont RL, McLellan AT, White WL, et al. Setting the standard for recovery: physicians' health programs. J Subst Abuse Treat 2009;36:159–71.

160. Yellowlees PM, Campbell MD, Rose JS. Psychiatrists with substance use disorders: positive treatment outcomes from physician health programs. Psychiatr Serv 2014;65:1492–5.

161. Skipper GE, Cambell MD, Dupont RL. Anesthesiologists with substance use disorder: A 5-year outcome study from 16 state physician health programs. Anesth Analg 2009;109:891–6.

162. Rose JS, Campbell M, Skipper G. Prognosis for emergency physicians with substance abuse recovery: 5-year outcome study. West J Med 2014;15:20–5.

17

Ethical and Legal Considerations

Background

Providing care to patients with substance use disorders commonly creates ethical dilemmas. Even though these patients (like others) often make poor choices, they should receive medical care incorporating the principles of ethical care for all patients, including autonomy, beneficence, nonmaleficence, and justice.[1] Additionally, inherent in the practice of medicine are veracity and confidentiality.[2] Both the American Medical Association[3] and the American Psychiatric Association[4] provide guidance on issues of medical ethics, with the latter association providing specific guidance applicable to patients with substance use disorders.

Substance use disorders intersect with the law in a number of ways. The most obvious is that the use of many substances is illegal. Thus ethical dilemmas may inevitably arise in the provision of care to patients using an illegal drug; ethical considerations may at times exceed legal considerations. Additionally, confidentiality related to substance use disorders has more stringent legal requirements than in other areas of medicine. Clinicians must be aware of attitudes they may hold toward individuals with substance use disorders who may have engaged in criminal activities, and they must still provide unbiased, compassionate care.

Legal Issues

Regulation of Drugs

In the United States, the Harrison Narcotics Tax Act of 1914 was the first federal law that regulated psychoactive substances (opium and coca); it allowed a physician to prescribe narcotics "in the course of his professional practice only." What constituted proper "professional practice" was, of course, subject to interpretation. The use of alcohol was banned during the period of Prohibition in United States from 1920 to1933. In 1970, the Controlled Substances Act consolidated a number of laws regulating the manufacture and distribution of a variety of legal and illegal psychoactive substances; the Drug Enforcement Administration (DEA) was created in 1973 to enforce this law.

The Controlled Substances Act divides psychoactive substances into five "schedules"; Table 17.1 provides the schedule classification of selected agents. Schedule I includes those substances considered to be of high abuse potential and no accepted therapeutic

TABLE 17.1 Selected Scheduled Drugs*

Schedule	Opioids	Sedatives	Stimulants	Hallucinogens and Others
Schedule I (High potential for abuse, no currently accepted therapeutic use)	Diacetylmorphine (heroin)	Gamma-hydroxybutyrate (GHB); methaqualone	Cathinone (khat); methcathinone (cat)	MDMA (ecstasy); lysergic acid diethylamide (LSD); marijuana; mescaline; psilocyn
Schedule II (High potential for abuse, but does have accepted therapeutic use)	Codeine; fentanyl; hydromorphone; meperidine; methadone; morphine; oxycodone, hydrocodone	Pentobarbital (Nembutal); secobarbital (Seconal)	Amphetamines (dexedrine, methamphetamine); cocaine	Phencyclidine (PCP)
Schedule III (Moderate abuse potential)	Buprenorphine; codeine combination products	Butalbital (Fiorinal, Fioricet)		Anabolic steroids; dronabinol; ketamine

(continued)

TABLE 17.1 (Continued)

Schedule	Opioids	Sedatives	Stimulants	Hallucinogens and Others
Schedule IV (Low abuse potential)	Butorphanol (Stadol); carisoprodol; tramadol (Ultram)	Phenobarbital; benzodiazepines; chloral hydrate; dichloralphenazone; eszopiclone; zaleplon; zolpidem	Modafinil (Provigil); phentermine	
Schedule V (Lowest potential for abuse)	Codeine preparations— 100 mg/100 mL (cough syrups) diphenoxylate (Lomotil); opium preparations— 100 mg/100 mL			Pregabalin

*Not all substances are listed; selected brand or street names appear in parentheses (some brand names are combination products).

Source: U.S. Drug Enforcement Administration (www.dea.gov).

use. The other scheduled agents have acceptable therapeutic use, but also a potential for abuse, which declines from the schedule II to V category. It should be noted that this is a legal classification, not a medical one, and that the two most important substances of abuse, tobacco and alcohol, are not included in this schedule. The proper prescribing of controlled substances is covered further in Chapter 13.

As a practical matter, in the United States, schedule II medications can only be dispensed for a month at a time with a written prescription and practitioners cannot give refills on these prescriptions, although the Controlled Substances Act does allow for exceptions in "emergency situations" such as hospice care. Practitioners can prescribe up to 90 days of schedule II medications by giving up to three 30-day prescriptions, two of them future-dated for the subsequent months. Schedule III and IV substances, by contrast, can be dispensed with an oral or written prescription and can be refilled up to five times or for up to 6 months after the date of the original prescription. The Controlled Substances Act only requires that schedule V medications be used for a "medical purpose" and places no other limitations on their use.

Patient Confidentiality

Confidentiality related to patients with substance use disorder is expected. For federally funded treatment programs, 42 CFR Part 2 provides a legal framework for confidentiality that mandates a second level of permission needed to share medical information related to treatment of substance use disorders in certain programs. A sample release is shown in Box 17.1. Under this law, federal rules allow disclosure under nine specific situations:

1. When a patient signs a consent form that complies with the regulations requirements
2. When a disclosure does not identify a patient as having a substance use disorder
3. When treatment staff discuss the patient among themselves

BOX 17.1 Sample Consent for Release of Confidential Information Related to Substance Use Disorder Treatment

This notice accompanies a disclosure of information concerning a patient in alcohol/drug abuse treatment, made to you with the consent of such patient. This information has been disclosed to you from records protected by Federal confidentiality rules (42 CFR Part 2). Federal rules prohibit you from making any further disclosure of this information unless further disclosure is expressly permitted by the written consent of the person to whom it pertains or as otherwise specified by 42 CFR Part 2. A general authorization for the release of medical or other information is NOT sufficient for this purpose. The Federal rules restrict any use of the information to criminally investigate or prosecute any alcohol or drug abuse patient.

I, _____ (name of patient), authorize TREATMENT PROGRAM _____ (name or general designation of program making disclosure) to disclose _____ (name of person or organization to which disclosure is made) the following information:

_____ All records of addiction treatment.

The purpose of the disclosure authorized herein is to:

Coordinate medical and addiction care (purpose of disclosure, as specific as possible).

I understand that my records are protected under the Federal regulations governing Confidentiality of Alcohol and Drug Abuse Patient Records, 42 CFR Part 2, and cannot be disclosed without my written consent unless otherwise provided for in the regulations.

I also understand that I may revoke this consent at any time except to the extent that action has been taken in reliance on it, and that in any event this consent expires automatically as follows:

_____

(date, event, or condition upon which this consent expires)

_____

Signature of patient: _____

Signature of parent, guardian, or authorized representative when required: _____

Date: _____

4. When the disclosure is to a "qualified service organization" that provides service to the patient
5. When there is a medical emergency
6. When the law requires disclosure of child abuse
7. When a patient commits a crime at the treatment program
8. When the information is for audit or evaluation purposes
9. When a court issues an order authorizing disclosure

42 CFR Part 2 was passed during a time when most treatment of substance use disorders was provided in specialized centers; the law was intended to encourage individuals with substance use disorders to seek treatment and to prevent law enforcement from using records to arrest or prosecute drug users. While the intentions behind these protections are understandable, this law has created some problems, particularly with the move toward more integrated and collaborative care using shared electronic health records.[5] SAMHSA has provided some guidance on the application of this law on their website,[6] but questions still remain. It is important to note that this law applies to federally assisted programs; "programs" are defined as "an individual or entity that holds itself out as providing, *and* provides alcohol or drug abuse diagnosis, treatment or referral for treatment." According the SAMHSA website, primary

care practitioners who prescribe controlled substances to treat substance use disorders (e.g., buprenorphine for opioid use disorder) would not be considered a "program" unless their primary activity was the treatment of substance use disorders.

Ethical Principles

In this section we briefly review general ethical principles and their application to the treatment of individual with substance use disorders. For a more detailed discussion of this topic, we refer readers to the *ASAM Principles of Addiction Medicine*.[7]

Autonomy

Autonomy dictates that patients have personal liberty and can choose their own actions. Inherent to autonomy is patient acceptance of consequences related to decisions made. As clinicians, we should always start by assuming everyone to be autonomous and able to make his or her own decisions. This may be questioned with patients with substance use disorder, as they are deemed to be making poor choices by using drugs. Making a poor choice is distinctly different from lacking the capacity to make proper decisions.[8] For example, individuals with heart disease who smoke cigarettes are making a bad choice, but their competence is not questioned.

Another factor to consider when treating someone with a substance use disorder is whether or not a drug is directly impacting decision-making. While an intoxicated patient may not be deemed competent to make a healthcare decision, this does not necessarily justify forcing an intoxicated patient into treatment. Family members may ask that their loved one with a substance use disorder be "forced" into treatment, and this may lead to difficult discussions on patient autonomy. There is no evidence that forcing or coercing someone with a substance use disorder into treatment is effective.[9] Nevertheless, the legal system frequently mandates treatment as part of sentencing; for some individuals, mandated treatment is a welcome option and is generally preferable to incarceration.

There is mixed opinion on requiring individuals arrested for driving while under the influence of alcohol to attend Alcoholics Anonymous (AA) meetings or other treatment programs. Many people in recovery are against this use of AA, as they believe AA should never be viewed as punishment. In contrast, others view this as useful, with anecdotal stories of long-term recovery after being sentenced to attend AA. Additionally, some ethicists have argued that forced treatment enables acquisition of autonomy, as individuals with addiction are not autonomous but rather controlled by a drug.[9]

Beneficence

Beneficence implies an obligation on the part of the healthcare practitioner to deliver care to the full benefit of patients. For someone with a substance use disorder, this means teaming up with the patient and using shared decision-making to develop a plan that will hopefully lead to recovery. Rapport-building skills are needed to strengthen the clinician–patient relationship and help create consensus for a care plan.

Nonmaleficence

Nonmaleficence simply means "do no harm." Treatments offered should be effective. Modalities of treatment without evidence of benefit should not be offered, and certainly treatment that can cause harm (i.e., rapid opioid detoxification under anesthesia) should not be prescribed. Less clear-cut, but still in the realm of nonmaleficence, is not prescribing a controlled substance to someone at high risk of misuse.

Justice

Justice mandates that patients with a substance use disorder be treated as any other patient might. For example, an elderly person at risk for falls should be treated the same in physical therapy whether the fall risk is related to a stroke or an alcohol use disorder. Another example is the consideration for liver transplantation: this may mandate a period of sobriety, but patients cannot be discriminated against on the basis of the cause of their liver failure. Inherent in justice is an obligation on the part of those taking care of patients with substance use disorder to be advocates for their patients, helping them avoid discrimination and assisting them in accessing services they need.

Fidelity

Fidelity focuses on the obligation of providers to be truthful to patients and maintain patient confidentiality. Treatment options must be presented to patients on the basis of evidence. Fidelity includes the expectation that providers will adhere to all ethical principles. As noted earlier, the laws governing the confidentiality of medical records of patients in substance use disorder treatment programs are more stringent than in other settings.

Futility

Futility is a term that must be considered carefully, as it must be evidence based, not based on personal experience. Initiating cardiopulmonary resuscitation for a patient with end-stage metastatic cancer may be regarded as futile. In contrast, refusing to perform a valve replacement on an individual with endocarditis from injection drug use cannot solely be based on a surgeon's personal experience of having never cared for a patient who ceased injecting drugs.[10] In such a case, an argument might be put forth that medical resources would be wasted. However, in this instance, an artificial valve is not a limited resource, and the ethical principles of patient autonomy, beneficence, and justice supersede an opinion of futility. In the inpatient setting, a hospital-based ethics committee is often available to assist in medical decisions that encompass issues of futility. Such committees are usually multidisciplinary, with legal, religious, medical (physicians, nurses, and social workers), and lay representation.

Dealing with Difficult Patients

Ideally, patients and clinicians are allied in a mutually agreed-upon quest for common goals. However, there are times when this does not occur; in some of these cases, the patient may evoke feelings of frustration and even anger in those caring for them. These individuals are often called "difficult" (or "problem") patients and frequently consume a great deal of clinicians' time and energy ("the thick chart syndrome"). There are a number of conditions associated with being a difficult patient, including somatoform disorder, anxiety or panic disorder, dysthymia or depression, and substance use disorders.[11] Unrecognized personality disorders appear to be quite common among these patients.[12] The higher prevalence of personality disorders among those with substance use disorders probably accounts for some of the association.

Although we may tend to view difficult interactions as the fault of the patient, it is clear that clinician characteristics play a role. In one survey, physicians who took care of a greater number of patients with substance use disorders were more likely to report frustration with their patients; other physician characteristics associated with greater frustration included younger age, longer work hours, higher stress, and practice in a medicine subspecialty.[13]

There are few empirical data on how best to manage difficult patients, but there are some common-sense strategies that we feel are helpful. First, it is important to establish rapport and to win the trust of the patient. This means listening and showing empathy for the patient's problems, no matter how trivial they may seem. Trying to downplay or dismiss their complaints is a setup for an adversarial relationship. It is also important to understand the patient's goals and expectations. This does not mean that you have to acquiesce to all their demands, but you cannot come up with a mutually acceptable plan of action unless you address their concerns. One recent study reported on a structured intervention that helped improve clinician satisfaction with difficult visits. This intervention included reflecting on one's own biases and assumptions and on why the patient was being considered difficult.[14]

Managing Manipulative Behavior

All patients should be treated with honesty and respect. It is natural for patients to bring certain expectations and desires to their interactions with healthcare professionals, and there is nothing wrong with them pursuing these goals, especially when this is done through open and honest dialogue. In general, manipulative behavior by patients is when they use inappropriate tactics to achieve their goals, such as lying, deception, or threats (or flattery). Generally, this occurs when patients feel that their goals and agenda are at odds with those of the clinicians who are caring for them. Most clinicians are trained to work with patients and do what is best for them but are less prepared to deal with situations in which the patient appears to be working at odds with their goals.

While manipulative behavior is probably more common among those with substance use disorders, these individuals should not be stereotyped in this fashion. Manipulative behavior is a characteristic of individuals with personality disorders (particularly borderline, narcissistic, and antisocial personality disorders)[15] and, as noted earlier, substance use is also associated with these disorders. There are probably a number of other reasons why individuals with substance use disorders may resort to manipulative behavior. Addiction is a powerful force, and the compulsion to continue such behavior leads individuals to act in ways they probably would not otherwise choose. As a result, individuals with substance use disorders may employ lying and deception in their interactions with others, either to obtain their substance of choice or to hide their problem. Furthermore, there is often a mistrust of healthcare professionals among these individuals and they may feel that they can only get the care they need through manipulative behaviors. It is important to remember that manipulative behavior may be appropriate at times, and is a normal response for persons who are dealing with a system that they view as hostile and unjust.

As with any problem, prevention is the best strategy. We feel that a number of measures can help prevent this kind of behavior. The first preventive measure is to address substance use disorders and their complications in a nonjudgmental and compassionate manner; this will help patients to be honest and forthright about their problems and should help lower barriers for them to seek help when they need it. The second preventive measure is to be honest and up front with the patient; this will help to foster trust. While this approach may seem obvious and many clinicians would argue that they are always honest, we have observed many situations where this has not been the case. When dealing with individuals who appear to be making unreasonable demands, some practitioners find it easier to avoid the patient and make decisions without speaking to them. We have even seen situations where patients have been deceived about the medications they are receiving. We believe that this approach just increases mistrust and encourages further manipulative behavior. As noted earlier, manipulation is a natural and normal response to a hostile and authoritarian system, so creating that sort of environment will only foster manipulative behavior.

However, even when treated with respect and honesty, some patients may still choose to use manipulative behavior to get what they want. This sort of behavior often creates feelings of anger among clinicians. It is important to always remain focused on the best interests of the patient, even when upset or frustrated with them, and to resist the temptation to punish them. The first step in dealing with a manipulative or demanding patient is to step back and consider whether the patient may have legitimate unmet needs; this does not condone the behavior, but these needs should be addressed. For example, a patient who demands more pain medication and is labeled "drug-seeking" may, in fact, be undertreated. When dealing with patients who are being manipulative, it is best to directly identify the specific problem behavior and tell them why you find it unacceptable, then try to develop a mutually acceptable plan for their subsequent treatment and how their problems will be dealt with in the future. It may be helpful to write down your agreement with the patient to document this discussion and reinforce its importance with them. It is also important that members of the healthcare team be in agreement with one another about the treatment plan and that one person be responsible for important decisions (to avoid splitting of the team).

At times, the level of behavior may be such that it would be appropriate to terminate your relationship with the patient (for example, when there are personal threats); however, it is important that this be done only when there is no other option and not just to get rid of a difficult or unpleasant patient. In these situations, it is essential that the patient be given assistance to find another source of care and be provided continued care until that transfer can occur.

Refusal of Care

Sometimes the disagreement between clinicians and patients can lead to situations where the patient refuses to comply with the recommended treatment. A number of studies indicate that patients with substance use disorders are less likely to comply with recommended treatment.[16] Furthermore, alcohol- and drug-related problems are associated with leaving hospitals against medical advice.[17,18] This is of particular concern during situations in which the patient has an acute life-threatening illness and refuses to comply with a potentially life-saving treatment. One example is an individual with injection drug use hospitalized for endocarditis who wishes to leave the hospital and refuses to complete a course of intravenous antibiotics. The first step should be to try to understand why the patient wishes to leave and to see if (reasonable) accommodations can be made so that the patient can complete the treatment. Very often, refusal of care occurs during times of conflict or disagreement between the patient and clinicians. In these instances the temptation to simply rid oneself of a problem patient must be resisted. In addition, it is important to assess whether the patient is competent to make this decision and able to understand the risks and options. If so, the patient should be informed of the risks he or she is taking, and this discussion should be carefully documented. If the patient still insists on leaving, the patient should not be abandoned; alternative treatment should be offered (for example, oral antibiotics) and the patient given the option to return for further treatment.

Assessment of a patient's competence or decision-making capacity is always difficult; there is no clear line that separates competence from incompetence or, for that matter, treatment from non-treatment. Moreover, there are issues particular to those with substance use disorders that further complicate these decisions. The first problem is acute intoxication or delirium, which is particularly an issue for those with an alcohol use disorder. In these situations, it may be best to hold the patient until the acute phase has cleared, especially if the person has an acute medical problem. The second problem is the ability of someone who has a substance use disorder to make rational and appropriate choices, even when they are not intoxicated or delirious. Some have argued that an individual with a substance use disorder who wishes to leave against medical advice when under treatment for a life-threatening illness is, almost by definition, incompetent, since their addiction prevents them from making rational choices.[19] On the other hand, we all make choices that may seem irrational to others or that may be motivated by forces beyond our control. For example, we generally respect the wishes of those who refuse blood transfusion on religious grounds, even though this may not seem rational to some of us. Nonetheless, involuntary commitment may be an option if it is felt that the patient is at great risk and is not competent to make decisions regarding their care, or it may be used when an individual is a potential hazard to others—for example, a person with tuberculosis who does not comply with treatment. However, involuntary commitment should always be the last resort and must be balanced with consideration for patient autonomy.

Other Issues

Drug Testing

Drug testing does not require a signed consent, but drug testing without a patient's knowledge raises ethical concerns. In general, it is recommended that the ordering of any test be discussed with a patient. Patients should be engaged in the decision to order a test and clinicians should provide an explanation for why a test is clinically indicated. Patient concerns related to issues such as cost and privacy should be considered. Exceptions may occur in some clinical settings, such as trauma where legal concerns may take precedent, or when a patient has a change in mental status with unclear cause.

Employment

If a patient with a substance use disorder is receiving employer-mandated treatment and requires an assessment in order to maintain his or her job, clinicians are bound to be truthful regarding treatment adherence. Ideally, practitioners should have a conversation with patients in advance and inform them of the ramifications of nonadherence to treatment. It should also be clear what medical information employers are able to obtain about their employee.

Pregnancy

The care of pregnant women with a substance use disorder is discussed in Chapter 16. Medical professionals frequently display particularly negative views when providing care to pregnant women with a substance use disorder.[20] Ethical issues may arise based on societal views of potential harm to an innocent fetus from substance use by the mother. A positive drug test in a mother or infant may lead to a Child Protective Services (CPS) evaluation of the situation. Some states mandate clinicians to report pregnant women with a substance use disorder. CPS evaluation occurs independent of the clinician, who should remain an advocate for the mother.

Fear of being judged harshly and of legal ramifications may prevent a pregnant woman with a substance use disorder from seeking medical care. As a result, most states have avoided criminalizing drug use by pregnant women and most recent attempts to criminalize such use have been overturned in court cases. In South Carolina, a woman who used cocaine in her third trimester of pregnancy was sentenced to prison for 8 years, and from 1989 to 1994, the Medical University of South Carolina tested pregnant women for cocaine, reporting those who tested positive to the police.[21] In 2001, the U.S. Supreme Court found the policy to be unconstitutional. In December 2014, the New Jersey Supreme Court unanimously ruled that the state's civil child abuse statute could not be used to charge patients who receive medically prescribed methadone treatment while pregnant. The decision in the case of *New Jersey Division of Child Protection & Permanency v. Y.N.* overturned a lower court finding that a mother may be charged with civil child abuse and neglect because her newborn exhibited temporary and treatable withdrawal from methadone that the woman received as treatment for opioid use disorder during pregnancy. A failure to overturn the initial lower court ruling would have been ethically wrong and devastating to the provision of substance use disorder treatment to pregnant women.

Notes

1. Page K. The four principles: can they be measured and do they predict ethical decision making? BMC Med Ethics 2012;13:10.

2. Jonsen AR, Siegler M, Winslade WJ. *Clinical Ethics: A Practical Approach to Ethical Decisions in Medicine*, 6th ed. New York: McGraw Hill; 2006.

3. American Medical Association. Code of Medical Ethics. Chicago, IL: AMA. http://www.ama-assn.org/ama/pub/physician-resources/medical-ethics/code-medical-ethics.page

4. American Psychiatric Association. The Principles of Medical Ethics with Annotations Especially Applicable to Psychiatry, 2013 Edition. http://www.psychiatry.org/practice/ethics/resources-standards

5. Manuel JK, Newville H, Larios SE, Sorenson JL. Confidentiality protections versus collaborative care in the treatment of substance use disorders. Addict Sci Clin Pract 2013;8:13.

6. Substance Abuse and Mental Health Services Administration, SAMHSA-HRSA Center for Integrated Health Solutions. Confidentiality. http://www.integration.samhsa.gov/operations-administration/confidentiality#general. Accessed January 17, 2015.

7. Clark HW, Bizzell AC, Campbell A. Ethical issues in addiction practice. In Ries RK, Fiellin DA, Miller SC, Saitz R, eds. *The ASAM Principles of Addiction Medicine*, 5th ed. Philadelphia: Wolters Kluwer; 2014:1685–93.

8. Geppert CMA, Bogenschutz MP. Ethics in substance abuse treatment. Psychiatr Clin North Am 2009;32:283–97.

9. Caplan AL. Ethical issues surrounding forced, mandated or coerced treatment. J Subst Abuse Treat 2006;31:117–20.

10. DiMaio JM, Salerno TA, Bernstein R, et al. Ethical obligation of surgeons to noncompliant patients: can a surgeon refuse to operate on an intravenous drug-abusing patient with recurrent aortic valve prosthesis infection? Ann Thorac Surg 2009;88:1–8.

11. Hahn SR, Kroenke K, Spitzer RL, et al. The difficult patient: prevalence, psychopathology, and functional impairment. J Gen Intern Med 1996;11:1–8.

12. Schafer S, Nowlis DP. Personality disorders among difficult patients. Arch Fam Med 1998;7:126–9.

13. Krebs EE, Garrett JM, Konrad TR. The difficult doctor? Characteristics of physicians who report frustration with patients: an analysis of survey data. BMC Health Serv Res 2006;6:128.

14. Edgoose JYC, Regner CJ, Zakletskaia LI. BREATH OUT: a randomized controlled trial of a structured intervention to improve clinician satisfaction with "difficult" visits. J Am Board Fam Med 2015;28:13–20.

15. Bowers L. Manipulation: searching for an understanding. J Psychiatr Ment Health Nurs 2003;10:329–34.

16. Gebo KA, Keruly J, Moore RD. Association of social stress, illicit drug use, and health beliefs with nonadherence to antiretroviral therapy. J Gen Intern Med 2003;18:104–11.

17. Saitz R, Ghali WA, Moskowitz MA. Characteristics of patients with pneumonia who are discharged from hospitals against medical advice. Am J Med 1999;107:507–9.

18. Anis A, Sun H, Guh DP, et al. Leaving hospital against medical advice among HIV-positive patients. CMAJ 2002;167:633–7.

19. Treisman GJ, Angelino AF, Hutton HE. Psychiatric issues in the management of patients with HIV infection. JAMA 2001;286:2857–64.

20. French A. Substance abuse in pregnancy: compassionate and competent care for the patient in labor. Clin Obstet Gynecol 2013;56:172–7.

21. Annas GJ. Testing poor pregnant women for cocaine—physicians as police investigators. N Engl J Med 2001;344:1729–32.

Index

Page numbers followed by an italicized f, n, or t indicate a figure, note, or table on the designated page.